Lookingbill & Marks'
PRINCIPLES *of* DERMATOLOGY

SEVENTH EDITION

James G. Marks Jr, MD
Professor
Department of Dermatology
Pennsylvania State University College of Medicine
Penn State Health
Hershey, PA

Jeffrey J. Miller, MD
Chair of Dermatology
Professor
Department of Dermatology
Pennsylvania State University College of Medicine
Penn State Health
Hershey, PA

L. Claire Hollins, MD
Vice Chair of Diversity, Equity & Inclusion
Assistant Professor
Department of Dermatology
Pennsylvania State University College of Medicine
Penn State Health
Hershey, PA

ELSEVIER

Elsevier
1600 John F. Kennedy Blvd.
Ste 1800
Philadelphia, PA 19103-2899

LOOKINGBILL & MARKS' PRINCIPLES OF DERMATOLOGY, SEVENTH EDITION   ISBN: 978-0-323-93424-4

Cover images from left to right: severe acne with post inflammatory hyperpigmentation, superficial spreading melanoma, atopic dermatitis, frontal fibrosing alopecia, hidradenitis suppurativa.

Previous editions copyrighted 2019, 2013, 2006, 2000, 1993 and 1986.

Content Strategist: Charlotta Kryhl
Senior Content Development Specialist: Suddha Sen
Content Development Manager: Somodatta Roy Choudhury
Publishing Services Manager: Shereen Jameel
Project Manager: Haritha Dharmarajan
Design Direction: Margaret Reid

Printed in India

Last digit is the print number: 9   8   7   6   5   4   3   2   1

To Donald P. Lookingbill, MD, friend, colleague, mentor, and inspiration for this text.

PREFACE

The primary goal of this seventh edition has not changed from that of the first edition; it is to facilitate dermatologic diagnosis through a morphologic approach to skin disease. Unlike most other introductory manuals, each chapter in our text is based on the appearance of the primary skin process (e.g., pustules) rather than on the etiology (e.g., infection). This arrangement helps to reflect the way in which most patients present in the clinical setting.

We are grateful to our many students and residents who have used our previous editions and provided us with thoughtful feedback over the years. Their suggestions have been incorporated into this new seventh edition of *Lookingbill and Marks' Principles of Dermatology*. It includes more skin of color illustrations, more diseases, key points, differential diagnosis algorithms, updated treatments, and pathogenesis that should be of use to medical students, primary care physicians, and physician extenders who peruse this book.

PREFACE TO THE FIRST EDITION

Skin diseases affect virtually everyone sometime during life. Because changes in the skin are so easily recognized by the patient, medical attention is frequently sought. Skin reacts in a limited number of ways, but the neophyte is often bewildered by the appearance of rashes that superficially look alike. This text is meant to be an introduction to cutaneous disorders. It is aimed toward medical students so that they may develop a logical approach to the diagnosis of common cutaneous diseases with an understanding of the underlying clinicopathologic correlations. It has been a most rewarding experience for us to see students on our clinical service at the M.S. Hershey Medical Center grasp the basic principles of skin disease in the short time they spend with us. Their questions, learning experience, and suggestions have been incorporated into this book.

We have purposely not tried to make this an encyclopedia of skin diseases, but have chosen those diseases that are most commonly seen. Uncommon diseases are discussed only to illustrate dermatologic principles or important diseases that should not be missed. There are several up-to-date large textbooks available for those who want to delve into the field more deeply.

We are grateful for the contribution of artwork and clinical slides from audiovisual programs in the series, A Brief Course in Dermatology, produced and distributed by the Institute for Dermatologic Communication and Education, San Francisco, California, as follows: From Skin Lesions Depicted and Defined, Part One, Primary Lesions, and Part Two, Secondary and Special Lesions, by Richard M. Caplan, M.D., Alfred W. Kopf, M.D., and Marion B. Sulzberger, M.D., and from Techniques for Examination of the Skin, by David L. Cram, M.D., Howard I. Maibach, M.D., and Marion B. Sulzberger, M.D.

We wish to acknowledge those people whose efforts contributed greatly to producing this book. Our secretaries, Dianne Safford, Joyce Zeager, and Sharon Smith, spent many hours typing the drafts and final manuscript. Nancy Egan, M.D. and Ronald Rovner, M.D., proofread much of the book and gave many worthwhile suggestions. Schering Corporation supported the cost of the illustrations which were so handsomely drawn by Debra Moyer and Daniel S. Beisel. Lastly, and most importantly, our families gave us the support and time necessary to write this volume.

ACKNOWLEDGMENTS

We acknowledge our families for again giving us the time to produce this book.

CONTENTS

Introduction

Algorithm for Diagnosis of Skin Diseases

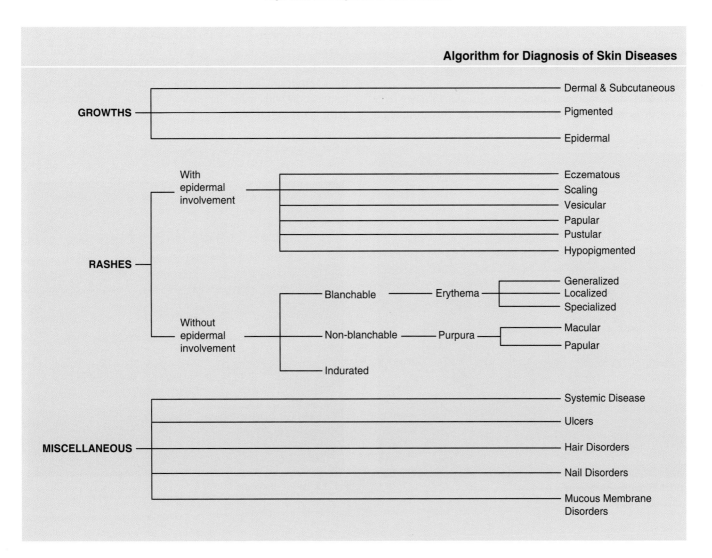

Algorithm for Diagnosis of Skin Diseases

- **GROWTHS**
  - Dermal & Subcutaneous
  - Pigmented
  - Epidermal

- **RASHES**
  - With epidermal involvement
    - Eczematous
    - Scaling
    - Vesicular
    - Papular
    - Pustular
    - Hypopigmented
  - Without epidermal involvement
    - Blanchable — Erythema
      - Generalized
      - Localized
      - Specialized
    - Non-blanchable — Purpura
      - Macular
      - Papular
    - Indurated

- **MISCELLANEOUS**
  - Systemic Disease
  - Ulcers
  - Hair Disorders
  - Nail Disorders
  - Mucous Membrane Disorders

Skin diseases are common, and a significant number of outpatient visits are for dermatologic complaints. A minority of these patients are seen by dermatologists; most of the remainder are seen by primary care physicians and physician extenders. In a survey of the family practice clinic at the Pennsylvania State University College of Medicine, we found that dermatologic disorders constituted 8.5% of diagnoses. The incidence is higher in a pediatric practice, in which as many as 30% of children are seen for skin-related conditions.

Although thousands of skin disorders have been described, only a small number account for most patient visits. The primary goal of this book is to familiarize the reader with these common diseases. Some uncommon and rare skin disorders are covered briefly in this book to expand the readers' differential diagnosis.

Our diagnostic approach divides skin diseases into two large groups: growths (Fig. 1.1) and rashes (Fig. 1.2). This grouping is based on both the patient's presenting complaint (often a concern about either a skin growth or a symptom from a rash) and the pathophysiologic process (a growth represents a neoplastic change and a rash is an inflammatory reaction in the skin). Furthermore, the correlation between the clinical appearance of the disorder and the pathophysiologic processes responsible for the disease facilitates making the diagnosis and selecting the proper treatment.

Growths and rashes are then subdivided according to the component of skin that is affected. Growths are divided into epidermal, pigmented, and dermal proliferative processes. Rashes are divided into those with and without an epidermal component. We also have chapters dedicated to ulcers, disorders of the hair, nails, mucous membranes, and skin signs of systemic disease. Self-assessment cases are presented at the end of every chapter to provide the learner an opportunity to reinforce diagnostic and treatment principles. New illustrations and photographs have been added to show the variations in color from light to dark skin. Algorithm here and at the beginning of each disease chapter will help the reader think through the differential diagnoses and arrive at the proper disease(s) to prescribe the appropriate laboratory tests and treatments. Our focus on frameworks will enable the reader to see the "big" picture before getting lost in the "weeds."

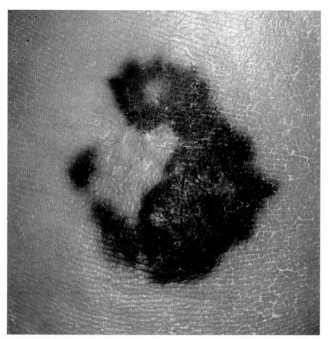

Fig. 1.1 Growth—melanoma.

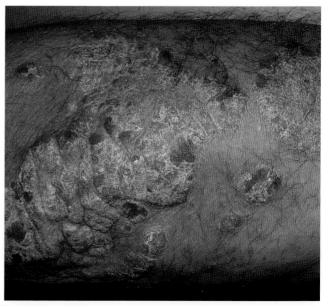

Fig. 1.2 Rash—psoriasis.

Structure and Function of the Skin

CHAPTER CONTENTS

ABSTRACT

The skin is a large organ, weighing an average of 4 kg and covering an area of 2 m². Its major function is to act as a barrier against an inhospitable environment to protect the body from the influences of the outside world and maintain internal homeostasis. The importance of the skin is well illustrated by the high mortality rate associated with extensive loss of skin from burns.

The major barrier is provided by the epidermis. Underlying the epidermis is a vascularized dermis that provides support and nutrition for the dividing cells in the epidermis. The dermis also contains nerves and appendages: sweat glands, hair follicles, and sebaceous glands. Nails are also considered skin appendages. The third and deepest layer of the skin is the subcutaneous fat. Loss of or defects in skin structure impair skin function. Skin diseases illustrate the loss of skin structure and resulting dysfunction of skin components (Table 2.1).

KEY POINTS

1. The major function of the skin is to act as a barrier to maintain internal homeostasis.
2. The epidermis is the major barrier of the skin.

COMPONENTS OF SKIN:
1. Epidermis
2. Dermis
3. Subcutaneous fat

EPIDERMIS

KEY POINTS

1. Keratinocytes are the principal cells of the epidermis.
2. Layers in ascending order: basal cell, stratum spinosum, stratum granulosum, stratum corneum.
3. Basal cells are undifferentiated, proliferating cells.
4. Stratum spinosum contains keratinocytes connected by desmosomes.
5. Keratohyalin granules are seen in the stratum granulosum.
6. Stratum corneum is the major physical barrier.
7. The number and size of melanosomes, not melanocytes, determine skin color.
8. Langerhans cells are derived from bone marrow and are the skin's first line of immunologic defense.
9. The basement membrane zone is the substrate for attachment of the epidermis to the dermis.
10. The four major ultrastructural regions of the basement membrane zone include the hemidesmosomal plaque of the basal keratinocyte, lamina lucida, lamina densa, and anchoring fibrils located in the sublamina densa region of the papillary dermis.

The epidermis is divided into four layers, starting at the dermal junction with the basal cell layer and eventuating at the outer surface in the stratum corneum. The dermal side of the epidermis has an irregular contour. The downward projections are called *rete ridges*, which appear three-dimensionally as a Swiss cheese–like matrix with the holes filled by dome-shaped dermal papillae. This configuration helps to anchor the epidermis physically to the dermis. The pattern is most pronounced in areas subject to maximum friction, such as the palms and soles.

The cells in the epidermis undergo division and differentiation. Cell division occurs in the basal cell layer, and differentiation occurs in the layers above it.

Cell division occurs in the basal cell layer.

Structure
Basal Cell Layer

The basal cells are the undifferentiated, proliferating cells. Skin stem cells are located in the basal layer in the interfollicular epidermis, and they give rise to keratinocytes. For normal skin homeostasis, daughter cells from the basal cell layer migrate upward and begin the process of differentiation. In normal skin, cell division does not take place above the basal cell layer. It takes about 2 weeks for the cells to migrate from the basal cell

TABLE 2.1   Skin Structure Correlated With Their Function and Illustrative Disease Dysfunction

Structure	Function	Disease Dysfunction
Epidermis		
Keratinocyte	Barrier	Pemphigus vulgaris
Melanocyte	Photoprotection	Oculocutaneous albinism
Langerhans cell	Immune protection	Allergic contact dermatitis
Dermal–epidermal junction	Structure Integrity	Bullous pemphigoid
Dermis		
Collagen	Foundation	Ehlers–Danlos syndrome
Nerves	Sensation	Leprosy
Blood vessels	Nutrition	Vasculitis
Sweat glands	Thermoregulation	Hypohidrotic ectodermal dysplasia
Sebaceous glands	Lubrication	Acne
Nails	Grasp	Tinea
Hair	Decorative	Alopecia areata
Subcutaneous fat	Insulation	Obesity
Nails	Grasp	
Hair	Decorative	
Sebaceous glands	Unknown	
Subcutaneous fat	Insulation from cold and trauma	
Subcutaneous fat	Calorie reservoir	

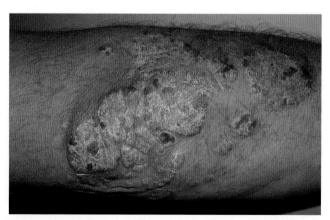

Fig. 2.1 Psoriasis—an autoinflammatory disorder characterized by thickened epidermis and increased scale.

layer to the top of the granular cell layer and a further 2 weeks for the cells to cross the stratum corneum to the surface, where they finally are shed. Injury and inflammation increase the rate of proliferation and maturation as illustrated by the increased epidermal thickness and transit time in lesions of psoriasis (Fig. 2.1).

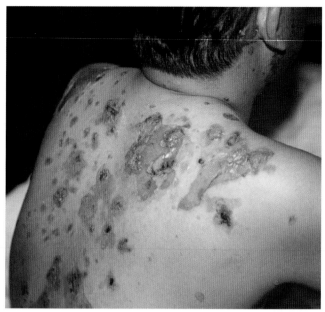

Fig. 2.2 Pemphigus vulgaris—an autoimmune blistering disease wherein antibodies directed against desmosomes result in keratinocyte separation in stratum spinosum.

Stratum Spinosum

The stratum spinosum lies above the basal layer and is composed of *keratinocytes*, which differentiate from the basal cells beneath them. The keratinocytes produce keratin, a fibrous protein that is the major component of the horny stratum corneum. The stratum spinosum derives its name from the "spines," or intercellular bridges, that extend between keratinocytes and are visible with light microscopy. Ultrastructurally, these are composed of desmosomes, which are extensions from keratin within the keratinocyte; functionally, they hold the cells together. Autoantibodies to desmoglein 3, a protein in the desmosome, result in the loss of cohesion between keratinocytes, bullae formation, and erosions as seen in pemphigus vulgaris (Fig. 2.2).

Keratinization begins in the stratum spinosum.

Stratum Granulosum

The process of differentiation continues in the stratum granulosum, or granular cell layer, in which the cells acquire additional keratin and become more flattened. In addition, they contain distinctive dark granules, seen easily on light microscopy, that are composed of keratohyalin. Keratohyalin contains two proteins, one of which is called *profilaggrin*, the precursor to filaggrin. As its name suggests, filaggrin plays an important role in the aggregation of keratin filaments in the stratum corneum. The other protein is called *involucrin* (from the Latin for "envelope") that plays a role in the formation of the cell envelope of cells in the stratum corneum. Ichthyosis vulgaris (*ichthys*, Greek for "fish") is an inherited dry skin condition secondary to deficient filaggrin production, as noted on light microscopy of a skin biopsy by a reduced or absent granular layer (Fig. 2.3).

Granular cells also contain lamellar granules, which are visualized with electron microscopy. Lamellar granules contain polysaccharides, glycoproteins, and lipids that extrude into the intercellular space and ultimately are thought to help form the "cement" that holds together the stratum corneum cells. Degradative enzymes also are found within the granular cells; these are responsible for the eventual destruction of cell nuclei and intracytoplasmic organelles.

Granular cells contain keratohyalin and lamellar granules.

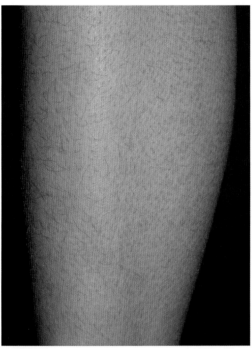

Fig. 2.3 Ichthyosis vulgaris—a loss-of-function filaggrin gene mutation causing a generalized dry skin condition. Note "fish-like" scale on the anterior shin.

Stratum Corneum

A remarkably abrupt transition occurs between the viable, nucleated cells at the top of the granular cell layer and the dead cells of the stratum corneum (Fig. 2.4). The cells in the stratum corneum are large, flat, polyhedral, plate-like envelopes filled with keratin. They are stacked in vertical layers that range in thickness from 15 to 25 layers on most body surfaces to as many as 100 layers on the palms and soles. The cells are held together by a lipid-rich cement in a fashion similar to "bricks and mortar." The tightly packed, keratinized envelopes in the stratum corneum provide a semi-impenetrable layer that constitutes the major physical barrier of the skin.

The stratum corneum is the major physical barrier.

The skin microbiome could be considered another outermost layer of the epidermis. With the better sequencing and metagenomics technologies, the role of the microbiome in human health and disease states is being actively investigated. It plays an active role in modulating the host's immune response to pathogens.

The epidermis, then, is composed of cells that divide in the basal cell layer (basal cells), keratinize in the succeeding layers (keratinocytes), and eventuate into the devitalized, keratin-filled cells in the stratum corneum.

Other Cellular Components

In addition to basal cells and keratinocytes, three other cells are located in the epidermis: melanocytes, Langerhans cells, and Merkel cells.

Melanocytes

Melanocytes are dendritic, pigment-producing cells located in the basal cell layer (Figs. 2.4 and 2.5). They protect the skin from ultraviolet radiation. Individuals with little or no pigment

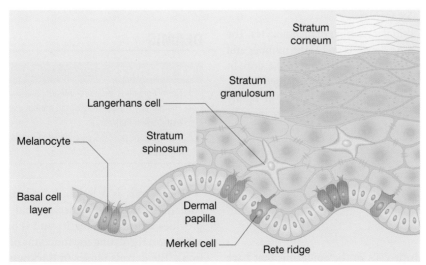

Fig. 2.4 Epidermis.

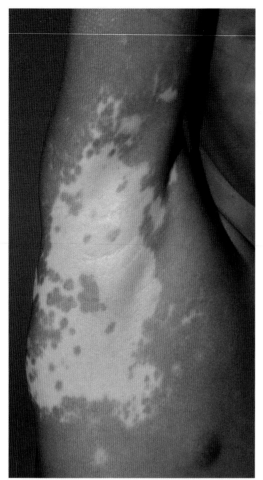

Fig. 2.5 Vitiligo—an autoimmune disease that results in loss of melanocytes.

develop marked sun damage and numerous skin cancers. The dendrites extend into the stratum spinosum and serve as conduits, through which pigment granules are transferred to their neighboring keratinocytes. The granules are termed *melanosomes*, and the pigment within is *melanin*, which is synthesized from tyrosine. Melanosomes are preferentially situated above the nucleus to protect the DNA.

People of all races have a similar number of melanocytes. The difference in skin pigmentation depends on (1) the number and size of the melanosomes and (2) their dispersion in the skin. In darkly pigmented skin, melanosomes are darker, larger in size, and more numerous compared with melanosomes in lightly pigmented skin. Sunlight stimulates melanocytes to increase pigment production and disperse their melanosomes more widely.

> Difference in skin color is due to the size, number, pigmentation, and dispersion of melanosomes.

Langerhans Cells

Langerhans cells are dendritic cells in the epidermis that have an immunologic function (Fig. 2.4). They are derived from the

bone marrow and constitute about 5% of the cells within the epidermis. On electron microscopic examination, characteristic "tennis racket"-shaped granules are seen. Langerhans cells are identical to tissue macrophages and present antigens to lymphocytes, with which they interact through specific surface receptors. As such, Langerhans cells are important components of the immunologic barrier of the skin.

> Langerhans cells are the first line of immunologic defense in the skin.

Merkel Cells

Merkel cells are located in the basal cell layer. They are more numerous on the palms and soles and are connected to keratinocytes by desmosomes. Merkel cells function as mechanoreceptors. Merkel cell carcinoma is a rare skin cancer with a high mortality rate, as discussed in Chapter 5.

Dermal–Epidermal Junction—The Basement Membrane Zone

The interface between the epidermis and dermis is called the *basement membrane zone*. With light microscopy, it is visualized only as a fine line. However, electron microscopic examination reveals four regions: (1) keratin filaments in the basal keratinocytes attach to hemidesmosomes (electron-dense units), which in turn attach to anchoring filaments in (2) the *lamina lucida*. The lamina lucida is a relatively clear (lucid) zone traversed by delicate anchoring filaments that connect hemidesmosome of basal cells to (3) the *lamina densa*; the lamina densa is an electron-dense zone composed primarily of type IV collagen derived from epidermal cells, and (4) *anchoring fibrils*, which are thick fibrous strands, composed of type VII collagen, and located in the sublamina densa region of the papillary dermis. The basement membrane zone serves as the "glue" between the epidermis and dermis and is the site of blister formation in some bullous diseases (Fig. 2.6). Hence, the structure, composition, and immunologic makeup of the basement membrane zone are under continuous, intense investigation.

DERMIS

> **KEY POINTS**
> 1. Dermis provides structural integrity and is biologically active.
> 2. The primary components of the dermal matrix are collagen, elastin, and extrafibrillar matrix.
> 3. Collagen, the principal component of the dermis, represents 70% of skin's dry weight.

The dermis is a tough, but elastic, support structure that contains blood vessels, nerves, and cutaneous appendages. It provides structural integrity and is biologically active by interacting and regulating the functions of cells (i.e., tissue regeneration). The dermis ranges in thickness from 1 to 4 mm, making it much thicker than the epidermis, which in most areas is only

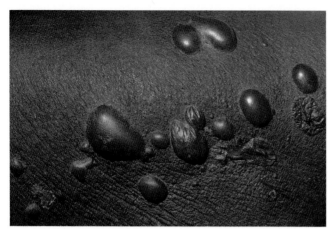

Fig. 2.6 Bullous pemphigoid—the most common autoimmune blistering disease in the elderly secondary to immune disruption of the hemidesmosome. Note bullae on inner thigh, a characteristic location.

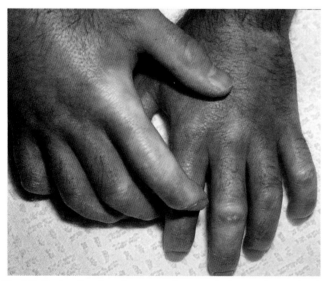

Fig. 2.7 Systemic scleroderma—an increase in the number and activity of fibroblasts produces excessive collagen and results in dermal thickening.

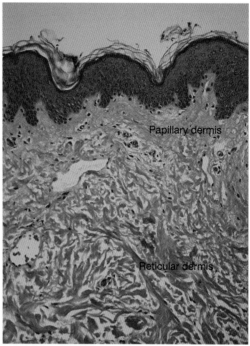

Papillary dermis

Reticular dermis

Fig. 2.8 Papillary dermis—fine, loose collagen strands. Reticular dermis – thick and dense collagen strands.

STRUCTURAL COMPONENTS OF THE DERMIS:
1. Collagen
2. Elastic fibers
3. Extrafibrillar matrix

Nerves and blood vessels course through the dermis, and a layer of subcutaneous fat lies below it (Fig. 2.9).

Free nerve endings are the most important sensory receptors.

Nerves

The skin is a major sensory receptor. Without the sensations of touch, temperature, itch, and pain, life would be less interesting and more hazardous. Sensations are detected in the skin by both free nerve endings and more complicated receptors that are corpuscular in structure. The free nerve endings are more widespread and appear to be more important. The nerve supply of the skin is segmental (dermatomal), with considerable overlap between segments (Fig. 2.10).

Blood Vessels

The blood vessels in the skin serve two functions: nutrition and temperature regulation. The epidermis has no intrinsic blood supply and therefore depends on the diffusion of nutrients and oxygen from vessels in the papillary dermis. Blood vessels in the dermis also supply the connective tissue and appendageal structures located therein.

about as thick as a piece of paper (Fig. 2.7). The dermal matrix is composed primarily of collagen fibers (principal component), elastic fibers, and ground substance (now called extrafibrillar matrix), which are synthesized by dermal fibroblasts. Collagen accounts for 70% of the dry weight of skin. Collagen and elastic fibers are fibrous proteins that form the strong, yet compliant skeletal matrix. In the uppermost part of the dermis (papillary dermis), collagen fibers are fine and loosely arranged. In the remainder of the dermis (reticular dermis), the fibers are thick and densely packed (Fig. 2.8). Elastic fibers are located primarily in the reticular dermis, where they are thinner and more loosely arranged than collagen fibers. The extrafibrillar matrix fills the space between fibers. It is a nonfibrous material made up of several different mucopolysaccharide molecules, collectively called *proteoglycans* or *glycosaminoglycans*. The extrafibrillar matrix imparts to the dermis a more liquid quality, which facilitates movement of fluids, molecules, and inflammatory cells.

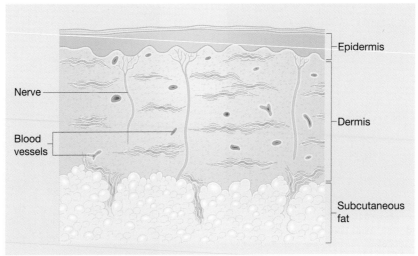

Fig. 2.9 Dermis and subcutaneous fat.

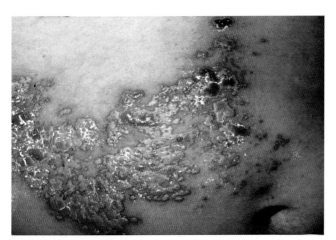

Fig. 2.10 **Herpes zoster**—reactivation of varicella-zoster virus in sensory nerve ganglia results in a painful, vesicular, dermatomal eruption.

FUNCTIONS OF BLOOD VESSELS:
1. To supply nutrition
2. To regulate temperature

The vasculature of the skin is arranged into two horizontal plexuses that are interconnected. The superficial plexus is located at the lower border of the papillary dermis, and the deep plexus is located in the reticular dermis. Temperature regulation is achieved through shunts between the plexuses. Increased blood flow in the superficial plexus permits heat loss, whereas shunting of blood to the deep plexus conserves heat.

SKIN APPENDAGES

KEY POINTS

1. Eccrine glands help to regulate body temperature.
2. Apocrine sweat glands depend on androgens for their development.
3. The stem cells of the hair follicle reconstitute the nonpermanent portion of the cycling hair follicle.
4. Sebaceous glands are under androgen control.
5. Nails, like hair, are made of keratin.

The skin appendages are the eccrine and apocrine sweat glands, hair follicles, sebaceous glands, and nails. They are epidermally derived but, except for nails, are located in the dermis.

Eccrine Sweat Glands

For physically active individuals and for people living in hot climates, the eccrine sweat glands are physiologically the most important skin appendage providing thermoregulation. They are activated by emotional and thermal stimuli. Cholinergic innervation is responsible for physiologic eccrine secretion. Botulinum toxin type A (Botox) injected intradermally or glycopyrrolate orally can treat hyperhidrosis by blocking acetylcholine action. Eccrine sweat glands help to regulate body temperature by excreting sweat onto the surface of the skin, from which the cooling process of evaporation takes place. Two to three million eccrine sweat glands are distributed over the entire body surface, with a total secretory capacity of 10 L of sweat per day. The secretory portion of the sweat apparatus is a coiled tubule located deep in the dermis. The sweat is transported through the dermis by a sweat duct, which ultimately twists a path through the epidermis (Fig. 2.11). Sweat secreted in the glandular portion is isotonic to plasma but becomes hypotonic by the time it exits the skin as a result of ductal reabsorption of electrolytes. Hence, the sweat apparatus is similar to the mechanism in the kidney, that is, glandular (glomerular) excretion is followed by ductal reabsorption.

Eccrine sweat glands help to regulate temperature and are under cholinergic innervation.

Apocrine Sweat Glands

In humans, apocrine sweat glands are androgen dependent for their development and serve no known useful function, although they are responsible for body odor. The odor actually results from the action of surface skin bacteria on excreted apocrine sweat, which itself is odorless. Apocrine sweat glands are located mainly in the axillary and anogenital areas. The

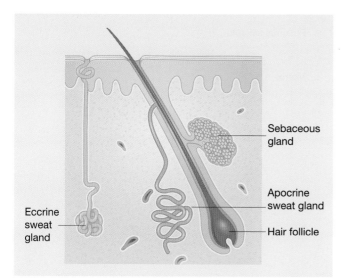

Fig. 2.11 Sweat gland, apocrine gland, and hair follicle with sebaceous gland.

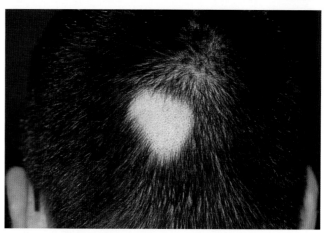

Fig. 2.12 **Alopecia areata**—autoimmune condition resulting in nonscarring circular patches of alopecia.

secretory segment of an apocrine gland is also a coiled tubule located deep in the dermis. However, unlike in eccrine glands, in which the secretory cells remain intact, in apocrine glands the secretory cells "decapitate" their luminal (apical) portions as part of the secretory product (Fig. 2.11). The apocrine duct then drains the secreted sweat into the midportion of a hair follicle, from which it ultimately reaches the skin surface.

Bacterial action on apocrine sweat causes body odor.

Hair Follicle

In most mammals, hair serves a protective function, but in humans it is mainly decorative.

Hair follicles are distributed over the entire body surface, except the palms and soles. Hair comes in two sizes: (1) vellus hairs, which are short, fine, light colored, and barely noticeable; and (2) terminal hairs, which are thicker, longer, and darker than the vellus type. Terminal hairs in some locations are hormonally influenced and do not appear until puberty (e.g., beard hair in males, and pubic and axillary hair in both sexes).

TYPES OF HAIR:
1. Vellus (light and fine)
2. Terminal (dark and thick)

A hair follicle can be viewed as a specialized invagination of the epidermis (Fig. 2.11), with a population of cells at the bottom (hair bulb) that are replicating even more actively than normal epidermal basal cells. These cells constitute the hair matrix. As with basal cells in the epidermis, the matrix cells first divide and then differentiate, ultimately forming a keratinous hair shaft. Melanocytes in the matrix contribute pigment, the amount of which determines the color of the hair. As the matrix cells continue to divide, hair is pushed outward and exits through the epidermis at a rate of about 1 cm/month. Hair

growth in an individual follicle is cyclical, with a growth (anagen) phase, a transitional (catagen) phase, and a resting (telogen) phase. The duration of the phases vary from one area of the body to another. On the scalp, for example, the anagen phase lasts for about 3 years, the catagen phase for about 3 weeks, and the telogen phase for about 3 months. The duration of the anagen phase varies from individual to individual, explaining why some persons can grow hair longer than others.

Hair growth cycles through growth (anagen), transitional (catagen), and resting (telogen) phases.

At the end of the anagen phase, growth stops and the hair follicle enters the catagen and telogen phase, during which the matrix portion and lower two-thirds of the hair follicle shrivels and the hair within the follicle is shed. Subsequently, through mesenchymal interaction with the hair follicle stem cells, a new hair matrix is formed at the bottom of the follicle, and the cycle is repeated (Fig. 2.12). At any time, 80%–90% of scalp hair is in the anagen phase and 10%–20% is in the telogen phase, thus accounting for a *normal* shedding rate of 25–100 hairs per day.

Normally, 25–100 hairs are shed from the scalp each day.

As shown in Fig. 2.11, the hair follicle is situated in the dermis at an angle. Not shown is an attached arrector pili muscle. When this muscle contracts, the hair is brought into a vertical position, giving a "goose flesh" appearance to the skin. The stem cells of the hair follicle are located in the "bulge" area of the follicle, where the arrector pili muscle inserts into the hair follicle, and in the dermal papilla. The stem cells are important for reconstituting the nonpermanent portion of the cycling hair follicle and play a role in reconstituting the epidermal cells.

Sebaceous Glands

Sebaceous glands produce an oily substance termed *sebum*, the function of which provides lubrication, hydration, and innate

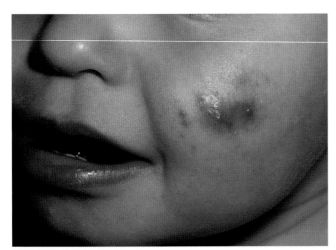

Fig. 2.13 **Infantile acne**—a common disorder affecting the pilosebaceous unit. Maternal androgens are influential.

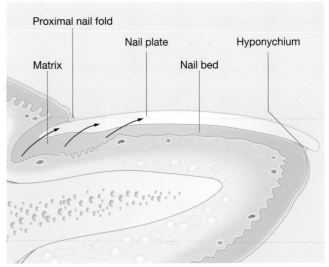

Fig. 2.14 Normal nail.

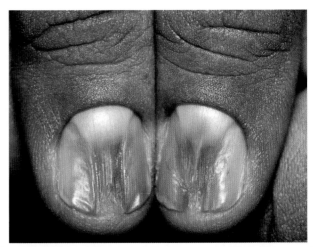

Fig. 2.15 **Lichen planus**—an inflammatory condition that normally affects the skin and mucous membranes but can affect the nail matrix and cause dystrophic nails.

immunity. However, the skin of children and the palmar and plantar skin of adults function well without sebum.

Sebaceous glands are part of the *pilosebaceous unit* and so are found wherever hair follicles are located. In addition, ectopic sebaceous glands are often found on mucous membranes, where they may form small yellow papules called *Fordyce spots*. In the skin, sebaceous glands are most prominent on the scalp and face and are moderately prominent on the upper trunk. The size and secretory activity of these glands are under androgen control. The sebaceous glands in newborns are enlarged owing to maternal hormones, but within months, the glands shrink (Fig. 2.13). They enlarge again in preadolescence from stimulation by adrenal androgens and reach full size at puberty, when gonadal androgens are produced.

Sebaceous glands are androgen dependent.

The lipid-laden cells in the sebaceous glands are wholly secreted (holocrine secretion) to form sebum. Triglycerides compose the majority of the lipid found in sebaceous gland cells. From the sebaceous glands, sebum drains into the hair follicle (Fig. 2.11), from which it exits onto the surface of the skin.

Nails

Nails, like hair, are made of keratin, which is formed from a matrix of dividing epidermal cells (Fig. 2.14). Nails, however, are hard and flat and lie parallel to the skin surface. Located at the ends of fingers and toes, they facilitate fine grasping and pinching maneuvers.

Nail is made of keratin produced in the matrix.

The *nail plate* is a hard, translucent structure composed of keratin. It ranges in thickness from 0.3 to 0.65 mm. Fingernails grow at a continuous rate of about 0.1 mm/day and toenails at a slightly slower rate.

1. Four epithelial zones are associated with the nail: The *proximal nail fold* helps to protect the matrix. The stratum corneum produced there forms the cuticle.

2. The *matrix* produces the nail plate from its rapidly dividing, keratinizing cells. Most of the matrix underlies the proximal nail fold, but on some digits (especially the thumb), it extends under the nail plate, where it is grossly visible as the white lunula. The most proximal portion of the matrix forms the top of the nail plate; the most distal portion forms the bottom of the nail plate. Inflammation of the matrix as found in lichen planus causes nail dystrophy (Fig. 2.15).

3. The epithelium of the *nail bed* produces a minimal amount of keratin, which becomes tightly adherent to the bottom of the nail plate. The pink color of a nail is due to the vascularity in the dermis of the nail bed.

4. The epidermis of the *hyponychium* underlies the free distal edge of the nail plate. Stratum corneum produced there forms a cuticle to seal the junction of the distal nail bed and nail plate.

Subcutaneous Fat

A layer of subcutaneous fat lies between the dermis and the underlying fascia. It helps to insulate the body from cold,

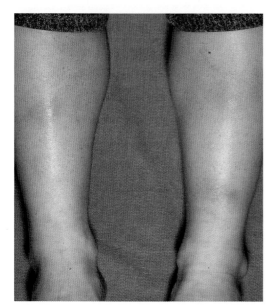

Fig. 2.16 **Erythema nodosum**. Subcutaneous nodules most commonly seen on shins of women after starting birth control pills; results from inflammation concentrated in the fibrous septa that separate the aggregated fat cells or lobules.

cushions deep tissues from blunt trauma, and serves as a reserve source of energy for the body. Biologically active fat cells play a role in hormone messaging, as evidenced by metabolic disturbances in obese children and adolescents with peripheral insulin resistance. Recent evidence supports the role of adipose-derived stem cells in wound healing, hair follicle support/growth, and protection against photoaging. Within the subcutaneous fat layer, aggregates of fat cells (lipocytes) are separated by fibrous septa that are traversed by blood vessels and nerves. Erythema nodosum is the result of subcutaneous inflammation concentrated in the fibrous septa (Fig. 2.16).

SUBCUTANEOUS FAT:
1. Insulates
2. Absorbs trauma
3. Is a reserve energy source
4. Is biologically active

3

Principles of Diagnosis

CHAPTER CONTENTS

ABSTRACT

The approach to a patient with skin disease does not differ markedly from the approach to any other patient. Data are collected from a history and physical examination (and sometimes from the laboratory), a differential diagnosis is generated, and the best diagnosis is selected.

KEY POINTS

1. Morphologic appearance is critical in making the diagnosis.
2. Skin diseases can be divided into growths and rashes.

Steps in dermatologic diagnosis:
1. History
2. Physical: identify the morphology of the basic lesion
3. Consider clinicopathologic correlations
4. Configuration or distribution of lesions (when applicable)
5. Laboratory tests

In history taking, a modified format is suggested. Instead of beginning with an exhaustive interrogation, it is more efficient to divide the history into a preliminary and a follow-up format. You should sit, face the patient, let the patient talk, listen, show empathy, and then clarify questions (location, duration, symptoms, and prior treatment).

The most important part of the physical examination is inspection. Dermatology is a visual specialty, and diagnosis rests heavily on skin inspection. Unfortunately, although the skin is the most visible organ of the body, in a routine physical examination it often is the one most overlooked. Skin lesions need to be looked *for*, not *at*. Just as the examiner hears only the subtle heart sounds for which he or she listens, so will a clinician see on the skin only the lesions for which he or she searches. We need to train our eyes to see the skin lesions before us and ultimately be able to recognize them.

Dermatologic diagnosis depends on the examiner's skill in skin inspection.

We have divided skin disorders into two broad categories: growths and rashes. A *growth* is a discrete lesion resulting from the proliferation of one or more of the skin's components. A *rash* is an inflammatory process that usually is more widespread than a growth. For both skin growths and rashes, the most important task is to characterize the clinical appearance of the basic lesion, that is, to identify its morphology. The pathophysiologic processes responsible for the clinical lesion must then be considered. These clinicopathologic correlations are emphasized in the diagnostic approach presented in this book. For skin rashes, important diagnostic information can sometimes also be obtained by noting the manner in which the lesions are arranged or distributed.

After the history and physical examination have been completed, laboratory tests may be indicated. In dermatology, these are usually simple office procedures that can provide valuable information needed either to confirm or to establish a diagnosis in selected disorders.

HISTORY

KEY POINTS

1. Establish rapport. Be seated.
2. Let the patient talk uninterruptedly in the beginning.
3. Clarify location, duration, symptoms, and prior treatment.
4. Expand the history based on the differential diagnosis.

In medicine, the traditional approach is to take the history before performing the physical examination. Some dermatologists prefer to reverse this order. We find it most useful to ask questions both before and after the examination. With this approach, a preliminary history is taken, in which several general questions are asked of all patients. Depending on the physical findings, more selective questions may be asked subsequently. For example, a history of sexual contact would be inappropriate for a 92-year-old severely disabled person complaining of an itching scalp, but would be indicated for a patient with an indurated ulcer on the penis.

PRELIMINARY HISTORY

In addition to its diagnostic value, a preliminary history also helps to establish rapport with the patient. The shortcut of examining the skin without expressing an interest in the person will often be found wanting, especially by the patient. This initial history is composed of two parts that correlate with the chief complaint and the history of the present illness in the standard history format.

> The initial history can be abbreviated by asking four general questions:
> 1. How long?
> 2. Where affected?
> 3. Does it itch or other symptoms?
> 4. How have you treated it?

Chief Complaint

In eliciting the chief complaint, one can often learn much by asking an open-ended question, such as, "What is your skin problem?" This is followed by four general questions regarding the history of the present illness.

History of the Present Illness

The general questions concern the onset and evolution of the condition, distribution, symptoms, and treatment to date.

Onset and Evolution

"When did it start? Has it gotten better or worse?" Answers to these questions determine the duration of the disorder and how the condition has evolved over time. For most skin conditions, this is important information.

Symptoms

"Does it bother you?" is an open-ended way of asking about symptoms. For rashes, the most common symptom is itching. If the patient does not respond to the general symptom question, you may want to ask specifically, "Does it itch?" Questions concerning systemic symptoms (e.g., "How do you feel otherwise?") are not applicable to most skin diseases and are more appropriately reserved until after the physical examination.

Treatment to Date

The question, "How have you treated it?" results in an incomplete response from almost all patients. For skin disease, one is particularly interested in learning what topical medications have been applied. Many patients do not consider over-the-counter preparations important enough to mention. The same applies to some systemic medications. Providing the patient with specific examples of commonly used topical and systemic medications,

such as calamine lotion and aspirin, may jog a patient's memory enough to recall similar products that they may have used. It is important to inquire about medications, not only because they cause some conditions but also because they may aggravate many others. For example, contact dermatitis initially induced by poison ivy may be perpetuated by contact allergy to an ingredient in one of the preparations used in treatment.

After the skin examination, one may need to return to the treatment question if any suspicion exists that a medication is causing or contributing to the disorder. Interestingly, a patient often recalls using pertinent medication only when the question is asked again to them.

> Persistence is often required in eliciting a complete medication history.

Finally, at the end of the visit, when one is ready to prescribe medications for the patient, it is helpful to know what medications have already been used. This approach avoids the potentially awkward situation in which a patient replies to your enthusiastic recommendation of your favorite therapy with, "I've already tried that and it didn't work!"

FOLLOW-UP HISTORY

After the initial history and physical examination, it is hoped that a diagnosis, or at least a differential diagnosis, has been formulated. With a diagnosis in mind, more focused questions may be necessary. This questioning may include obtaining more details about the history of the present illness or may be directed toward eliciting specific information from other categories of the traditional medical history, including previous medical history, review of systems, family history, and social history. The following serve only as examples for the use of focused questions.

Previous Medical History

After the physical examination, one may want to learn more about the patient's general health. For example, in a patient with suspected herpes zoster, a previous history of chickenpox would be of interest. We have discussed how topically applied and systemically administered medications often contribute to skin conditions. Skin findings may encourage further pursuit of these possibilities. For example, in a patient with a generalized rash or hives, systemic drugs should be high on the list of possible causes. Because drugs can cause virtually any type of skin lesion, it is useful to consider drug eruptions in the differential diagnosis of almost any skin disease. It may also be helpful to ascertain whether the patient has any known allergies to determine whether any medications are currently being used that could produce a cross-reaction.

> Drugs can cause all types of skin rash.

Review of Systems

In a patient with a malar rash, a diagnosis of systemic lupus erythematosus should be considered, and the examiner will want to question the patient further for symptoms of additional skin or other organ involvement, including Raynaud phenomenon, photosensitivity, hair loss, mouth ulcers, and arthritis. In a patient with a generalized maculopapular eruption, the two most common causes are drugs and viruses, so the physician will want to inquire about both medication use and viral symptoms, such as fever, malaise, and upper respiratory or gastrointestinal symptoms.

Family History

In certain cutaneous conditions, some knowledge of the family history may help in diagnosis. Innumerable inherited disorders have dermatologic expression. The following serve only as examples:

- In a child with a chronic itching eruption in the antecubital and popliteal fossae, atopic dermatitis is suspected. A positive family history of atopic diseases (atopic dermatitis, asthma, hay fever) supports the diagnosis.
- In a young person with multiple café-au-lait spots, a diagnosis of neurofibromatosis is considered. A positive family history for this disorder, substantiated by examination of family members, helps to support the diagnosis of this dominantly inherited disease.

> Inherited disorders have numerous skin findings.

Knowledge of the family's present health is also important when considering infectious diseases. For example, impetigo can occur in several family members, and this knowledge may help in considering the diagnosis; it would certainly be important for treatment. Likewise, in a patient with suspected scabies, it is important to know, for both diagnostic and therapeutic purposes, whether other family members are itching.

Social History

In some disorders, knowledge of the patient's social history may be important. For example, a chronic skin ulcer from persistent herpes simplex infection is a sign of immunosuppression, particularly acquired immune deficiency syndrome (AIDS). Therefore a patient with such an ulceration should be asked about high-risk factors for acquiring AIDS, including sexual behavior, intravenous drug abuse, and exposure to blood products.

> For persistent skin infections, consider the possibility of undiagnosed AIDS.

Another common occasion for probing into a patient's social history is when the patient is suspected of having contact dermatitis; this aspect of the social history could be subtitled the *skin exposure history*. Patients encounter potentially sensitizing materials both at work and at play. Industrial dermatitis is a leading cause of workers' disability. For chronic hand dermatitis, questions about occupational exposure are important and should be directed particularly to materials and substances the patient contacts either by handling or by immersion. Similarly, a patient presenting with an acute eruption characterized by streaks of vesicles should be queried regarding recent outdoor activities resulting in exposure to poison ivy or poison oak. Contact dermatitis is a common and challenging problem. On the part of the physician, it often requires painstaking efforts in a detective-type search to elicit from the patient an exposure history that fits the dermatitis.

> A complete "skin exposure history" is required whenever contact dermatitis is suspected.

Some harbor the misconception that in dermatology, one needs only to glance at the skin to arrive at a diagnosis and that talking with the patient is superfluous. Although this is occasionally true, we hope that the previous examples serve to illustrate that this frequently is not the case. In fact, in some instances (and contact dermatitis is a good example), detailed historical information is essential to establish a diagnosis.

PHYSICAL EXAMINATION

> ### KEY POINTS
> 1. A complete skin examination is recommended at the first visit.
> 2. Good lighting is critical.
> 3. Describe the morphology of the eruption.

The physical examination follows the preliminary history. For the skin to be inspected adequately, three essential requirements must be met: (1) an undressed patient, clothed in an examining gown; (2) adequate illumination, preferably bright overhead fluorescent lighting; and (3) an examining physician prepared to see what is there.

> One should practice thorough hand hygiene prior to and after touching the patient.

Examine the entire mucocutaneous surface, but patients will be more firmly convinced of your sincere interest in their particular problems if you start by examining the affected areas before proceeding with the more complete examination.

At least for the initial examination, the patient needs to be disrobed so that the entire skin surface can be examined. Busy physicians who tend to overlook this rule will miss much. An occasional patient may be reluctant to comply, saying, "My skin problem is only on my hands; why do you need to look at the rest of my skin?" We tell such patients that we have at least two reasons: other lesions may be found that "go along with" the lesions on the hands and help to confirm the diagnosis. For example, in a patient with sharply demarcated plaques on the palms, the finding of a few scaling plaques on the knees or a sharply marginated intergluteal plaque will help to substantiate a suspicion of psoriasis.

1. An important incidental skin lesion may be found. The finding of a previously undetected malignant melanoma on a patient's back is an example. We studied the yield from a complete skin examination in 1,157 consecutive new dermatology patients and found an incidental skin malignancy in 22. Some 20 of these patients had basal cell carcinoma, 1 had melanoma, and

1 had Kaposi sarcoma that served as the presenting manifestation of AIDS. A subsequent study of 874 patients reported an incidental skin cancer detection rate of 3.4%.

> The entire skin surface is examined for:
> 1. Lesions that may accompany the presenting complaint
> 2. Unrelated but important incidental findings

For the skin to be examined adequately, it must be properly illuminated. Natural lighting is excellent for this purpose but is difficult to achieve in most offices and hospital rooms. The alternative is bright overhead fluorescent lighting, supplemented with a movable lamp that is usually wall mounted. One additional illuminator that is often useful is a simple penlight. Either this or the movable lamp can be used as side lighting to detect whether a lesion is subtly elevated. For this technique, the light is directed onto the lesion from an angle that is roughly parallel to the skin. If the lesion is elevated, a small shadow will be thrown, and the relief of the skin will be appreciated. The penlight also is useful for examining the mouth, an area that is sometimes overlooked but in which one may detect lesions that are helpful in diagnosing a cutaneous disorder.

Another piece of examination equipment that is occasionally useful is the Wood's light, a long-wavelength ultraviolet "black" light. Contrary to some popular misconceptions, this light does not enable one to diagnose most skin fungal infections, it detects fluorescence of affected hairs only in some, now uncommon, types of tinea capitis. The Wood's light is, however, still used to accentuate pigmentary alterations in the skin, such as vitiligo.

Except for provision of adequate illumination, minimal equipment is needed for examining the skin. A simple handheld lens can be helpful. Enlarging the image may improve diagnostic accuracy. However, on some occasions, such as clarifying a burrow in scabies or detecting Wickham striae in a lesion of lichen planus, a handheld lens can be useful. For diagnosing pigmented growths, dermatologists often employ a dermatoscope. This is an illuminated handheld magnifying device intended to help the clinician to diagnose melanoma and other growths clinically.

> A dermatoscope is useful in diagnosing growths, especially melanoma.

An adequate examination of the skin should actually be called a mucocutaneous examination so that one is reminded to include an examination of the mouth. Similarly, the scalp and nails should not be overlooked. Because both cutaneous and systemic diseases may be expressed in the nails and nail beds as well as in the mouth, these areas should be inspected in every cutaneous examination.

> The scalp, mouth, and nails should not be overlooked.

Physical examination depends largely on inspection, but one should not neglect the opportunity to palpate the skin as well. The two major purposes for this are (1) to assess the texture, consistency, and tenderness of the skin lesions and (2) to reassure patients that we are not afraid to touch their skin lesions—that they do not have some dreadful contagious disease.

Nothing is more disquieting to a patient than to be cautiously approached with a gloved hand. For anogenital, mucosal, and all weeping lesions, gloving is necessary and expected, but for most other lesions, the physician learns more and the patient is less frightened if the touching is done without gloves. Palpation is the major method by which we evaluate not only the consistency (e.g., softness, firmness, fluctuance) but also the depth of a lesion.

> Palpation helps to:
> 1. Assess texture and consistency
> 2. Evaluate tenderness
> 3. Reassure patients that they are not contagious

After the patient is properly gowned and perfectly illuminated, for what do we inspect and palpate? The first and most important step is to characterize the appearance (i.e., identify the morphology) of each skin lesion. After the morphology of a lesion is identified, its clinicopathologic correlation can be considered.

> The most important task in the physical examination is to characterize the morphology of the basic lesion.

TERMINOLOGY OF SKIN LESIONS

KEY POINTS

1. Primary lesions include macule, patch, papule, plaque, nodule, cyst, vesicle, pustule, ulcer, wheal, telangiectasia, burrow, and comedo.
2. Secondary lesions include scale, crust, oozing, lichenification, induration, fissure, and atrophy.

A special vocabulary is used in describing the morphologic appearances of skin lesions. These terms are illustrated and defined in Fig. 3.1.

CLINICOPATHOLOGIC CORRELATIONS

KEY POINTS

1. Envisioning the gross and microscopic morphology together helps to make the diagnosis.
2. Rash or growth?
3. Epidermal, dermal, or subcutaneous?

The lesions defined in Fig. 3.1 result from alterations in one or more of the skin's structural components. For clinical diagnostic purposes, we try to envision what pathologic changes are associated with each clinical lesion (Table 3.1). Scale, lichenification, vesicles, bullae, pustules, and crusts represent epidermal alterations, whereas erythema (red in lighter skin, purple or dark brown in darker skin), purpura, and induration reflect

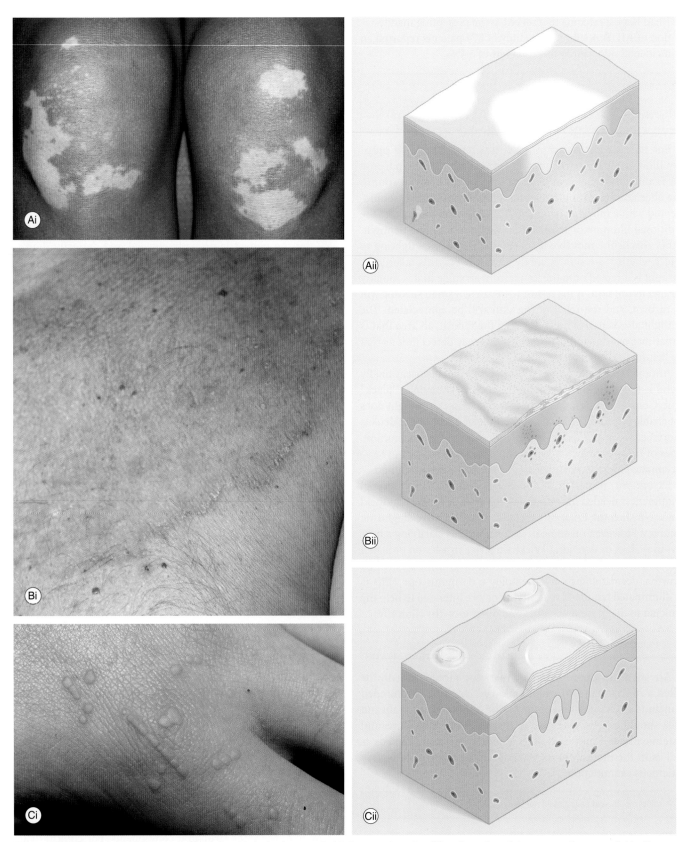

Fig. 3.1 **Skin lesions**. (A) Vitiligo—**macule**. A flat skin lesion is recognizable because its color differs from that of the surrounding normal skin. The most common color changes are white (hypopigmented), brown/black (hyperpigmented), and red/purple (erythematous and purpuric). (B) Tinea corporis—**patch**. A macule with some surface change, either slight scale or fine wrinkling. (C) Flat warts—**papules**. Small elevated skin lesions <0.5 cm in diameter.

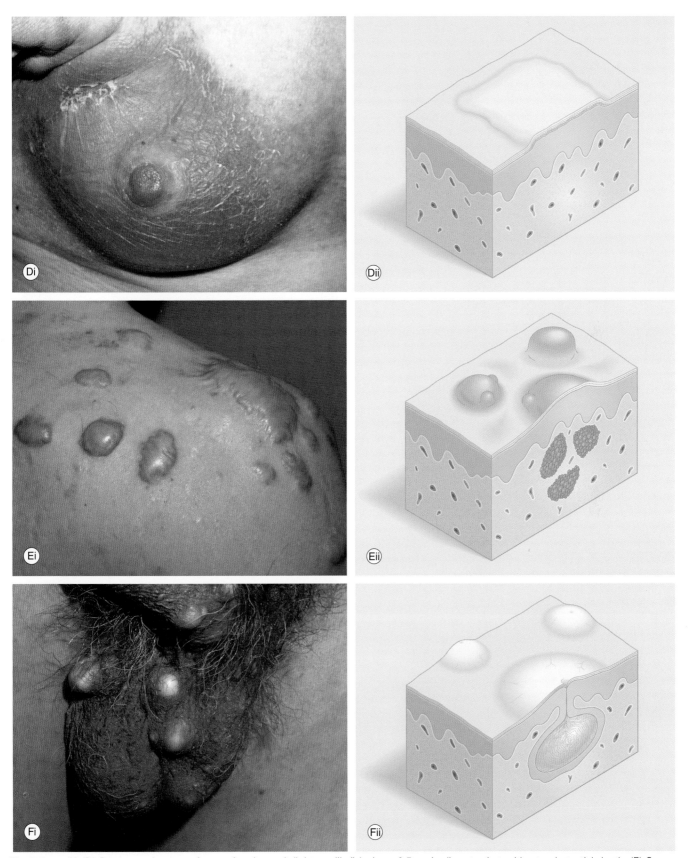

Fig. 3.1 cont'd (D) Breast carcinoma—**plaque**. An elevated, "plateau-like" lesion >0.5 cm in diameter but without substantial depth. (E) Scars—**nodules**. Elevated, "marble-like" lesions >0.5 cm in both diameter and depth. (F) Epidermal inclusion—**cysts**. Nodules filled with expressible material that is either liquid or semisolid.

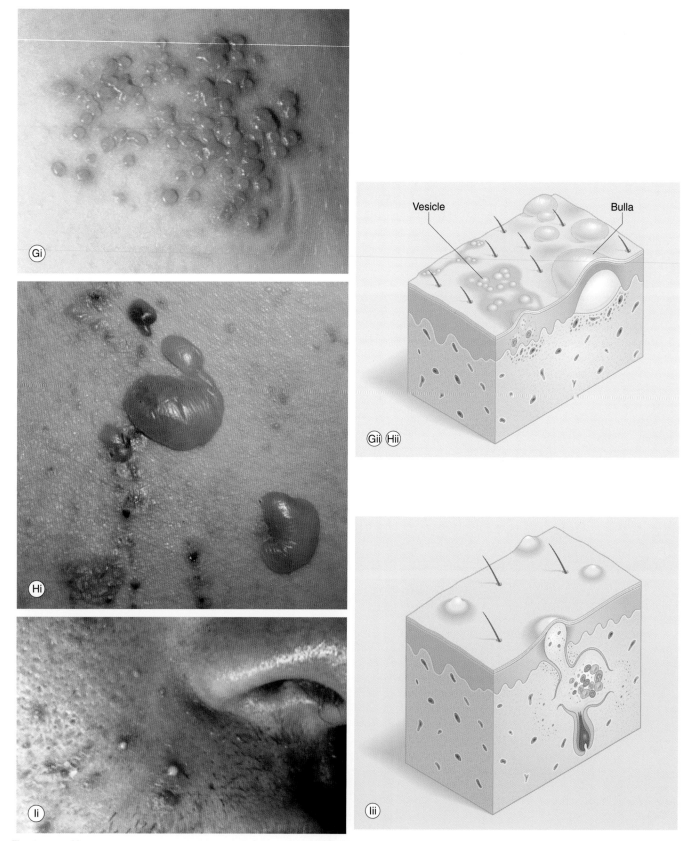

Fig. 3.1 cont'd (G) Herpes simplex—**vesicles**. (H) Bullous pemphigoid—**bullae**. Blisters are filled with clear fluid. Vesicles are <0.5 cm in diameter, and bullae are >0.5 cm in diameter. (I) Acne—**pustules**. Vesicles filled with cloudy or purulent fluid.

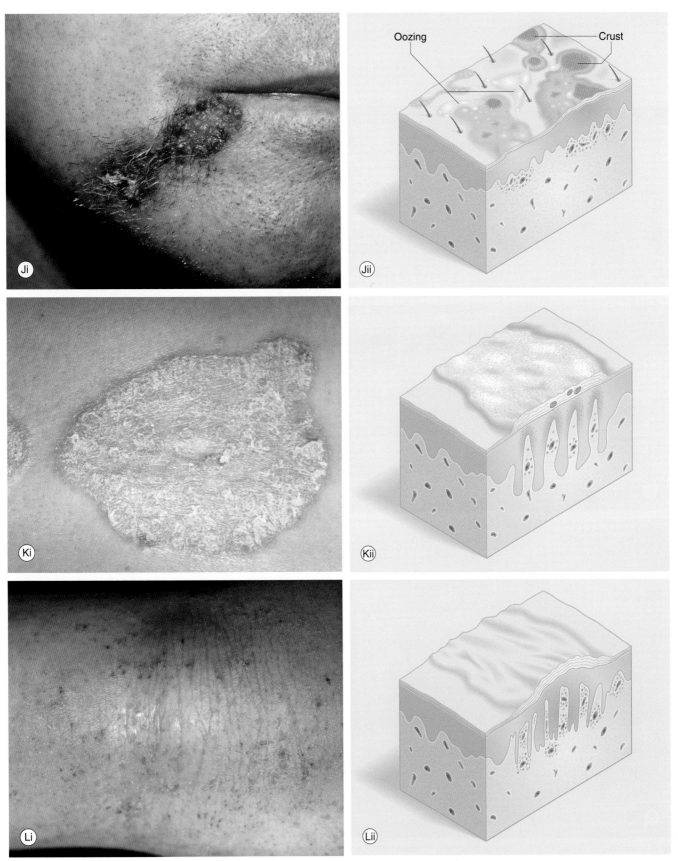

Fig. 3.1 cont'd (J) Chronic herpes simplex—**crust**. Liquid debris (e.g., serum/blood or pus) that has dried on the surface of the skin. Crust most often results from the breakage of vesicles, pustules, or bullae. (K) Psoriasis—**scale**. Visibly thickened stratum corneum. Scales are dry and usually whitish. These features help to distinguish scales from crusts, which are often moist and usually yellowish, brown, or red. (L) Atopic dermatitis—**lichenification**. *Epidermal thickening* characterized by (i) visible and palpable thickening of the skin with (ii) accentuated skin markings.

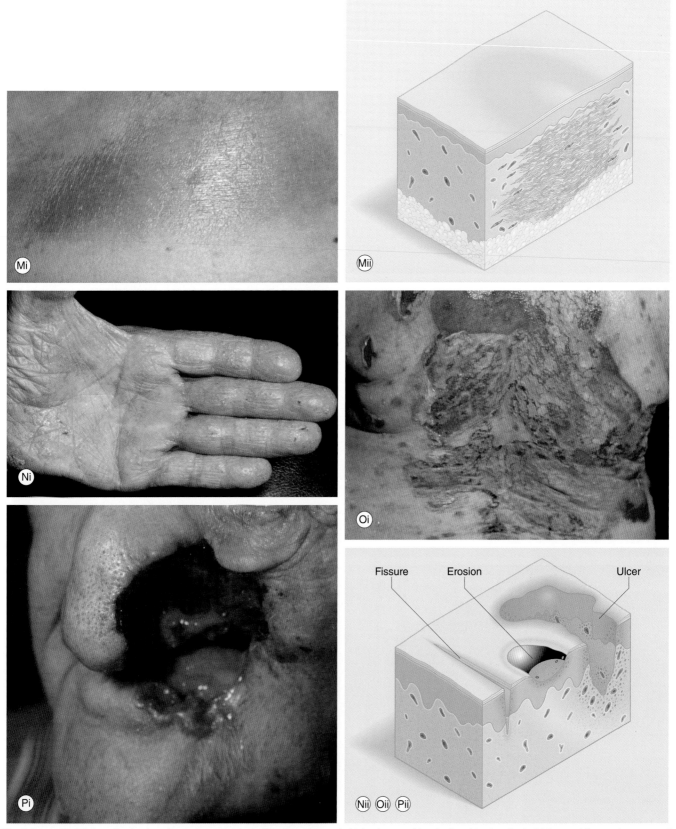

Fig. 3.1 cont'd　(M) Localized scleroderma (morphea)—**induration**. *Dermal thickening* resulting in the skin that *feels* thicker and firmer than normal. (N) Hand dermatitis—**fissures**. A fissure is a thin, linear tear in the epidermis. (O) Pemphigus vulgaris—**erosion**. An erosion is limited in depth, confined to loss of the epidermis and superficial dermis. (P) Basal cell carcinoma—**ulcer**. An ulcer is a deeper defect devoid of epidermis, as well as part or all of the dermis.

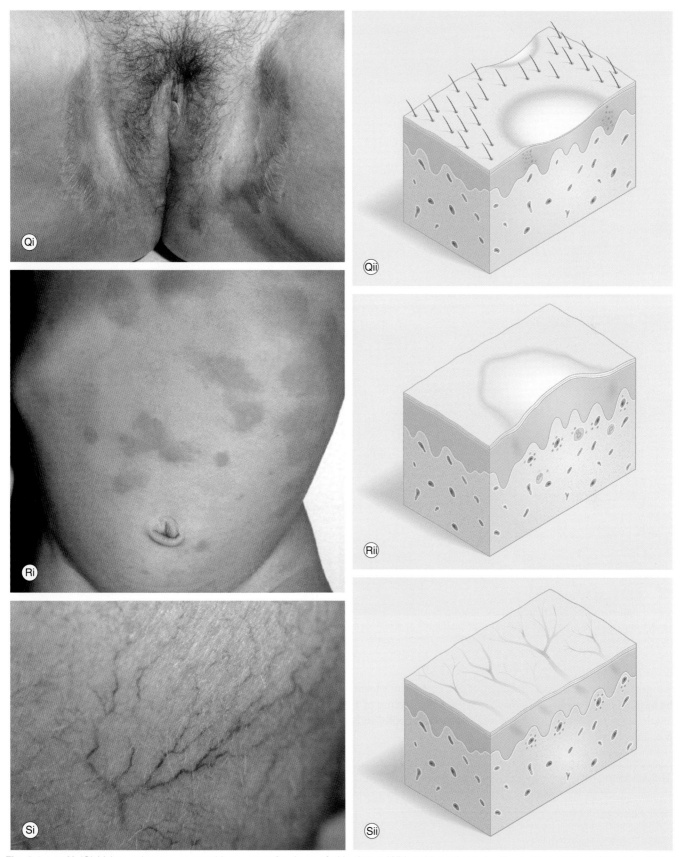

Fig. 3.1 cont'd (Q) Lichen sclerosus et atrophicus—**atrophy**. Loss of skin tissue. With epidermal atrophy, the surface appears thin and wrinkled. Atrophy of the much thicker dermal layer results in a clinically detectable depression in the skin. (R). Urticaria—**wheal**. A papule or plaque of dermal edema. Wheals (or *hives*) often have central pallor and irregular borders. (S) Sun damage/aging—**telangiectasia**. Superficial blood vessels enlarged sufficiently to be clinically visible.

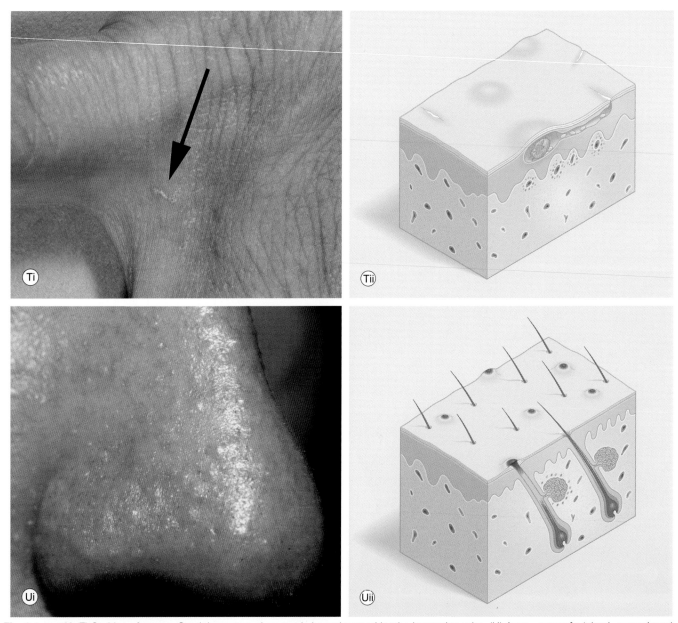

Fig. 3.1 cont'd (T) Scabies—**burrow**. Serpiginous tunnel or streak *(arrow)* caused by the burrowing mite. (U) Acne—**comedo** (plural, *comedones*). The noninflammatory lesions of acne that result from keratin impaction in the outlet of the pilosebaceous canal.

changes in the dermis. Such clinicopathologic correlations form the basis of the diagnostic approach. For example, scaling of a nodule suggests hyperkeratosis of the stratum corneum and, thus, an epidermal growth.

> Erythema appears red in lighter skin and purple or dark brown in darker skin.

> Determine which of the skin components are involved in the clinical lesion to make a clinicopathologic correlation.

Most skin disorders can be categorized first as proliferative "growths" (neoplasms) or inflammatory "rashes" (eruptions). The growths and rashes are then subdivided, depending on how they appear clinically and which structural component is involved pathologically.

> Growths are hyperplastic lesions; rashes are inflammatory.

GROWTHS

Growths are subdivided into epidermal, pigmented, and dermal or subcutaneous proliferative processes.

> Growths are subdivided into one of three categories:
> 1. Epidermal
> 2. Pigmented
> 3. Dermal or subcutaneous

TABLE 3.1 Clinicopathologic Correlations

Skin Component	Pathologic Alteration	Clinical Manifestation
Epidermis		
Stratum corneum	Hyperkeratosis	Scale
Subcorneal epidermis	Hyperplasia	Lichenification
	Hyperplasia	Papules, plaques, and nodules
	Disruptive inflammatory changes	Vesicles, bullae, and pustules
	Dried serum/blood	Crusts
Melanocytes	Increased number or function	Pigmented macules, papules, and nodules
	Decreased number or function	White spots
Dermis		
Blood vessels	Hyperplasia or inflammation	Macules, papules, and nodules
	Vasodilation	Erythema
	Hemorrhage	Purpura
	Vasodilation with edema	Wheals
Nerves	Hyperplasia	Papules, nodules
Connective tissue	Hyperplasia	Induration, papules, nodules, and plaques
	Loss of epidermis	Erosion
	Loss of epidermis and dermis	Ulceration
Dermal appendages		
Pilosebaceous units	Hyperplasia	Hirsutism
	Atrophy	Alopecia
	Hyperplasia or inflammation	Comedones, papules, nodules, and cysts
Sweat glands	Hypersecretion	Hyperhidrosis
	Hyperplasia or inflammation	Vesicles, papules, pustules, and cysts
Subcutaneous fat	Hyperplasia or inflammation	Induration and nodules

Epidermal growths result from hyperplasia of keratinocytes; many of these neoplasms have scaling surfaces. *Scale* accumulates when the rate of stratum corneum production exceeds the rate of shedding. *Hyperkeratosis* is another term used to describe an excessive accumulation of keratin, the fibrous protein that makes up the stratum corneum. The term "hyperkeratosis" is most often used with skin growths (e.g., seborrheic keratoses); "scaling" is used to describe both growths and rashes.

> Scale and hyperkeratosis are both terms for excess stratum corneum.

Because the normal function of the epidermis is to produce the keratotic stratum corneum, hyperkeratosis may be expected in epidermal neoplasms. These proliferative processes may be benign (e.g., seborrheic keratoses), premalignant (e.g., actinic keratoses), or malignant (e.g., squamous cell carcinoma).

Hyperplasia of the subcorneal epidermis results in elevated lesions of the skin papules, plaques, and nodules. Benign growths originating in the epidermis often appear superficial. Malignant epidermal growths, by definition, have invaded the dermis, and they therefore feel or appear *indurated*, a term used to designate thickening of the dermis.

> Malignant epidermal growths usually are indurated, except for superficial basal and squamous cell carcinomas, which are patches.

Pigmented lesions result from increased melanin production or increased numbers of melanin-producing cells, and so may be either macular or papular. Freckles are common examples of hyperpigmented macules that result from increased melanin production. Nevi and melanomas are examples of growths characterized by increased numbers of melanin-producing cells. Nevi that are sufficiently cellular to impart a mass effect are elevated, and so appear clinically as hyperpigmented papules, plaques, or even nodules.

Dermal and subcutaneous growths result from *focal* proliferative processes in the dermis or subcutaneous fat. They appear most often as nodules, which are most fully appreciated by palpation. The proliferative elements that form nodules may be either endogenous (e.g., a dermatofibroma that results from the proliferation of dermal fibroblasts) or exogenous (e.g., a metastasis from an internal malignant disease) to the skin. Because often no surface markers exist to differentiate one dermal nodule from another, the definitive diagnostic test frequently must be a biopsy. This clinical point deserves emphasis: for undiagnosed skin nodules, particularly firm lesions, malignancy must be suspected, and a biopsy must be performed.

> A skin biopsy is often required for the diagnosis of a dermal nodule.

RASHES

For rashes, the first diagnostic step is to determine whether the epidermis is involved. Types of epidermal involvement are listed in Table 3.2. Although some rashes produce several epidermal changes, usually one change is distinctive or predominant.

Acute dermatitis (eczema) is histologically characterized by epidermal intercellular edema (spongiosis), which is manifested clinically by vesicles, or "juicy" papules. Chronic dermatitis has lichenification as its hallmark. *Lichenification* represents epidermal hyperplasia clinically expressed as thickened skin with accentuated skin markings.

Epidermal rashes:
1. Eczematous
2. Scaling
3. Vesicular
4. Papular
5. Pustular
6. Hypopigmented

Scaling eruptions are the result of thickened stratum corneum. Scaling rashes can involve either focal areas or the entire cutaneous surface. Examples of the former are more common and are represented by the so-called papulosquamous diseases. These disorders are characterized by scaling (squamous) papules and plaques and patches. Psoriasis and fungal infections serve as examples. Ichthyosis (fish skin) is an example of generalized scaling.

Scale is usually white or light tan and flakes off rather easily. These features help to distinguish scale from crust. *Crust* is dried serum/blood and debris on the skin surface; it is usually darker, most often dark red, yellow, or brown; it is adherent and, when removed, a weeping base is revealed. The distinction between scale and crust is important because the differential diagnoses are entirely different. Crusts are associated with vesicles, bullae, pustules, and malignant growths.

> Scale (keratin) must be distinguished from crust (dried serum/blood).

Vesicles and bullae occur when fluid accumulates within or beneath the epidermis. They characterize a relatively small number of important dermatologic disorders, so are extremely helpful diagnostic findings. Vesicles and bullae occur either intraepidermally or subepidermally. The differential diagnoses are different for intraepidermal and subepidermal blisters, so it is important to try to distinguish them. Clinically, one clue is the fragility of the blister. Because of their more substantial roof, fresh subepidermal blisters are tense and less easily broken, whereas intraepidermal bullae are flaccid and easily ruptured. A biopsy of the *edge* of an early lesion confirms the clinical impression.

> Vesicles and bullae are important diagnostic findings and occur intraepidermal or subepidermal.

Pruritic papules are produced by inflammation, predominantly in the dermis. Pustules occur when inflammatory cells aggregate within the epidermis. Pustules may be located superficially in the epidermis, or they may arise from superficial locations in appendageal structures. With purulence, one usually thinks of bacterial infection. This is an appropriate reflex, and Gram staining or culture of the contents of a pustule is indicated if a bacterial infection is suspected. However, not all pustular processes are bacterial in origin; viral and fungal infections can also result in pustules, and acne is a common example of a noninfectious cause.

> Pustules often (but not always) indicate an infection.

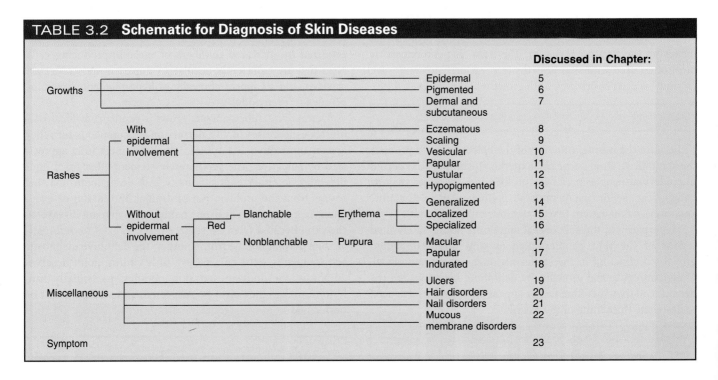

TABLE 3.2	Schematic for Diagnosis of Skin Diseases			Discussed in Chapter:
Growths			Epidermal	5
			Pigmented	6
			Dermal and subcutaneous	7
Rashes	With epidermal involvement		Eczematous	8
			Scaling	9
			Vesicular	10
			Papular	11
			Pustular	12
			Hypopigmented	13
	Without epidermal involvement	Red — Blanchable — Erythema	Generalized	14
			Localized	15
			Specialized	16
		Nonblanchable — Purpura	Macular	17
			Papular	17
			Indurated	18
Miscellaneous			Ulcers	19
			Hair disorders	20
			Nail disorders	21
			Mucous membrane disorders	22
Symptom				23

When melanin pigment is lost from the epidermis, white spots result. Because no associated increase in cellular mass occurs, hypopigmented lesions can be expected to be macular (not papular) white spots. Hypopigmentary changes are accentuated under Wood's light examination, whereby previously unnoticed lesions may become apparent and the degree of pigment loss can be roughly assessed. The more pronounced the pigment loss, the whiter the lesion appears under the scrutiny of the Wood's light.

> Hypopigmentary changes are accentuated with Wood's light examination.

Dermal rashes without epidermal involvement are either inflammatory or infiltrative; most are inflammatory. Inflammatory eruptions appear red because of vasodilation of *dermal* blood vessels (the epidermis is devoid of vasculature). Redness in skin lesions can be caused by either *erythema* or *purpura*. It is extremely important to differentiate between the two. With erythema, the increased blood in the skin is contained within dilated blood vessels. Therefore erythema is *blanchable* (Fig. 3.2). With purpura, blood has extravasated from disrupted blood vessels into the dermis, and the lesion is nonblanchable (Fig. 3.3). The test for blanchability is called *diascopy*. It is

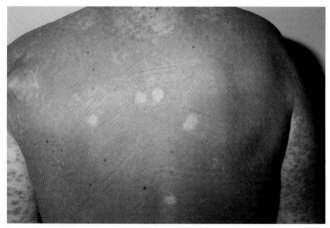

Fig. 3.2 Erythema is red and blanchable, as demonstrated with fingertip pressure on the midback in this patient with a drug eruption.

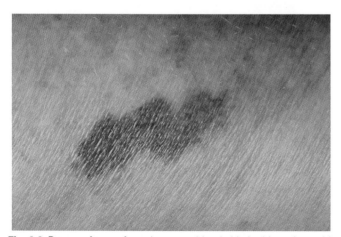

Fig. 3.3 Purpura is purple and was not blanchable in this patient with fragile skin that had been injured.

performed by simply applying pressure with a finger or glass slide and observing color changes. Depending on the skin color, red (erythema and purpura) may not be easily appreciated. For example, red appears as dark purple or brown in darker-skinned individuals.

Erythematous rashes are subdivided into generalized, localized, and specialized (e.g., hives) types. A *wheal*, or hive, is a special type of blanchable, transient, erythematous lesion of the skin. Blood vessels in a wheal are dilated, and fluid leaks from them, causing edema in the surrounding dermis. This fluid is not compartmentalized as in vesicles or bullae, but rather is dispersed evenly throughout the dermal tissue. The result is an elevated erythematous lesion, often with central pallor that is due to the intense edema.

Purpuric rashes are subdivided into macular and papular categories. *Macular purpura* is flat and nonpalpable, whereas *papular purpura* is elevated (sometimes subtly) and palpable. This clinical distinction is important because the differential diagnoses and clinical implications are different for the two types. Macular purpura occurs in two settings: (1) conditions associated with increased capillary fragility and (2) bleeding disorders. Macular hemorrhage is not accompanied by inflammation. In papular or palpable purpura, inflammatory changes are present in the vessel walls and are responsible for the elevation of the lesions. Disruption and necrosis of the blood vessels caused by an inflammatory reaction are called *necrotizing vasculitis*. This condition is usually immunologically mediated and can occur in numerous settings, such as sepsis, collagen vascular diseases, and, occasionally, drug reactions. In the diagnosis of a patient with palpable purpura, such systemic processes must be excluded.

> Macular purpura is usually a sign of a bleeding disorder or vascular fragility; papular purpura indicates a necrotizing vasculitis, often systemic.

Rashes resulting from *infiltrative processes* in the dermis are much less common than inflammatory disorders. Clinically, they feel indurated. Induration, resulting from increased amounts of collagen, is also called *sclerosis*. Scleroderma, an idiopathic disorder of increased collagen deposition, is an example.

MISCELLANEOUS CONDITIONS

Skin ulcers and disorders of hair, nails, and mucous membranes are easily recognizable and grouped as miscellaneous.

An *ulcer* is totally devoid of epidermis, and some or all of the dermal tissue is missing. Ulcers may extend down to underlying bone (e.g., in advanced decubitus ulcers). An *erosion* can be considered a "superficial ulcer" just missing epidermis and minimal dermis. Both ulcers and erosions are characterized by weeping and crusting. Malignant processes can result in ulcerations that do not heal. For this reason, all chronic ulcers should be biopsied.

> A chronic ulcer/erosion should undergo biopsy to rule out malignancy.

TABLE 3.3   Some Examples of Configuration

Configuration	Morphology	Disease	Illustration
Linear	Vesicles Papules	Contact dermatitis[a] Psoriasis[b] Lichen planus[b] Flat warts	Fig. 3.4
Grouped	Vesicles Papules	Herpes (simplex and zoster) Insect bites Leiomyomas	Fig. 3.5
Annular	Scaling	Tinea corporis	Fig. 3.6
		Secondary syphilis	
		Subacute cutaneous lupus erythematosus	
	Dermal plaque	Granuloma annulare Sarcoid	
Geographic	Wheals Plaques	Urticaria Mycosis fungoides	Fig. 3.7

[a]Typical for contact dermatitis from a plant resin (e.g., poison ivy).
[b]The Koebner reaction.

Too little hair is a much more common dermatologic complaint than too much hair. *Alopecia* means hair loss. For diagnostic purposes, it is helpful to classify alopecia as either *nonscarring* or *scarring*. Clinically, the distinction depends on whether follicular openings are visible. The differential diagnoses are different for each of these two categories.

> For alopecia, first determine whether it is scarring or nonscarring.

Most nail disorders are inflammatory and can affect the nail matrix, nail bed, or periungual skin (paronychia). Inflammation and scaling in the nail bed result in separation of the nail plate from the bed (onycholysis). Fungal infection and psoriasis are the most common causes.

The two most common manifestations of mucous membrane disorders are (1) erosions and ulcerations and (2) white lesions. On mucous membranes, whiteness represents hyperkeratosis, which is white because of maceration from continuous wetness.

> Mucous membrane disorders:
> 1. Erosions and ulcerations
> 2. White lesions

CONFIGURATION OF SKIN LESIONS

KEY POINTS
1. Configuration can help make the diagnosis.
2. Morphology is more important than configuration.

The diagnosis of rash is often aided by considering the configuration of the lesions or their distribution on the body surface. *Configuration* refers to the pattern in which skin lesions are arranged. The four most common patterns are listed in

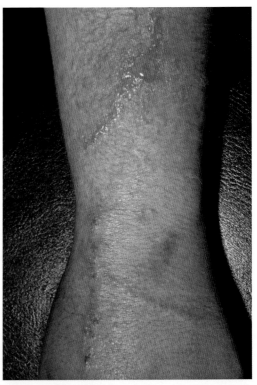

Fig. 3.4 Contact dermatitis from poison ivy, demonstrating linear streaks of papules and vesicles.

Table 3.3, along with examples of diseases that most often present in these configurations. Occasionally, a configuration is specific for a disease. For example, streaks of vesicles are characteristic of contact dermatitis from poison ivy or poison oak. More often, a configuration is not completely specific for a given disease but may still be helpful in the diagnosis. For example, in psoriasis, scaling papules sometimes develop in streaks as a result of the Koebner reaction, in which lesions of a disorder develop after trauma, such as scratching.

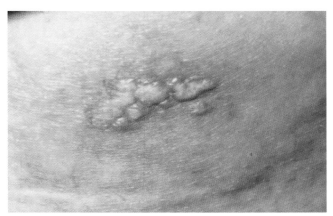

Fig. 3.5 **Herpes simplex**—grouped vesiculopustules.

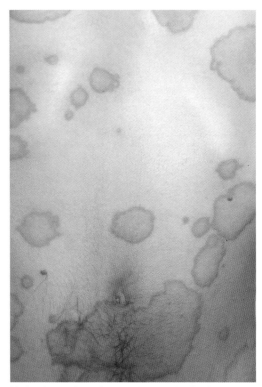

Fig. 3.7 **Urticaria**—typical wheals with central pallor from dermal edema and irregular red borders.

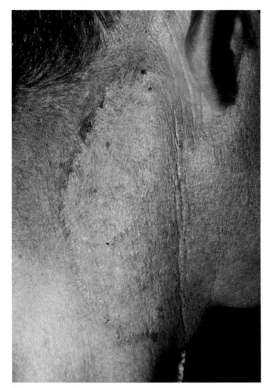

Fig. 3.6 **Tinea corporis**—annular scaling patch.

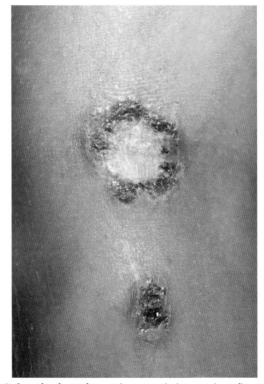

Fig. 3.8 **Annular impetigo**—when morphology and configuration (or distribution) appear to conflict, the morphology takes precedence.

As can be seen from Table 3.3 (Figs. 3.4–3.7), configuration considerations are sometimes diagnostically helpful, but morphology takes precedence. The annular impetigo shown in Fig. 3.8 illustrates this point. If the crust had been interpreted as scale, the annular lesions would almost certainly have been misdiagnosed as tinea corporis (ringworm). The honey-colored crust, however, should focus attention on the vesiculopustular nature of the primary process and raise the question of bacterial infection. So, for dermatologic diagnosis, the morphology of the primary lesion must be identified correctly before consideration is given to a specific configuration, if one is present. If a conflict appears to exist between the morphology and the configuration, more diagnostic weight should be given to the morphology.

TABLE 3.4 Regional Diagnoses

Growths	Rashes	Growths	Rashes
Scalp		**Groin (Inguinal)**	
Nevus	Seborrheic dermatitis (dandruff)	Skin tag	Intertrigo
Seborrheic keratosis	Psoriasis	Wart	Tinea cruris
Pilar cyst	Tinea capitis	Molluscum contagiosum	Candidiasis
	Folliculitis		Pediculosis pubis
			Hidradenitis suppurativa
Face			Psoriasis
Nevus	Acne		Seborrheic dermatitis
Lentigo	Acne rosacea	**Extremities**	
Actinic keratosis	Seborrheic dermatitis	Nevus	Atopic dermatitis
Seborrheic keratosis	Contact dermatitis (cosmetics)	Dermatofibroma	Contact dermatitis
Sebaceous hyperplasia	Herpes simplex	Wart	Psoriasis
Basal cell carcinoma	Impetigo	Seborrheic keratosis	Insect bites
Squamous cell carcinoma	Pityriasis alba	Actinic keratosis	Erythema multiforme
Flat wart	Atopic dermatitis	Xanthoma	Lichen planus (wrists and ankles)
Nevus flammeus	Lupus erythematosus		Actinic purpura (arms)
			Stasis dermatitis (legs)
Trunk			Vasculitis (legs)
Nevus	Acne		Erythema nodosum (legs)
Skin tag	Tinea versicolor	**Hands (Palmar)**	
Cherry angioma	Psoriasis	Wart	Essential dermatitis
Seborrheic keratosis	Pityriasis rosea		Atopic dermatitis
Epidermal inclusion cyst	Scabies		Psoriasis
Lipoma	Drug eruption		Tinea manuum
Basal cell carcinoma	Varicella		Erythema multiforme
Keloid	Mycosis fungoides		Secondary syphilis
Neurofibroma	Secondary syphilis	**Feet (Dorsal)**	
Genitalia		Wart	Contact dermatitis (shoe)
Wart (condyloma acuminatum)	Herpes simplex	**Feet (Plantar)**	
	Scabies	Wart (plantar)	Contact dermatitis (shoe)
Molluscum contagiosum	Psoriasis	Corn	Tinea pedis
Seborrheic keratosis	Lichen planus	Nevus	Essential dermatitis
	Syphilis (chancre)		Psoriasis
	Contact dermatitis		Atopic dermatitis

DISTRIBUTION OF SKIN LESIONS

KEY POINTS

1. The distribution of skin lesions and the region affected can suggest or confirm a diagnosis.

Many skin diseases have preferential areas of involvement, so the location of the eruption may help in diagnosis. A good example of this is herpes zoster, in which consideration of all three diagnostic criteria (morphology, configuration, and distribution) secures the diagnosis: vesicles in grouped configuration and dermatomal distribution are diagnostic for herpes zoster.

Many skin disorders have favored regional distributions (i.e., a propensity for a particular area of the body), such as the scalp, face, hands, groin, or feet. Sometimes, this propensity can be used as a starting point for developing a differential diagnosis. These "regional" diagnoses are outlined in Table 3.4. For rashes that affect widespread areas, the distribution *pattern* may also aid in the diagnosis. This is particularly true for contact dermatitis, in which the location of the rash on the skin may be helpful, not only in leading one to suspect a contact origin but also in providing a clue about the nature of the contactant. For example, a rash on the earlobes and around the neck should lead one to suspect allergic contact dermatitis caused by the nickel present in jewelry.

4

Dermatologic Therapy and Procedures

CHAPTER CONTENTS

ABSTRACT

Because the skin is so accessible, it can be treated with a variety of therapeutic options not available for use in diseases of internal organs. Drugs for dermatologic therapy can be administered topically, intralesionally, and systemically. In addition, physical modalities such as ultraviolet (UV) and ionizing radiation, surgery, laser, and cryotherapy can be easily administered.

At one time, dermatologic therapy was based largely on empiric approaches. However, much progress has been made in defining the scientific bases for numerous dermatologic treatments, resulting in a well-rounded rationale for choosing specific modalities.

The discussions in this chapter are limited to principles of external therapies unique to the skin. Other, more specific, topical therapies, such as those used for acne and for fungal diseases, as well as all systemic therapies, are discussed in chapters (5-22) concerning the diseases in which they are used.

PRINCIPLES OF TOPICAL THERAPY

KEY POINTS

1. Many drugs are available in topical preparation.
2. The vehicle is almost as important as the active ingredient.
3. Give enough volume to treat the area of disease involvement adequately.

A diverse group of medications is available in topical preparations, including antibiotics, antifungals, corticosteroids, acne preparations, sunscreens, cytotoxic agents, antipruritics, antiseptics, and pesticides. Topical therapy has the distinct advantage of delivering medications directly to the target organ. This route reduces the potential of systemic side-effects and toxicity seen with systemic therapy. The disadvantages of topical therapy are that it is time-consuming, it can require large volumes of medication, it requires patient education in the technique of using topical medications, and, at times, it is not esthetically pleasing because of staining or greasy preparations.

> Advantages of topical medication:
> 1. Direct delivery to target tissue
> 2. Reduced systemic side-effects

For a medication to be effective topically, it must be absorbed into the skin. The main diffusion barrier of the skin is the stratum corneum, which is responsible for most of the protection offered by the skin against toxic agents, microorganisms, physical forces, and loss of body fluids.

Percutaneous absorption is influenced by (1) physical and chemical properties of the active ingredient, (2) concentration, (3) vehicle, and (4) variations in the type of skin. Cutaneous penetration of an active ingredient is enhanced when it has a low molecular weight, is lipid soluble, and is nonpolar.

> Percutaneous absorption depends on:
> 1. Active ingredient
> 2. Concentration
> 3. Vehicle
> 4. Skin type

Substances move across the stratum corneum by passive diffusion and follow a dose–response curve. The higher the *concentration* applied, the greater the quantity of medication absorbed.

The *vehicle* is nearly as important as the active agent in the formulation of topical medications. This was realized when investigators found that the release of drugs varied greatly with different vehicles. The more occlusive the vehicle, the greater the hydration of the stratum corneum and penetration of the medication. In addition, occlusive vehicles increase local skin temperature and prevent mechanical removal and evaporation of the active agent. An ointment is the most occlusive vehicle.

Percutaneous absorption is also influenced by the *location of the skin* to which it is applied. Passive diffusion is slow through the stratum corneum but rapid through the viable epidermis and papillary dermis. Therefore absorption is generally low on the palm and sole, in which the stratum corneum is thick, and high on the scrotum, face, and ear, in which the stratum corneum is thin. Breakdown of the barrier function of the stratum corneum by disease, chemicals (soaps or detergents), and physical injury results in increased permeability.

The *selection of a topical preparation* must involve not only the active agent but also its other ingredients. The formulation of many topical medications is complex. A water-based preparation (cream), for example, is composed of numerous ingredients, including the active agent, vehicle, and preservative, as well as an emulsifier to bring together the oil and water components of the preparation. As a general rule, it is better to select a commercially formulated preparation that is scientifically compounded than an extemporaneous preparation. The most frequently used vehicles are creams, ointments, lotions, foams, and gels.

Creams are semisolid emulsions of oil in water that vanish when rubbed into the skin. They are white and nongreasy and contain multiple ingredients. Preservatives are added to prevent the growth of bacteria and fungi. *Ointments* (oil-based) are emulsions of water droplets suspended in oil that do not rub in when applied to the skin. They are greasy and clear and do not require preservatives. Ointments are selected when increased hydration, occlusion, and maximal penetration of the active ingredient are desired. *Lotions* are suspensions of powder in water that may require shaking before application. Calamine lotion is the classic example. Itching is relieved by the cooling effect of water evaporation, and a protective layer of powder is left on the skin. Other liquids such as solutions, sprays, aerosols, and tinctures are characterized by ingredients dissolved in alcoholic vehicles that evaporate to leave the active agent on the skin. These agents are particularly useful for hairy areas. *Gels* are transparent and colorless semisolid emulsions that liquefy when applied to the skin.

WRITING A DERMATOLOGIC PRESCRIPTION

Writing a prescription for a topical medication involves more than simply requesting the active ingredient. In addition to the medication, the vehicle, concentration, and amount must be indicated, as well as the instructions for use. Several concentrations and vehicles may be available for a given topical drug. The physician should indicate which vehicle the pharmacist is to dispense. Patient compliance is often directly related to personal preference of the vehicle. Greasy ointments on the face and hands can be unacceptable to the patient and on the trunk or extremities may soak through clothing.

Elements of a topical prescription:
1. Medication
2. Vehicle
3. Concentration
4. Amount
5. How to apply

The type of error most frequently made in prescribing a topical drug probably involves the volume of medication to be dispensed. The size of the area being treated, the frequency of application, and the time between appointments or before the predicted clearing of the eruption must all be taken into consideration when writing the prescription. An adequate quantity of medication is necessary to ensure the patient's compliance, successful therapy, and cost savings. Smaller volumes of medication are comparatively more expensive than larger volumes. One gram covers an area approximately 10×10 cm. A single application of a cream or ointment to the face or hands requires 2 g; for one arm or the anterior or posterior trunk, 3 g; for one leg, 4 g; and for the entire body, 30 g. Prescribing 15 g to be applied twice a day to an eruption that involves large portions of the trunk and extremities would be unreasonable; the patient would be required to return for refills twice daily.

Amount needed for one application:
1. Face or hands: 2 g
2. Arm: 3 g
3. Leg: 4 g
4. Whole body: 30 g

The physician needs to know the principles involved in writing a dermatologic prescription. For example, the patient's eruption is moderately severe and requires an intermediate-strength topical steroid such as triamcinolone acetonide. Triamcinolone acetonide is available in three concentrations: 0.025%, 0.1%, and 0.5%. A 0.1% concentration is effective for moderately severe eruptions and can generally be used without concern for local or systemic side-effects. In this example, it is dispensed in a cream vehicle because the patient prefers a nongreasy preparation that rubs into the skin. The patient is going to use the medication on extensive areas of skin, requiring approximately 10 g per application twice a day. A prescription for 454 g (1 lb) of cream will last almost 2 weeks, and two refills will allow more than enough medication until the next appointment in 4 weeks.

DRESSINGS AND BATHS

KEY POINTS
1. Dressing may be dry, wet, or occlusive.
2. Baths can be considered a form of wet dressing.

Dressings are useful as protective coverings over wounds. They prevent contamination from the environment, and many absorb serum and blood.

Dry dressings are used to protect wounds and to absorb drainage. They usually consist of absorbent gauze secured with adhesive tape. Adhesive tape can cause allergic contact dermatitis, in which case hypoallergenic tapes may be used. These are made of an acrylic plastic adhesive mass with a plastic or cloth backing. After surgery, the skin is often painted with an adhesive that contains benzoin, which may also be responsible for allergic contact dermatitis. Dry dressings may be nonadherent or adherent. *Nonadherent dressings* are used for clean wounds. When changed, they should not pull off newly formed epithelium. An example of a nonadherent dressing is petrolatum-impregnated gauze. *Adherent dressings* are used for the debridement of moist wounds. The dressings may be dry or wet at first. For dry dressings, gauze is applied and changed regularly. For wet-to-dry dressings, water, saline, or an antiseptic solution is added to the dressing and allowed to dry. Accumulated debris is removed, although removal may be painful. Discomfort can be reduced if adherent dressings are first moistened (i.e., remoistened) before removal.

Wet dressings are used to treat acute inflammation. They consist of gauze, pads, or towels soaked continuously with water, an *astringent* (drying agent), or an antimicrobial solution. They soothe, cool, and dry through evaporation. In addition, when changed, they remove crusts and exudate. Water is the most important ingredient of wet dressings, but astringents such as aluminum sulfate tetradecahydrate, calcium acetate monohydrate (Domeboro), and antiseptics such as povidone-iodine (Betadine) are frequently added. Impermeable covers such as plastic should *not* be placed over wet dressings because of the maceration that would ensue.

Occlusive dressings made of semipermeable plastic membranes (e.g., Duoderm) promote wound healing by maintaining a moist environment. They are frequently used on chronic ulcers (e.g., stasis ulcers). The moist environment allows the migration of keratinocytes over the ulcer base to proceed more rapidly. In addition, occlusive dressings allow autodigestion of necrotic tissue by the accumulation of inflammatory cells. For some wounds (e.g., donor graft sites), these dressings also significantly reduce pain.

Baths may be thought of as a form of wet dressing. They are effective in soothing, decreasing itching, cleansing, and relaxing. They are used for acute eruptions that are crusting and weeping. They hydrate dry skin, but only if a moisturizer is applied immediately after the bath. Routinely used baths include tar emulsions (Cutar), colloidal oatmeal (Aveeno), and bath oils. Baths are limited to 30 minutes to prevent maceration and are performed once or twice daily.

TOPICAL STEROIDS (GLUCOCORTICOSTEROIDS)

KEY POINTS

1. Potency depends on steroid structure, concentration, and vehicle.
2. Learn to use low (hydrocortisone 1%), moderate (triamcinolone 0.1%), high (fluocinonide 0.05%), and super-high (clobetasol 0.05%) potency steroids.

Perhaps no topical therapeutic modality is used more frequently than steroids because of their antiinflammatory effects. The use of glucocorticosteroids applied directly to diseased skin has resulted in a high therapeutic benefit with relatively little local and systemic toxicity. The mechanism of action of topical glucocorticosteroids is complex and is not thoroughly understood.

Potency

The potency of a topical glucocorticosteroid depends on its molecular structure. For example, triamcinolone acetonide is 100 times more potent than hydrocortisone. In addition, the vehicle carrying the steroid is important. For a steroid to be effective, it must be absorbed. Penetration of glucocorticosteroids through the stratum corneum (and, hence, increased activity) is optimized by using nonpolar, lipophilic glucocorticosteroid molecules compounded in vehicles that readily release the steroid.

Dozens of different topical glucocorticosteroids (Fig. 4.1) have been formulated for use in skin disease, with many of these developed on the basis of potency assays. Measurement of the ability of glucocorticosteroids to induce vasoconstriction or blanching of the skin, *vasoconstrictive assay*, is the most frequently used method of estimating relative potency. The results of the vasoconstrictive assay are in parallel with those found in clinical studies. Because this assay is much simpler to perform than complicated clinical studies, it is widely used to screen specific formulations before they are used in clinical trials.

> Vasoconstrictive assay is the most common method for measuring potency.

Table 4.1 lists some topical glucocorticosteroids with different potencies. The percentage of the steroid present is relevant only when comparing percentages of the same compound. Thus triamcinolone acetonide 0.5% is stronger than its 0.1% formulation, but hydrocortisone 1% is much weaker than triamcinolone

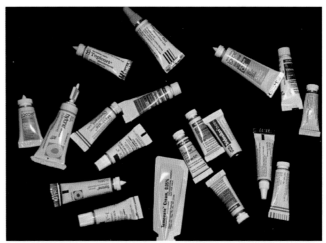

Fig. 4.1 Multiple steroids—choose and become familiar with a low, medium, high, and super-high potency steroid.

TABLE 4.1	Topical Steroids	
Potency	**Generic Name**	**%**
Low	Hydrocortisone	1.0
Medium	Triamcinolone acetonide	0.1
High	Fluocinonide	0.05
Super-high	Clobetasol propionate	0.05

acetonide 0.1%. In addition, potency depends on the vehicle. The same preparation tends to be more potent in an ointment base than in a cream base because of enhanced percutaneous penetration.

Side-Effects

Numerous hazards are involved with the use of topical gluco-corticosteroids. In general, the more potent the glucocorticosteroid, the greater the likelihood of an adverse reaction. However, when patients are educated on proper use, side-effects are uncommon.

> Topical side-effects: uncommon with proper use
> 1. Atrophy
> 2. Acne
> 3. Enhanced fungal infection
> 4. Retarded wound healing
> 5. Contact dermatitis
> 6. Glaucoma, cataracts

Systemic side-effects are worrisome but rarely occur. They include adrenal suppression, iatrogenic Cushing syndrome, and growth retardation in children. These complications have been reported with long-term, extensive use of potent topical steroids, particularly when these agents are used under occlusion. The recent introduction of super-high-potency topical steroids has increased the possibility of hypothalamic-pituitary-adrenal axis suppression. These steroids should be used cautiously for longer than 2 consecutive weeks, and the total dosage should not exceed 50 g/week.

> Systemic side-effects: worrisome but rare
> 1. Adrenal suppression
> 2. Cushing syndrome
> 3. Growth retardation

Guidelines for Topical Steroid Usage

A bewildering array of topical steroids is available in different vehicles. When prescribing a steroid preparation, one should consider several factors before making the selection of potency: vehicle, amount to be dispensed, and frequency of use. It is best to become familiar with one steroid in each class: lowest, medium, high, and super-high potency. By using only a few preparations, you will gain an enhanced appreciation of clinical efficacy, frequency of side-effects, available vehicles and volumes, and costs. Lowest potency topical steroids are recommended for dermatoses that are mild and chronic and involve the face and intertriginous regions. More potent steroids (medium and high) are used for dermatoses that are more severe and recalcitrant to treatment.

Once the appropriate potency has been selected, the vehicle (Fig. 4.2) should be chosen. Acute and subacute inflammations characterized by vesiculation and oozing are best treated with nonocclusive vehicles in a gel, lotion, or cream. Ointments, because of their occlusive properties, are better for treating chronic inflammation characterized by dryness, scaling, and

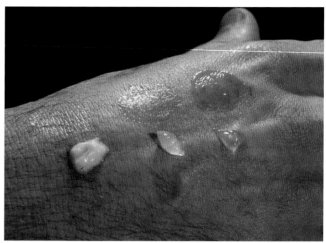

Fig. 4.2 **Steroid cream, ointment, and gel**—vehicles are important.

lichenification. Because of their greasy nature, ointments are less acceptable esthetically. However, they have less potential for irritation and allergic reaction. Lotions, solutions, foams, and gels are best used on hairy areas such as the scalp.

> Use creams on weeping eruptions, ointments on dry lichenified skin, and gels, foams, or solutions on hairy areas.

Another consideration in topical steroid therapy is the frequency of application. The stratum corneum acts as a reservoir and continues to release topical steroid into the skin after the initial application. Applications once or twice a day are usually sufficient. Investigators have observed that chronic dermatoses, especially psoriasis, may become less responsive after prolonged use of topical steroids. This phenomenon is called *tachyphylaxis*. This diminished responsiveness after repeated applications has also been observed in vasoconstrictive assays.

Finally, the physician should instruct the patient in proper application and dispense sufficient medication to ensure adequate treatment. The need for continued treatment should be reviewed periodically.

> A good rule is to use the smallest quantity and the weakest preparation that are effective for a particular eruption.

PHOTOTHERAPY

KEY POINTS

1. Positive effects are therapeutic.
2. Negative effects are sunburn, photoaging, and skin cancer.

Photobiology and Therapy

The sun emits a broad spectrum of electromagnetic radiation that is both ionizing (cosmic, gamma, and X-rays) and nonionizing (ultraviolet [UV], visible, infrared, and radio) (Fig. 4.3). The Earth's atmosphere absorbs one-third of the solar radiation. Of the radiation that reaches the Earth's surface, 60% is infrared,

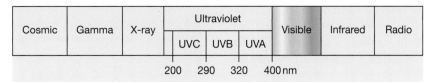

Fig. 4.3 Electromagnetic spectrum.

37% is visible, and 3% is in the UV range. The UV spectrum is between X-ray and visible light and composes the 200- to 400-nm wavelength band. It is subdivided into three groups based on physical and biologic properties: UVC (200–290 nm, germicidal spectrum), UVB (290–320 nm, sunburn spectrum), and UVA (320–400 nm). All the UVC radiation is filtered by the ozone layer, so only UVB and UVA rays reach the Earth's surface.

Because light has properties of waves and particles, two theories are used to describe its physics. The wave theory relates the speed of light to its wavelength and frequency; the light spectrum is divided according to its wavelength (in nanometers). The quantum theory is based on the existence of a particle of energy (photon) and relates light energy (in joules) directly to frequency and inversely to wavelength.

The positive effects of UV radiation include vitamin D metabolism and phototherapy of cutaneous diseases. Numerous diseases are responsive to UV radiation alone or in combination with a photosensitizing drug (photochemotherapy). These diseases include psoriasis, dermatitis, pityriasis rosea, pruritus, vitiligo, and mycosis fungoides. However, these beneficial effects must be weighed against the potential adverse effects, which include sunburn, aging, and skin cancer.

For therapeutic purposes, sunlight is the least expensive source of UV radiation. However, because of its varying intensity and availability, it is often not the optimal source. To overcome these disadvantages, artificial light sources were developed. Fluorescent bulbs are placed in a light box for office use or are combined in groups of two or four for self-treatment at home. The enhancement of phototherapy using tar is sometimes used to treat psoriasis. High-intensity UVA fluorescent bulbs were developed and combined with psoralens in the photochemotherapy of psoriasis (*PUVA* or *psoralens* plus *UVA*). PUVA is also used for selected patients with vitiligo, mycosis fungoides, and atopic dermatitis. Narrow band UVB has largely replaced PUVA because of efficacy, ease of administration, and decreased side-effects. However, close supervision, experience in use, and awareness of adverse effects are necessary for proper administration of UV radiation.

Sun Protection

Excessive exposure to solar irradiation results acutely in sunburn and chronically in premature aging (Fig. 4.4) and carcinogenesis. These adverse effects might be prevented with the use of topical sunscreens, protective clothing, shade, and by avoiding midday exposure when sunlight is most intense.

Sun protection includes: sunscreen with at least sun protective factor 30 (SPF 30) and reapplication after a couple hours, protective clothing, shade, and avoiding midday sun.

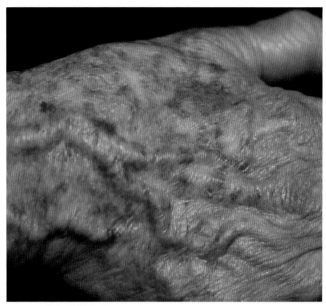

Fig. 4.4 **Photoaged skin**—note the actinic damage: brown macules, fragility, and purpura.

The amount of protection afforded by a sunscreen is measured by its SPF. In general, to provide adequate protection, a sunscreen should have an SPF of at least 30. The SPF is calculated by comparing the amount of time required to produce erythema (minimal erythema dose) in skin covered with a sunscreen divided by the time required to produce erythema in an unscreened control site. Thus a sunscreen with an SPF of 10 would allow a person who normally burns in 20 minutes to be exposed for as long as 200 minutes before burning occurs. Reapplication of sunscreen also enhances protection.

The two broad categories of sunscreens are chemical and physical. The most widely used chemical sunscreens contain *para*-aminobenzoic acid (PABA) esters, benzophenones, salicylates, anthranilates, and cinnamates and are available in cream, lotion, spray, or gel vehicles. Physical sunscreens contain titanium dioxide or zinc oxide in vehicles similar to the chemical sunscreens. Sunscreens with benzophenone combined with PABA esters are those most often used to protect against sunburn, which is primarily due to UVB radiation, and, to a lesser degree, to protect against UVA. Many moisturizers that are advertised as having "antiaging" properties contain sunscreens. Newer sunscreens containing avobenzone (Parsol) or ecamsule (Mexoryl) are particularly helpful for patients who have photosensitivities provoked by UVA and for those who are receiving PUVA therapy.

An additional measure of a sunscreen is its ability to remain effective when the person using it is sweating or swimming. This property is called *substantivity* and has been found to be a function of both the active sunscreen and its vehicle. At present, no universally accepted means of expressing substantivity exists, as there is with SPF. In choosing a sunscreen, phrases such as *water resistant* or *waterproof* indicate a preparation's substantivity.

Topical sunscreens are not without mild irritant cutaneous and ocular adverse reactions. However, allergic contact dermatitis or allergic photocontact dermatitis rarely occurs from sunscreen ingredients.

DIAGNOSTIC TESTS

KEY POINTS
1. Microscopic examination is frequently diagnostic.
2. Sample selection is critical in obtaining the proper diagnostic specimen.

In general, laboratory tests serve as important tools that are relied on, sometimes too heavily, diagnostic aids. Imaging studies and blood and urine tests are occasionally helpful for patients suspected of having a systemic disease. For example, an antinuclear antibody test should be ordered for a patient with skin lesions of lupus erythematosus. A serologic test for syphilis is appropriate for a patient with a skin rash in which syphilis is considered to be a possible cause. However, because most dermatologic diseases are limited to the skin, tests for systemic disease are less frequently indicated than are microscopic examinations, cultures, biopsies, and patch tests, which more specifically involve the skin.

As a highly accessible organ, the skin lends itself to direct laboratory examination. Specimen gathering is easy, minimally traumatic, and often highly rewarding diagnostically. Numerous tests can be performed in the office, with results immediately available. For other tests, specimens must be sent to the microbiology or pathology laboratory for further evaluation.

Diagnostic tests include:
- Microscopic examination
- Cultures
- Biopsy
- Patch testing

Potassium Hydroxide Mount for Dermatophytic Infections

For undiagnosed scaling lesions of the skin, a fungal origin must be excluded. The best way to do this is with a potassium hydroxide (KOH) preparation of the scale scraping. For experienced hands, this simple test is more sensitive than fungal culture. For those just learning to perform KOH examinations, hyphae are more easily said than seen. The following steps should be followed in performing this examination:

If it scales, scrape it!

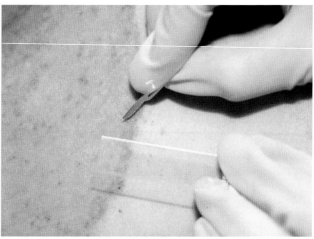

Fig. 4.5 **Obtain scales for fungal KOH** preparation at the inflammatory margin of the patch.

1. *Vigorously* scrape the scale from the edge of the scaling lesion onto a microscopic slide (Fig. 4.5). Use a no. 15 scalpel blade for scraping. Avoid extremely thick pieces of scale, because they are difficult to examine.
2. No more than 1 or 2 drops of 20% KOH with dimethylsulfoxide on the scale before applying the coverslip.
3. *Blot* out the excess KOH by firmly pressing a paper towel on top of the coverslip and slide. This important step achieves two purposes. First, it spreads the cells into a thin layer on the slide. A monolayer of cells is desired for the microscopic examination; grossly, this looks like a cloudy film under the coverslip. Second, the blotting removes excess KOH on and around the coverslip; the microscope objective can be permanently etched by contact with KOH.
4. When examining the preparation under the microscope, use *low illumination*. This is most easily achieved by racking the light condenser down all the way. Bright illumination "washes out" the preparation so that hyphae "disappear."
5. Scan the *entire* coverslip under low power (×10). In the cellular areas, look for the hyphae, which often appear as slightly refractile branching tubes (Fig. 4.6). When suspicious elements are seen, use the high-dry objective (×45) for confirmation.
6. Unlike mucous membrane preparations for candidiasis, in skin scrapings, hyphae are often sparse. *Careful search*, sometimes with multiple preparations, is indicated when there is a high index of suspicion that a lesion may be fungal.

Potassium Hydroxide Preparation for Candidal Infection

In addition to causing scale, candidal infections may cause pustules. Sometimes, the pustules predominate and are a good source of material for KOH examination. The specimen is prepared and examined exactly as outlined above. KOH preparations are particularly useful for diagnosing candidal infections because the finding of hyphae or pseudohyphae is diagnostic of *infection* with this organism. Spores are inadequate for the

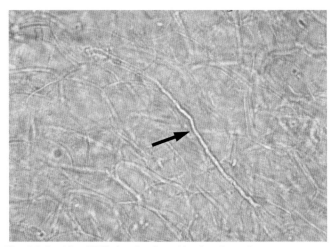

Fig. 4.6 **Positive KOH** showing fungal hyphae (*arrow*).

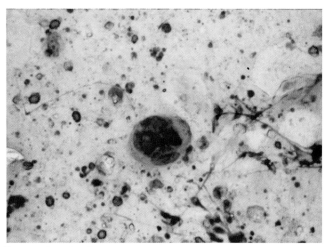

Fig. 4.8 **Positive Tzanck preparation** showing multinucleated giant cell typical of a herpes virus infection.

Scabies Scraping

Finding a scabies mite under the microscope confirms the diagnosis as well as ensuring treatment compliance, should the patient be skeptical. Burrows produce the highest yield, but because their presence alone is diagnostic, scraping a burrow serves to confirm the diagnosis. On close inspection of the burrow, the adult scabies mite is sometimes barely visible as a tiny black speck (see Fig. 11.24). Under the microscope, the mite appears more impressive (Fig. 11.25). Scraping may be more helpful when definite burrows are not found, in which case small papules or questionable burrows are scraped. However, scraping anything other than the black dot at the end of the burrow is frequently negative. The scraping is done with a no. 15 scalpel blade moistened with oil (any oil) so that the scraped skin adheres to the blade, from which it can be easily transferred to a drop of oil on a glass slide, covered with a coverslip, and examined microscopically. In scraping, the scalpel blade is held perpendicular to the skin surface. The key to a successful test is to scrape *vigorously*. Alternatively, *KOH* can be used on the slide without the use of oil at all.

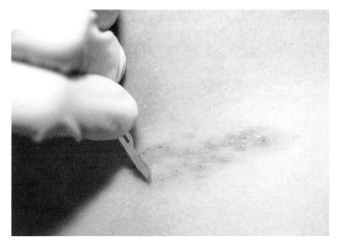

Fig. 4.7 **Scrape the base** of the blisters for a Tzanck preparation.

diagnosis of infection; yeast organisms, including *Candida albicans*, can colonize skin without infecting it. For this reason, a culture growing *C. albicans* does not necessarily implicate infection, whereas finding hyphal forms on KOH examination does.

Hyphae, not spores, are the diagnostic findings in candidal infections.

Scraping the black dot at the end of a burrow yields the highest number of mites.

Tzanck Preparation

The Tzanck preparation provides an opportunity to make an immediate diagnosis of a herpes simplex or varicella-zoster infection. The preferred specimen is the scraping of the contents and base of a freshly opened vesicle (Fig. 4.7). This material is placed on a glass slide, air-dried, methanol fixed, and then stained for 10 seconds with toluidine blue. Inclusion bodies are not well seen, but the finding of multinucleate giant cells is diagnostic for infection with either herpes simplex or varicella-zoster virus (Fig. 4.8). The Tzanck preparation is less sensitive than polymerase chain reaction (PCR) assay, which is the best method to confirm a herpes infection.

Culture

The microbiology laboratory can confirm and further characterize bacterial, viral, and fungal pathogens, some of which may initially be identified in an office microscopic examination.

Organisms for both superficial and deep fungal infections can be isolated from an appropriate skin specimen. For a superficial fungal (dermatophyte) infection, this specimen is simply a collection of scales scraped or vigorously swabbed from the surface of the lesion. For deep fungal infections, skin tissue is needed and obtained most easily with a punch biopsy from the active border of the lesion. Tissue should simultaneously be sent to the pathology laboratory for histologic examination to include special fungal stains. If the specimen is sufficiently large (6 mm punch), it may be bisected; otherwise, two biopsy specimens should be collected.

Material for bacterial culture should be obtained from intact pustules, bullae, or abscesses. If only crusts are present, they should first be removed so that the underlying exudate can be swabbed and cultured. More invasive procedures are required for deeper bacterial infections. For bacterial cellulitis, the responsible organisms can sometimes be retrieved from the involved site by injecting and aspirating 0.5–1 mL of nonbacteriostatic saline. However, cellulitis is usually treated and not cultured. Cultures of skin biopsies may also be rewarding, especially for mycobacterial infections of the skin. Some atypical mycobacteria grow only at room temperature, so to handle the skin tissue properly, the laboratory needs not only the specimen but also the clinician's diagnostic considerations.

> Intact pustules, bullae, or abscesses are the source of specimen for bacterial cultures.

Viral cultures must be transported in a viral transport medium, which can be obtained from the viral laboratory. For herpes cultures, a vesicle is opened or a crust is unroofed, and the underlying serum is swabbed. The swab is placed in the transport medium, and the container is returned to the laboratory for processing. Herpes simplex cultures have a high yield, but herpes varicella-zoster grows either slowly (7–10 days) or not at all. An immunofluorescent staining technique for herpes varicella-zoster produces a much higher yield in a much faster time (same day). The test is performed on a vesicle fluid smeared on a special slide, which is returned to the virology laboratory for testing. More recently, PCR assay is the preferred method to diagnosis herpes infections, being rapid, specific, and sensitive.

> PCR of vesicle fluid is an effective and efficient diagnostic test for herpes viral infections.

Skin Biopsy

In no other organ-based specialty is tissue so easily available for histologic examination as in dermatology. Although a biopsy is not necessary to diagnose the majority of skin disorders, in certain circumstances its value cannot be overemphasized. The following serve only as examples. Already mentioned is the mandate that skin nodules of uncertain origin must undergo a biopsy to rule out malignancy. For plaques with unusual shapes and colors, a diagnosis of mycosis fungoides, a cutaneous T-cell lymphoma, may be confirmed with a skin biopsy, but sometimes only after multiple biopsies have been taken serially over time. A skin biopsy is usually necessary to secure the exact diagnosis of a primary blistering disorder. In lupus erythematosus, the information obtained from a skin specimen may help to establish the diagnosis.

> A skin biopsy done properly is often an indispensable diagnostic test.

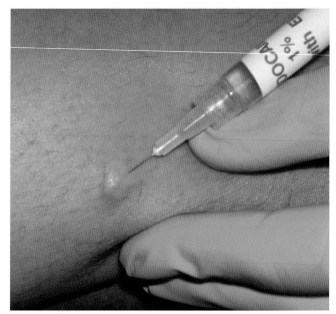

Fig. 4.9 Use 1% lidocaine, usually with epinephrine (less bleeding) and a 30-gauge needle (less pain), to raise a wheal for local anesthesia.

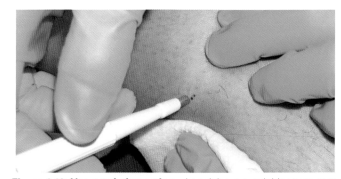

Figure 4.10 Use a twisting action when doing a punch biopsy to sample epidermal and deeper dermal tissue.

Occasionally, excisional biopsies may be preferred (e.g., for melanoma), but for most skin lesions a punch or shave biopsy is more convenient to perform. For a punch biopsy, a 3-mm instrument is standard, but punches are available in sizes ranging from 2 to 8 mm. The procedure is simple. After the skin is infiltrated with a local anesthetic (Fig. 4.9), the punch tool is pushed into the skin while twisting through all layers of tissue (Fig. 4.10). The specimen is then *gently* lifted and snipped off at the subcutaneous fat level. Hemostasis can be achieved simply with pressure or absorbable gelatin (Gelfoam) packing. Occasionally, the skin defect is closed with a suture to stop bleeding.

Note that, in the foregoing procedure, gentleness is emphasized. A biopsy specimen will be artifactually damaged, sometimes to the point of being histologically uninterpretable, if it is squeezed too firmly with the tissue forceps. To avoid this problem, either lift the specimen gently from below or grasp it by the very edge. With nodules and other dermal processes, it is particularly important that the specimen be of full thickness.

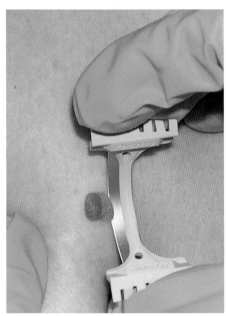

Fig. 4.11 **Shave biopsy** is the most common technique for obtaining a superficial biopsy.

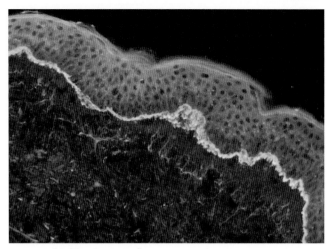

Fig. 4.12 **Positive immunofluorescence** showing a linear deposit of immunoglobulin G at the dermal-epidermal junction, characteristic of bullous pemphigoid.

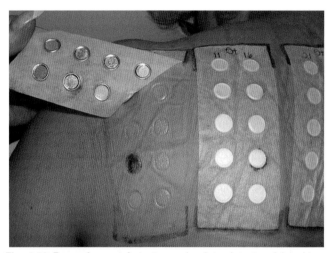

Fig. 4.13 **Removing patch tests** on day 2 to detect a delayed-type hypersensitivity reaction.

For processes involving the subcutaneous fat, even deeper and larger specimens may need to be obtained with a larger punch or an excision.

Superficial lesions can undergo biopsy or be removed with a shave technique. A wheal is raised with the anesthetic injection, after which the area is shaved with a scalpel blade maneuvered either parallel to the surface or in a slight "scooping" fashion (Fig. 4.11). Deep scoop shave biopsies can be accomplished for malignant lesions such as a melanoma.

For most skin lesions, adjacent normal skin is not needed, so the biopsy should be obtained from the center of the lesion. The exception is with blistering disorders, in which case the biopsy should be taken from the edge of an early lesion to include a portion of the adjacent, nonblistered skin. This is needed to identify the exact histologic origin of the blister: intraepidermal versus subepidermal.

For routine histologic processing and for most special stains, the specimen is placed in formalin. For electron microscopy, buffered glutaraldehyde is used. With immunofluorescence testing, the specimen is placed in a special buffered transport solution.

Immunofluorescence Test

For the diagnosis of blistering disorders such as pemphigus, bullous pemphigoid, and dermatitis herpetiformis, immunofluorescence tests on skin (direct) and, sometimes, serum (indirect) are invaluable and widely used (Fig. 4.12). These techniques detect autoantibodies directed against portions of skin. For example, immunoglobulin (Ig) G antibodies deposited at the basement membrane in pemphigoid are detected by direct immunofluorescence testing using the patient's skin and fluorochrome-labeled anti-IgG antibodies. The presence of IgM, IgA, complement, and fibrin can also be detected with appropriate reagents.

Patch Testing

Patch testing is a valuable tool for identifying responsible allergens in patients with allergic contact dermatitis. These tests detect delayed (type IV) hypersensitivity responses to contact allergens. Patch test reactions take several days to develop and hence differ from scratch/prick tests, which evoke immediate (type I) hypersensitivity responses (within minutes). Either specifically suspected substances may be tested, or an entire battery of allergens may be screened. For either purpose, standardized trays of common sensitizing chemicals are available, each appropriately diluted in water or petrolatum. These test materials are applied to the skin under occlusive patches that are left in place for 48 hours. The patches then are removed, the sites inspected, and positive reactions noted (Fig. 4.13). Because these delayed hypersensitivity responses sometimes take more than 48 hours, a final reading at 72–96 hours is recommended. If positive tests are found, the last and most important step is to determine their clinical relevance. In itself, a positive patch test does not prove that agent to be the cause of dermatitis. Clinical correlation with an appropriate exposure history is required. Patch testing should not be done with unknown chemicals because severe irritant reactions with residual scars can result. Contact dermatitis and patch testing are discussed further in Chapter 8.

> Patch testing is used to detect relevant contact allergens and confirm allergic contact dermatitis.

DERMATOLOGIC SURGERY

KEY POINTS

1. Know the surgical options
2. Know how to handle complications
3. Obtain informed consent and do a safety time out

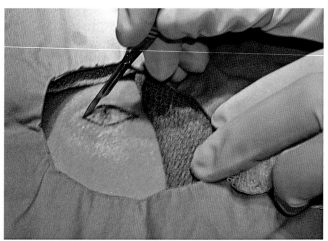

Figure 4.14 Excision demonstrating that the length is three times greater than the width, and the cut is perpendicular to the skin surface.

Numerous techniques are available for surgery of the skin. The three most common and simplest procedures are elliptical excision, curettage and electrodesiccation, and cryosurgery. For defects that cannot be closed primarily, skin flaps or grafts may be used. A specialized, precise technique for treating skin cancer is called Mohs surgery, which involves serial excisions of tissue that are systematically mapped and microscopically examined to define the extent of cancerous invasion and to ensure that surgical margins are free of tumor. This technique is the most successful means of treating basal cell and squamous cell carcinomas. Using immunostaining, Mohs surgery has also been used to excise selected melanomas.

> Mohs technique is the most effective surgery for basal and squamous cell carcinoma. It is most frequently used for recurrent and facial carcinomas. In selected cases, using immunostaining, Mohs surgery can treat melanoma.

Before surgery, the patient should be informed of the procedure chosen, why it is necessary, and what to expect and do after surgery. The potential complications of the procedure, including excessive scar formation, infection, bleeding, and nerve injury, should be explained. A safety time out is used to confirm the correct patient, the procedure, and the correct surgical site. When properly selected and technically well performed, simple excision, curettage and electrodesiccation, and cryosurgery usually have no significant complications.

> Surgery explanation includes procedure, potential complications, and what to do after the operation.

Excision

The simple elliptical excision is used to obtain tissue for biopsy and for the removal of benign and cancerous lesions. The axis of the lesion, cosmetic boundaries (e.g., the vermilion border of the lip), and skin lines should be taken into consideration when planning the excision. Most procedures require a minimal number of instruments, including a needle holder, small

forceps, skin hook, small clamp, small pointed scissors, syringe, and needle (30 gauge), and a no. 15 scalpel blade plus handle. Disposable sterile gloves, drape gauze, and cautery are also necessary.

Numerous antiseptics are available for preoperative preparation of the skin, including 70% isopropyl alcohol, povidone-iodine (Betadine), and chlorhexidine gluconate (Hibiclens). The boundaries of the excision are marked. This is done before injection of local anesthesia because the volume of anesthetic distorts the normal skin contours. The preferred local anesthetic is 1% lidocaine because of the rarity of allergic reactions. In addition, lidocaine, an amide, does not cross-react with procaine hydrochloride (Novocain), an ester. Transdermal anesthesia with a topical anesthetic cream can be applied under an occlusive dressing 1–2 hours before the procedure to reduce the pain associated with injection.

> Lidocaine (Xylocaine) does not cross-react with procaine hydrochloride (Novocain).

Normal saline or diphenhydramine hydrochloride (Benadryl) may be used for local anesthesia if lidocaine cannot be used. The addition of epinephrine to lidocaine prolongs its anesthetic effect and reduces operative bleeding.

The length of the ellipse should be three times the width to ensure easy closure. The cut should be made perpendicular to the surface and through the dermis into the subcutaneous tissue (Fig. 4.14). Hemostasis is achieved with pressure, electrodesiccation, or suture ligation. Repair of the wound is easy if an adequate ellipse has been formed, the edges are perpendicular, and skin lines are followed. If the defect is large, the edges may be undermined to reduce closure tension. Buried absorbable suture is used to close deeper layers. Numerous methods are used for skin closure: interrupted sutures with monofilament nylon is the simplest method. In most cases, 5-0 or 4-0 sutures are adequate for both subcuticular and skin closure. The removal of skin sutures depends on the site, wound tension, and whether buried

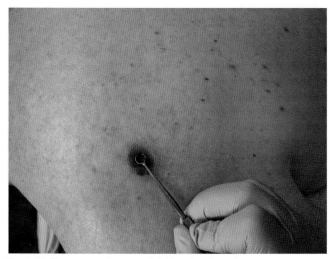

Fig. 4.15 **Curettage** of a superficial basal cell carcinoma.

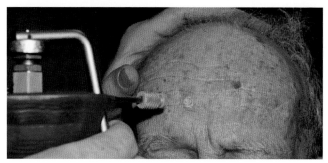

Fig. 4.16 **Cryotherapy of a seborrheic keratosis**—using a spray unit; the white freeze cycle should last about 10 seconds.

sutures have been used. In general, facial sutures are removed in 5 days, and trunk and extremity sutures are removed in 1–2 weeks. Alternatively, absorbable sutures may be used which do not require removal. Most wounds are dressed with either sterile adherent bandages or gauze secured with tape. Paper tape should be used in patients with a history of adhesive sensitivity. Topical antibiotics are not necessary after surgery. The patient is instructed to keep the wound dry for 24 hours, to change the dressings daily, and to return to the clinic if bleeding, purulent drainage, or excessive pain or swelling occurs. Postoperative pain is usually negligible and at its worst the first night after surgery, and typically requires only acetaminophen. Worsening pain days after surgery should prompt a clinic visit to inspect the surgical site for infection.

> The length of elliptical excision is three times its width.
>
> Suture removal:
> • Face: 5 days
> • Trunk and extremities: 1–2 weeks

Curettage and Electrodesiccation

The procedure of curettage and electrodesiccation is used most often for the treatment of selected small basal cell and squamous cell carcinomas. It is a deceptively simple procedure that requires proper selection of tumor and a skilled practitioner. Otherwise, the recurrence rate is unacceptably high. The tumor is prepared and anesthetized with a local anesthetic. The *curette*, an oval instrument with a cutting edge (Fig. 4.15), is used to remove the soft cancerous skin. The tumor margins are determined by "feel," with normal skin having a firm and gritty consistency. After curettage, the base and borders of the wound may be electrodesiccated to destroy residual tumor and to provide hemostasis. The wound heals by secondary intention over several weeks.

> Curettage and electrodesiccation require experience to avoid a high recurrence rate.

Cryosurgery

Keratoses and warts are frequently treated with cryosurgery. Liquid nitrogen (−195.6°C) is the standard agent because it is inexpensive, rapid, and noncombustible. Tissue destruction is caused by intercellular and extracellular ice formation, by denaturing lipid-protein complexes, and by cell dehydration. This treatment usually requires no skin preparation or anesthesia. Liquid nitrogen application is accomplished with direct spray and usually requires <30 seconds (Fig. 4.16). A repeat freeze-thaw cycle results in more cellular damage than a single cycle.

During the procedure, the patient feels a stinging or burning sensation. Subsequently, burning occurs along with tissue swelling. Within 24 hours, a blister may occur in the treated area. If the blister is excessively large or painful, the fluid should be removed in a sterile manner, keeping the roof of the blister intact to act as a biologic bandage. Otherwise, it is allowed to heal spontaneously.

> Avoid overzealous cryotherapy which can cause excessive tissue destruction.

Treatment of skin cancers with cryotherapy requires an operator experienced with thermocouple devices to ensure adequate freezing for tissue destruction. Postoperative morbidity includes significant tissue edema and necrosis.

PATIENT EDUCATION

> **KEY POINTS**
> 1. Verbal and written communication is important.
> 2. Education enhances understanding and compliance.

A dialog must be established between the physician/advanced practice clinician and the patient. This is begun during the history and physical examination. Once a diagnosis is established, the patient should be told what the disease is, what its cause is if known, and what to expect from treatment. Patients are frequently hesitant to ask certain questions because they are either afraid or embarrassed. It is important that these unasked questions be answered: Is my disease contagious? Is it cancer? Do I have something wrong internally that is causing my skin problems?

Answer the unasked questions:
- Contagious?
- Cancer?
- Internal?

For therapy to be successful, patient cooperation and compliance are necessary. To ensure this goal, therapeutic options, expected outcome, and potential side-effects should be explained. Instructions on how to use topical medications must be demonstrated. All too frequently, too much medication is applied, and it is not rubbed in sufficiently. For example, when applying a white cream, patients should be instructed to apply sparingly and rub it in until it "disappears." If white cream remains on the surface, either too much has been applied or it has not been rubbed in sufficiently. Dressings may be either too wet or too dry, or left on too long, resulting in maceration. These pitfalls are avoided when the medication or dressing is applied to the area of dermatitis as a demonstration while the patient is in the office.

Patient instruction sheets supplement the spoken word. They inform and instruct patients. Frequently, medical problems and therapies are complex, and the patient fails to understand them. Instruction sheets save time, reinforce what has been told to the patient, answer unasked questions, and provide a reference for the patient to read.

Epidermal Growths

CHAPTER CONTENTS

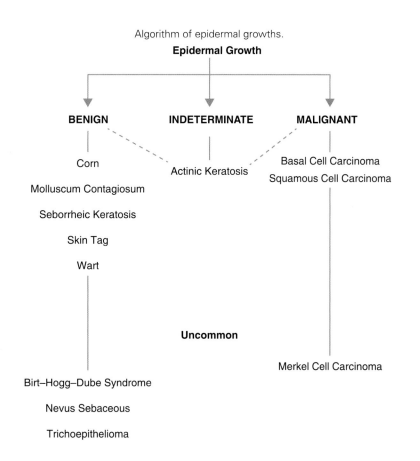

Algorithm of epidermal growths.

Epidermal Growth

BENIGN — INDETERMINATE — MALIGNANT

Corn

Molluscum Contagiosum

Seborrheic Keratosis

Skin Tag

Wart

Actinic Keratosis

Basal Cell Carcinoma
Squamous Cell Carcinoma

Uncommon

Birt–Hogg–Dube Syndrome

Nevus Sebaceous

Trichoepithelioma

Merkel Cell Carcinoma

ABSTRACT

Neoplasms of the epidermis (Table 5.1) are derived from the proliferation of basal cells or keratinocytes. Epidermal growths are recognized clinically by a localized thickening of the epidermis that often is accompanied by thickening of the stratum corneum, which is called *hyperkeratosis* or *scale*. Large, indurated, rapidly growing, crusted, or ulcerated tumors suggest a malignant process and should undergo biopsy. Unless injured or irritated, benign growths do not bleed or become crusted or ulcerated.

KEY POINTS

1. Proliferation of keratinocytes or basal cells.
2. Scaling is usually prominent.
3. Bleeding, crusting, or pain suggests cancer.

ACTINIC KERATOSIS

KEY POINTS

1. Precancerous, but low potential
2. Prevent with sun protection

Definition

Actinic (solar) keratosis can be a precancerous neoplasm of the epidermis caused by the ultraviolet (UV) portion of sunlight. The abnormal keratinocytes in actinic keratoses are confined to the epidermis and constitute a potentially premalignant change. The proliferation of these abnormal cells clinically manifests as a rough, scaling patch or papule (Fig. 5.1). Their clinical course is often indeterminant: spontaneous involution, staying stable, or progression into carcinoma.

> Although considered premalignant, most actinic keratoses do not progress to skin cancer.

Incidence

The incidence of actinic keratoses varies with (1) skin pigmentation, (2) geographic location, and (3) the amount of sun exposure. Thus the incidence of actinic keratoses is high in white patients who have light skin, live in the southern United States where there is an abundance of natural sunlight, and engage in frequent outdoor activity. In the authors' clinic, 1.7% of new patients were seen because of actinic keratoses, although the incidence would be higher in the "Sunbelt." Moreover, in many patients, actinic keratoses are an incidental finding.

> Light skin and abundant sun exposure may result in actinic keratoses.

History

Risk factors can usually be elicited in the history. The patient may have a genetic predisposition. Fair-skinned white patients have the least amount of protective pigment. A family history of skin cancer or an Irish or Anglo-Saxon heritage is frequently obtained. Second, the geographic location where the patient has lived directly influences the amount of UV light exposure. As one moves toward the equator, the UV light intensity increases dramatically, as does human melanin production. Lastly, the occupational and recreational activities of the patient with reference to sun exposure provide another clue. Farmers, sailors, and others with occupations that require working outdoors have a high amount of UV light exposure. Similarly, persons who spend many hours at the poolside or on the beach are at higher risk.

Physical Examination

Actinic keratoses are 1- to 10-mm, pinkish, ill-marginated patches and papules that have a rough, yellowish brown, adherent scale. Their ill-defined margins make them indistinct to the casual observer. Their rough-textured surface is often easier to feel than to see. Actinic keratoses occur in sun-exposed areas: the face, dorsum of the hands and forearms, neck, upper back, chest, and lower legs. They generally are found on UV-damaged skin that has a yellowish hue, wrinkles, and freckled pigmentation.

> An actinic keratosis is rough, scaling, and ill-marginated; it is often easier felt than seen.

Differential Diagnosis

An actinic keratosis must be differentiated from other epidermal tumors. Most often, it is confused with a *seborrheic keratosis*. The well-demarcated, "pasted on" appearance of a seborrheic keratosis differentiates it from an actinic keratosis. In situ squamous cell carcinoma is a larger patch or thin plaque with margins that are usually well defined, in contrast to the margins of an actinic keratosis. Hypertrophic or indurated actinic keratosis (Fig. 5.1) cannot be differentiated with certainty from *squamous cell carcinoma* and should undergo biopsy. *Superficial basal cell carcinoma*, which resembles in situ squamous cell carcinoma clinically, is occasionally confused with actinic keratosis. Lichenoid keratosis should also be considered in the differential diagnosis. A lichenoid keratosis is an inflamed lentigo or thin seborrheic keratosis, which is well-demarcated with some residual tan/brown coloration within the pink inflamed lesion.

DIFFERENTIAL DIAGNOSIS OF ACTINIC KERATOSIS

- Seborrheic keratosis
- Squamous cell carcinoma
- Superficial basal cell carcinoma
- Lichenoid keratosis

Laboratory and Biopsy

Actinic keratosis is characterized histologically by a partial-thickness dysplasia of the epidermis (Fig. 5.1B). Hyperkeratosis with underlying irregular hyperplasia of mildly dysplastic keratinocytes is seen. A chronic inflammatory response is present in the dermis. All thick and indurated actinic keratoses should undergo biopsy to rule out squamous cell carcinoma, as well as lesions that have not responded to previous treatment.

> Indurated and therapeutically unresponsive actinic keratoses should undergo biopsy to rule out carcinoma.

TABLE 5.1 Epidermal Growths

	Frequency (%)[a]	Etiology	Physical Examination	Differential Diagnosis	Laboratory Test (Biopsy)
Actinic keratosis	1.7	Sunlight	Ill-marginated, reddish, rough, scaling patch or papule	Squamous cell carcinoma Seborrheic keratosis Superficial basal cell carcinoma Lichenoid keratosis	When thick scale or indurated base
Basal cell carcinoma	1.7	Sunlight			Yes
Nodular			Pearly nodule with telangiectasia, often has central depression or ulcer	Molluscum contagiosum Squamous cell carcinoma Sebaceous hyperplasia Nevus Merkel cell carcinoma Trichoepithelioma	
Pigmented			Blue-black plaque or nodule with pearly border	Malignant melanoma Nevus Seborrheic keratosis	
Superficial			Red, scaling, crusted eczematous appearing patch	Psoriasis Eczema Bowen disease Lichenoid keratosis	
Sclerosing			Whitish, slightly depressed, sometimes crusted pink plaque/patch	Squamous cell carcinoma Nonhealing scar	
Corn	0.4	Friction	Hyperkeratotic papule or nodule with compact clear core	Wart	No
Molluscum contagiosum	0.3	Poxvirus	Translucent papule with umbilicated center	Comedo Nodular basal cell carcinoma	No
Seborrheic keratosis	1.6	–	Tan-brown, greasy, pasted on papule or plaque	Wart Actinic keratosis Nevus Malignant melanoma Pigmented basal cell carcinoma	No
Skin tag	0.5	–	Soft, skin-colored, pedunculated papule	Neurofibroma nevus	No
Squamous cell carcinoma	0.2	Sunlight Viruses Chemicals	Flesh-colored, hard, crusted or scaling nodule, often ulcerated	Basal cell carcinoma Wart Lichenoid keratosis Actinic keratosis Merkel cell carcinoma Trichoepithelioma Nevus sebaceous	Yes
Wart	5.2	Papillomavirus			No
Common			Flesh-colored, scaling, vegetative papule or nodule, skin lines interrupted, studded with black puncta	Corn Squamous cell carcinoma	
Flat			Reddish, smooth, flat, well-demarcated papule	Lichen planus Comedo Corn	
Plantar			Solitary, grouped, or mosaic scaling papules, skin lines interrupted, studded with black puncta	Squamous cell carcinoma	
Genital			Soft, moist, cauliflower-appearing papules or nodule	Squamous cell carcinoma Secondary syphilis Seborrheic keratosis	No

[a]Percentage of new dermatology patients with this diagnosis seen in the Hershey Medical Center Dermatology Clinic, Hershey, Pennsylvania.

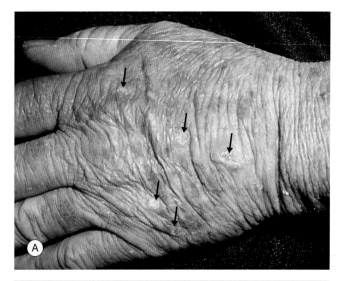

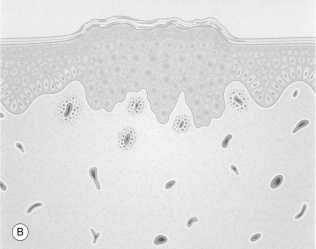

Fig. 5.1 **Actinic keratosis**. (A) Rough, scaling, ill-marginated, pink-ish patches and papules on markedly sun-damaged skin (arrows). (B) Epidermis—atypical keratinocytes in the lower epidermis. Dermis—chronic inflammation.

Therapy

Prevention by reducing sunlight exposure is the most effective form of therapy. Patients who are sensitive to the sun or have developed actinic keratoses should wear protective clothing such as broad-brimmed hats and long-sleeved shirts when outside. Sunscreens with a sun protective factor (SPF) of 30 or greater should be used on exposed skin and reapplied after a couple of hours. The regular use of sunscreens prevents the development of new actinic keratoses, as well as hastening the resolution of those that already exist. Avoidance of sun exposure at midday (from 10:00 a.m. to 2:00 p.m.), when UV radiant energy is most intense, is recommended. Patient awareness and education should begin in childhood.

Nicotinamide, a B vitamin, given 500 mg twice daily has been shown to reduce actinic keratosis. It is nonprescription, inexpensive, has minimal side-effects, and does not interact with other medicines.

> Use sun protection to prevent more actinic damage.

Cryosurgery with liquid nitrogen is the most common treatment for actinic keratoses and is most useful when a few lesions are present. Thick, hypertrophic, actinic keratoses are also better treated in this way. Freezing can be accomplished in a manner similar to that described for warts.

> Avoid overzealous liquid nitrogen treatment of actinic keratoses because of possible scarring.

Topical chemotherapy with 5-fluorouracil cream 5% is the most common means of treating multiple actinic keratoses. 5-Fluorouracil inhibits DNA synthesis by blocking the enzyme thymidylate synthase. When 5-fluorouracil is applied to normal skin, little reaction occurs, but when it is applied to sun-damaged skin, those areas with actinic keratoses become inflamed. The medication is applied to the involved areas twice daily. Redness develops within several days. Subsequently, within 1–4 weeks, the actinic keratoses become painful, crusted, and eroded, at which time the medication is stopped. Patients need to be warned about the discomfort and cosmetically unsightly effects of 5-fluorouracil, which are temporary and resolve several weeks after discontinuing treatment. Because of the marked amount of inflammation that can occur, small regions may be treated at a time in patients with extensive actinic keratoses. A few patients may become allergic to 5-fluorouracil. Patients with severe actinic damage can be expected to require retreatment every couple of years.

> Warn patients about the marked inflammation, crusting, and pain that is caused by 5-fluorouracil.

Alternative agents include (1) diclofenac gel 3% (Solaraze), a nonsteroidal antiinflammatory drug, applied twice daily for 3 months; (2) imiquimod cream 5%, a topical immune response modifier, applied twice weekly for 4 months; (3) tirbanibulin ointment 1%, a microtubule inhibitor, applied daily for 5 days; and (4) photodynamic therapy, chemical peel.

THERAPY FOR ACTINIC KERATOSIS

Prevention
- Sunscreen ≥SPF 30, reapply after a couple of hours
- Broad-brimmed hat, long-sleeved shirt, and pants
- Avoidance of intense midday sun (from 10:00 a.m. to 2:00 p.m.)
- Nicotinamide 500 mg twice a day

Initial
- Cryotherapy with liquid nitrogen

Alternative
- 5-Fluorouracil 5% cream twice daily for 1–4 weeks
- Diclofenac 3% gel twice daily for 3 months
- Imiquimod 5% cream twice weekly for 16 weeks
- Tirbanibulin ointment 1% daily for 5 days
- Photodynamic therapy, chemical peels

Course and Complications

In patients with chronically sun-damaged skin, the acquisition of more actinic keratoses can be expected. Some actinic keratoses spontaneously disappear (up to 26%), although others may develop into squamous cell carcinoma. The number that do develop into squamous cell carcinoma appears to be small, much less than 1%. Metastases from squamous cell carcinomas arising in actinic keratoses are very uncommon.

> Actinic keratosis has a small potential of developing into a squamous cell carcinoma.

Pathogenesis

Actinic keratoses are produced by UV radiation–induced damage to keratinocyte DNA. This results in unrepaired or error-prone repaired DNA. Abnormal replication occurs and results in epidermal cellular hyperplasia. The cells within an actinic keratosis are arranged in a disorderly way and have increased mitoses and an abnormal chromatin pattern. Other precancerous keratinocytic neoplasms similar to actinic keratoses are caused by artificial UV light, X-irradiation, or polycyclic aromatic hydrocarbons.

BASAL CELL CARCINOMA

KEY POINTS
1. Malignancy of the epidermal basal cell.
2. Very rarely metastasizes.
3. Different types have different appearances.

Definition

Basal cell carcinoma is a malignant neoplasm arising from the basal cells of the epidermis. Although these cancers rarely metastasize, their potential for local destruction attests to their malignant nature. UV radiation is the cause of most basal cell carcinomas in humans. Four clinically and histopathologically distinct types of basal cell carcinoma are recognized: nodular, pigmented, superficial, and scarring (sclerotic).

Incidence

Basal cell carcinoma is the most common human malignant disease; it affects more than 2 million persons annually in the United States. Of the new patients in the authors' clinic, 2% are seen for basal cell carcinoma. The increased frequency in adults with light skin is related to sun exposure.

> Basal cell carcinoma is the most common skin cancer, but it very rarely metastasizes.

History

The patient with basal cell carcinoma seeks medical attention because of a new growth, especially if it is a nonhealing, easily bleeding lesion. There may be a personal or family history of skin cancer. The risk of basal cell carcinoma is higher in patients with light skin, in those who live in southern latitudes, and in those who work or play outdoors. Frequently, these patients have a history of sunburning easily and tanning poorly. While it can happen, it is very uncommon in dark-skinned individuals.

Physical Examination

The usual patient with basal cell carcinoma has fair skin, blue eyes, blonde or red hair, and actinic-damaged skin manifested by freckles, yellow wrinkling, and actinic keratoses. Basal cell carcinoma occurs in sun-exposed skin, particularly the head and neck.

> A "pearly" appearance is the most characteristic feature of a nodular basal cell carcinoma.

The *nodular type* (Fig. 5.2) of basal cell carcinoma is the most common. It is a "pearly," semitranslucent papule or nodule that often has a central depression or crater, telangiectasia, and a rolled, waxy border. Ulceration and crusting can occur. Nodular basal cell carcinoma occurs most frequently on the face, especially the nose.

> Types of basal cell carcinoma:
> 1. Nodular
> 2. Pigmented
> 3. Superficial
> 4. Scarring (sclerotic)

Pigmented basal cell carcinoma (Fig. 5.3) is a shiny, blue-black papule, nodule, or plaque. The pigment is often speckled, and a pearly, rolled margin can be seen when the tumor is viewed from the side. This is the most common presentation on dark skin.

Superficial basal cell carcinoma (Fig. 5.4) occurs most frequently on the thorax. It is a red, slightly scaling, well-demarcated, eczematous appearing patch. Centrally, it may become slightly eroded and crusted, subsequently leaving an atrophic, slightly depressed center. Its shape is oval to round, with a characteristic thread-like, pearly, rolled border. It is often referred to as multicentric superficial basal cell carcinoma because it skips islands of normal skin, similar to the way a forest fire may surround a stand of trees yet leave it unburned.

The *scarring (sclerotic or morpheaform) basal cell carcinoma* (Fig. 5.5) is an atrophic, white, slightly eroded, or crusted plaque that often looks like a scar. It is frequently depressed and is the least common and most aggressive type of basal cell carcinoma.

Differential Diagnosis

Nodular basal cell carcinoma and *sebaceous hyperplasia* are sometimes difficult to differentiate clinically. Sebaceous hyperplasia is the proliferation of sebaceous glands surrounding a hair follicle that appears as a 1- to 3-mm, yellowish papule with overlying telangiectasia and a central pore. The yellowish coloration and central pore help to differentiate it from a basal cell carcinoma. Other epithelial growths that resemble a nodular basal cell carcinoma include a *nonpigmented nevus, molluscum contagiosum*, Merkel cell carcinoma, trichoepithelioma,

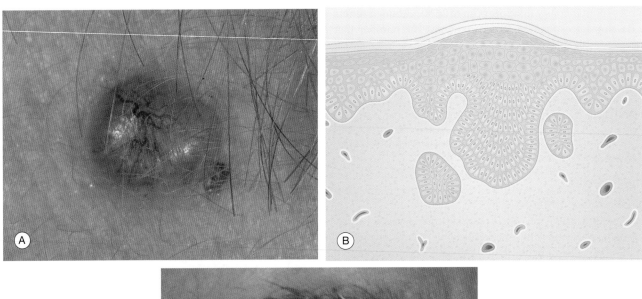

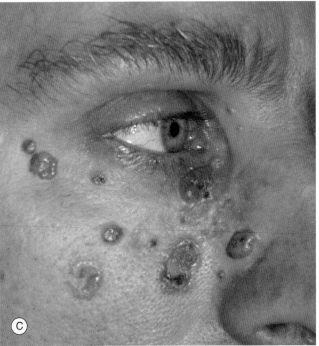

Fig. 5.2 (A) Nodular basal cell carcinoma. (B) Basal cell carcinoma. Epidermis—thickened. Dermis—invasive buds and lobules of basaloid cells. (C) Basal cell nevus syndrome—multiple pearly to flesh-colored papules and nodules with rolled border and telangiectasia and some crusting.

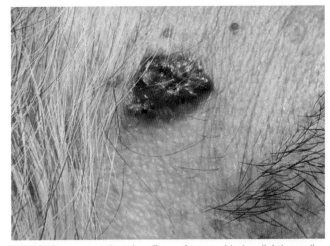

Fig. 5.3 **Pigmented basal cell carcinoma**—black, slightly scaling, translucent plaque.

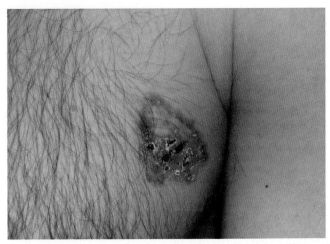

Fig. 5.4 **Superficial basal cell carcinoma**—red, slightly scaling and crusted patch.

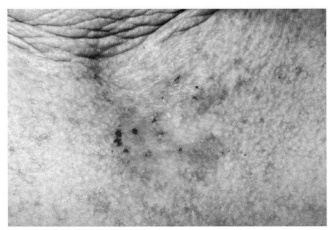

Fig. 5.5 Scarring basal cell carcinoma—pink, atrophic white, slightly crusted, ill-marginated patch.

fibrous papule of the nose, lichenoid keratosis, and *squamous cell carcinoma*.

Pigmented basal cell carcinoma can be confused with a *seborrheic keratosis, pigmented nevus*, and, most importantly, *malignant melanoma*. The pearly, rolled border of pigmented basal cell carcinoma helps to differentiate it from a malignant melanoma. If doubt exists, an excisional or deep shave biopsy should be performed.

Superficial basal cell carcinoma resembles a patch of *dermatitis*. It can be confused with *psoriasis, nummular dermatitis*, and *squamous cell carcinoma*. A persistent solitary lesion and lack of response to topical steroids clinically differentiate superficial basal cell carcinoma from dermatitis or psoriasis. A skin biopsy is the only way to differentiate it from squamous cell carcinoma in situ.

Any *nonhealing scar-like lesions* should undergo biopsy to rule out a scarring basal cell carcinoma.

DIFFERENTIAL DIAGNOSIS OF BASAL CELL CARCINOMA

Nodular
- Sebaceous hyperplasia
- Flesh-colored nevus
- Molluscum contagiosum
- Merkel cell carcinoma
- Trichoepithelioma
- Fibrous papule of the nose
- Squamous cell carcinoma

Pigmented
- Seborrheic keratosis
- Pigmented nevus
- Malignant melanoma

Superficial
- Dermatitis
- Lichenoid keratosis
- Squamous cell carcinoma

Scarring
- Scar

Laboratory and Biopsy

The diagnosis of basal cell carcinoma should be confirmed by a shave or punch biopsy. The technique of skin biopsy is reviewed in Chapter 4. The tumors are made up of uniform cells that resemble the basal layers of the epidermis (Fig. 5.3B). They have a uniform, large, oval, blue nucleus with indistinct cytoplasm. The tumor extends from the epidermis into the dermis as nodular or cystic structures, bands, or strands or as buds from the epidermis. The nodular areas have peripheral palisading with retraction from the surrounding stroma. The cells in some basal cell carcinomas have a "squamoid" appearance, which makes them difficult to differentiate from squamous cell carcinoma. The infiltrative, morpheaform, micronodular, and mixed histologic subtypes of primary basal cell carcinoma are more aggressive and more difficult to eradicate.

A chronic eczematous patch or nonhealing crusted lesion should be biopsied to rule out a superficial basal cell carcinoma.

Therapy

Sun protective measures, such as the use of sunscreens, protective clothing, and avoiding midday UV light exposure, are important for the prevention of future basal cell carcinomas. Nicotinamide 500 mg twice a day is also effective in reducing basal cell carcinoma.

Treatment of basal cell carcinoma should be individualized according to the location of the lesion, the histopathologic type, the age of the patient, the general health of the patient, the size of the basal cell carcinoma, and whether it is primary or recurrent. Recurrence of basal cell carcinoma is related particularly to location on the nose or ear, size more than 2 cm, and histologic pattern of micronodular, infiltrative, and morpheic types. Treatment modalities include scalpel excision, curettage and electrodesiccation, radiotherapy, cryotherapy, and topical 5-fluorouracil or imiquimod. Each treatment must be *properly* selected to achieve a high cure rate. Surgical modalities are those most frequently used and have the best cure rates. The surgical techniques are reviewed in Chapter 4.

Excision with primary suture closure, the most frequently used form of therapy, allows for histologic assessment of surgical margins. When the wound is large, grafts or tissue transposition flaps may be used to achieve closure. Excision is good for most basal cell carcinomas, but is *the treatment of choice* for large basal cell carcinomas, recurrent tumors, sclerosing types of basal cell carcinoma, basal cell carcinomas at sites of high recurrence such as the nose or ear, and basal cell carcinoma that extends into the subcutaneous tissue. A specialized form of excision using detailed mapping of the extent of the tumor with histologic orientation is the *Mohs micrographic surgical technique*. This meticulous procedure is most often used for basal cell carcinomas on the head and neck, recurrent basal cell carcinoma, and primary tumors with a high risk of recurrence.

> Mohs micrographic surgery has the highest cure rate and preserves the most normal skin. It is indicated for most facial/neck basal cell carcinomas and for recurrent basal cell carcinomas.

Curettage and electrodesiccation is a therapeutic modality frequently used by dermatologists. The clinical margins of the tumor are defined by vigorous curettage until the firm, fibrous consistency of normal dermis is felt. This is often followed by electrodesiccation. The entire procedure of curettage and electrodesiccation may be repeated to ensure the removal of the tumor. The resultant wound heals by secondary intention over a 2- to 3-week period, with excellent cosmetic results in most cases. Experience is needed to obtain good cure rates. Curettage and electrodesiccation should not be used for basal cell carcinomas with poorly defined clinical borders, for sclerosing basal cell carcinomas, for recurrent basal cell carcinomas, or in certain anatomic locations such as the nasolabial fold and eyelids.

Radiation therapy is reserved for elderly patients because the subsequent chronic radiodermatitis that occurs years after the therapy may be cosmetically unacceptable, and because of the potential for developing a new primary cancer in the radiotherapy site. Radiation therapy is used when the patient refuses surgical treatment or has a large tumor that would be difficult to treat surgically.

Cryosurgery with liquid nitrogen is reserved for those clinicians experienced in its use for cancer therapy. The margins and depth of the tumor must be estimated clinically. Cryoprobes are used to monitor the depth of the freeze. After surgery, marked tissue reaction occurs with edema, tissue necrosis, weeping, and crusting.

Topical chemotherapy with *5-fluorouracil* or imiquimod is, in general, inappropriate for treating skin cancer. It should not be used on deep or recurrent tumors. It is occasionally used in patients who have multiple, superficial, multicentric basal cell carcinomas that otherwise would require numerous surgical procedures. Treatment is continued for weeks until marked inflammation and erosion occur. Residual areas suspected to have tumor must undergo biopsy, and another therapeutic modality must be used if basal cell carcinoma persists.

Vismodegib and sonidegib are hedgehog pathway inhibitors targeting smoothened (SMO). They are indicated in the treatment of locally advanced, multiple, or metastatic basal cell carcinoma. Serious adverse side-effects, including birth defects, limit their use.

Cemiplimab, a programed death receptor-1 (PD-1) blocking antibody, is indicated for patients with locally advanced basal cell carcinoma previously treated with a hedgehog pathway inhibitor or for whom a hedgehog pathway inhibitor is not appropriate.

Prevention of further sun-induced damage to the skin is mandatory. Sun protection includes the regular use of sunscreens with an SPF of 30 or greater, protective clothing (wide-brimmed hat and long-sleeved shirt), and avoidance of midday sun (from 10 a.m. to 2 p.m.).

> Prevention with sun protection—sunscreen, clothing, and avoid midday sun.

THERAPY FOR BASAL CELL CARCINOMA

Prevention
- Sunscreen ≥SPF 30. Reapply after a couple of hours
- Broad-brimmed hat, long-sleeved shirt, and pants
- Avoidance of intense midday sun (from 10:00 a.m. to 2:00 p.m.)
- Nicotinamide 500 mg twice a day

Initial
- Excision
- Curettage and electrodesiccation
- Mohs micrographic surgery

Alternative
- Radiation
- Cryotherapy
- 5-Fluorouracil or imiquimod topically for multiple superficial basal cell carcinomas
- Vismodegib, sonidegib
- Immunotherapy

Course and Complications

Because its course is frequently indolent, a basal cell carcinoma is often ignored. It may enlarge locally and can invade underlying tissues, resulting in significant morbidity and mutilation. Vital structures, such as an eye, a nose, or an ear, may be totally lost.

Basal cell cancer rarely metastasizes, presumably because of stromal dependence. The metastatic rate is estimated to be less than 0.003% (1 in 52,000 cases in one series). The excessively large, ulcerated, locally destructive, and recurrent basal cell carcinoma is most likely to metastasize. Regional lymph nodes, lung, and bone are the most likely tissues involved. Routine follow-up every 6–12 months of patients with basal cell carcinoma is recommended because 35% of these patients will develop another basal cell carcinoma within 5 years.

Pathogenesis

The most common factor related to the development of basal cell carcinoma is UV radiation. Other factors to be considered are arsenic ingestion, genetic predisposition, X-irradiation, and chronic irritation. Mutations of the genes, SMO and patched (PTCH), in the hedgehog pathway are implicated in over 90% of basal cell carcinomas and in basal cell nevus syndrome. *Basal cell nevus syndrome* is a rare autosomal-dominant disorder characterized by early development of multiple basal cell carcinomas (Fig. 5.2C), jaw cysts, macrocephaly, palmar and plantar pits, increased risk of medulloblastoma, and other congenital abnormalities. The origin of basal cell carcinoma is a pluripotential primordial epithelial cell in the basal layer of the skin or, less often, a cutaneous appendage such as the hair follicle.

CORNS

KEY POINTS

1. Caused by pressure or friction
2. Do not interrupt skin lines

Definition

A corn is a localized thickening of epidermis secondary to chronic pressure or friction. It occurs most often on the feet. Synonyms are *clavus* and *heloma*.

Incidence

Corns are extremely common. Many patients treat themselves or see a podiatrist rather than a physician.

History

The patient seeks medical care because of painful feet when standing or walking. A history of ill-fitting footwear or foot injury may be obtained.

Physical Examination

Corns are white-gray or yellow-brown, well-circumscribed, horny papules or nodules. Paring the surface with a scalpel reveals a translucent core with the preservation of skin lines. Hard corns occur on the sole (Fig. 5.6) and external surface of the toes, where drying occurs. Soft corns occur between the toes, where sweating results in maceration.

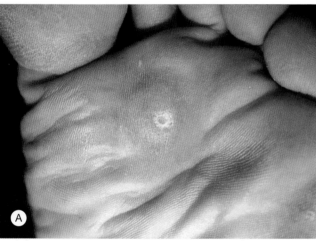

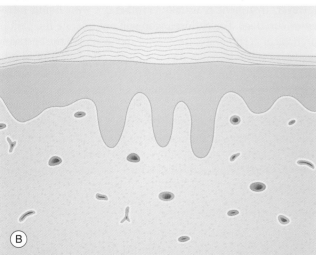

Fig. 5.6 Corn. (A) Thick, yellowish plaque with intact skin lines and compressed keratin center. (B) Epidermis—thickened, with hyperkeratosis.

> Corns have a clear center and intact skin lines.

Differential Diagnosis

Plantar warts and corns are commonly confused. The simple maneuver of paring the surface and identifying the presence of skin lines with a translucent core confirms that the lesion is a corn.

DIFFERENTIAL DIAGNOSIS OF A CORN

- Wart

Laboratory and Biopsy

A biopsy is unnecessary (Fig. 5.6B).

Therapy

The goal of treating corns is to provide immediate relief of pain and then to reduce the friction and pressure that have caused the corn. Immediate relief is provided by paring down the hyperkeratotic surface. Softening of hard corns may be accomplished with keratolytic agents such as 40% salicylic acid plasters. Changing ill-fitting footwear and shielding the sites with pads, rings, and orthotic devices reduce mechanical trauma. When these procedures fail, surgical correction of a foot deformity or removal of a bony prominence (exostosis) should be considered.

THERAPY FOR CORN

Initial
- Paring down with scalpel
- Softening with salicylic acid plaster
- Reduction of trauma—change of shoes, protective pads, rings, etc.

Alternative
- Surgery—correction of bony deformity

Course and Complications

Persistence of the corn can be expected unless the underlying mechanical problem is reduced or removed. Underlying bursitis from chronic inflammation and sinus formation with infection, osteomyelitis, and gangrene may occur and are particularly worrisome in patients with arteriosclerosis, diabetes mellitus, or peripheral neurologic disorders.

> A corn will persist unless friction and pressure are relieved.

Pathogenesis

Repeated pressure and trauma resulting extrinsically from ill-fitting shoes and intrinsically from an exostosis or other anatomic skeletal defects result in the formation of corns.

MOLLUSCUM CONTAGIOSUM

Definition

Molluscum contagiosum is caused by a DNA poxvirus, *molluscipoxvirus*, that infects epidermal cells. Clinically, the lesions appear as smooth, dome-shaped papules that often are umbilicated (Fig. 5.7).

Incidence

Molluscum contagiosum is a common childhood disease. Spread among family members occurs but is uncommon.

History

In adults, venereal transmission is suggested by a history of sexual exposure and the location of lesions in the genital region.

Physical Examination

The papules of molluscum contagiosum are 2- to 5-mm wide, hard, smooth, dome-shaped, and flesh colored or translucent.

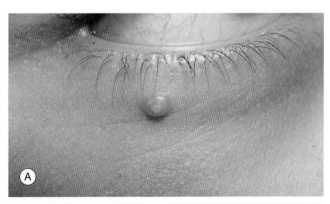

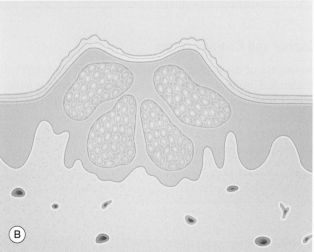

Fig. 5.7 Molluscum contagiosum. (A) Smooth, flesh-colored papule with umbilicated whitish center. (B) Epidermis—thickened, containing molluscum bodies.

The papules have a central umbilication from which a "cheesy" core can be expressed. They occur singly or in groups, most often on the trunk, face, and extremities of children and on the genitals of sexually active adults. Uncommonly, they become disseminated, resulting in hundreds of lesions. If inflamed, they are difficult to recognize because of secondary redness and crusting.

Differential Diagnosis

The translucent papule of molluscum contagiosum can resemble *nodular basal cell carcinoma* or a *comedo*. Nodular basal cell carcinomas usually have telangiectasia and occur in sun-exposed skin of older patients. Comedones lack umbilication. An inflamed molluscum contagiosum may appear to be a bacterial infection of the skin.

DIFFERENTIAL DIAGNOSIS OF MOLLUSCUM CONTAGIOSUM

- Nodular basal cell carcinoma
- Comedo

Laboratory and Biopsy

The diagnosis usually is clinically obvious. When doubt exists, a simple office procedure is confirmatory. The molluscum papule is removed by curettage and crushed onto a slide. This unstained material readily reveals numerous oval molluscum bodies when examined with a microscope. A biopsy usually is not necessary unless the typical features are masked by secondary inflammation (Fig. 5.7B).

> When in doubt, the diagnosis may be confirmed by expressing the cheesy core and smearing it onto a glass slide for microscopic examination.

Therapy

Treatment may be deferred awaiting spontaneous resolution. However, treatment is usually cryotherapy with liquid nitrogen or curettage. For children who will not tolerate the pain of curettage or cryotherapy, the careful application of the blistering chemical cantharidin can be used in the office, or topical salicylic acid preparations or tretinoin can be used at home, similar to the treatment of warts. The most reliable means of eradication is by curettage. The molluscum papule, composed of many molluscum bodies, is scraped off, with some discomfort and bleeding. The topical immune response modifier, imiquimod (Aldara) cream 5% applied daily has also been successful. Also, berdazimer gel 10.3%, which is a nitric oxide–releasing agent, has been an effective treatment.

Course and Complications

Spontaneous remission often occurs within 6–9 months, although lesions have been known to persist for many years, and more lesions may develop by autoinoculation. Individual lesions can become secondarily inflamed and may resemble

<table>
<tr><td>

THERAPY FOR MOLLUSCUM CONTAGIOSUM

Initial
- None
- Cryotherapy with liquid nitrogen
- Salicylic acid
- Tretinoin
- Cantharidin

Alternative
- Curettage
- Imiquimod cream 5%
- Berdazimer gel 10.3%

</td></tr>
</table>

furuncles. Involvement of the eyelids is uncommon but may result in chronic conjunctivitis. The development of hundreds of lesions with little tendency for involution should alert the clinician to consider immunocompromise. Molluscum contagiosum is one of the most common cutaneous findings in acquired immune deficiency syndrome (AIDS) and AIDS-related complex, infecting 9% of these individuals. In the patient with AIDS, molluscum contagiosum is often recalcitrant to treatment and causes significant morbidity and disfigurement.

Pathogenesis

Although it is difficult to produce lesions after experimental inoculation, molluscum contagiosum is certainly contagious. Intimate physical contact, such wrestling or sexual intercourse, or even sharing towels, has resulted in transmission of the disease.

The molluscum contagiosum virus replicates in the cytoplasm of the keratinocyte, with resulting large intracytoplasmic inclusion bodies (molluscum bodies) and proliferation of the epidermis. The center of the papule ultimately disintegrates, forming a crater and releasing molluscum bodies.

Spontaneous involution results from a host immune response that is presumed to be cell mediated. The stimulus that provokes this response after many months of inactivity is unknown, as with warts.

SEBORRHEIC KERATOSIS

KEY POINTS
1. Common in older adults
2. Flesh-colored, tan, brown, dark brown, well-demarcated, "pasted on" appearance
3. When in doubt, biopsy to rule out melanoma

Definition

A seborrheic keratosis is a benign neoplasm of epidermal cells that clinically appears as a scaling, "pasted on" papule or plaque. It is thought to be an autosomal-dominant inherited trait.

Incidence

Seborrheic keratoses usually appear in middle age, with at least a few lesions present in most elderly patients.

History

Many patients remember family members who had seborrheic keratoses. These neoplasms are gradually acquired in middle and later life, and grow slowly. They often scale or are scratched off by the patient only to recur.

Physical Examination

Seborrheic keratoses vary in size from 2 mm to 2 cm or larger and are slightly to markedly elevated (Fig. 5.8). Color ranges from flesh to tan or brown or, occasionally, black. The keratoses are oval to round, greasy-appearing, "pasted on," sharply marginated growths. The surface is often verrucous or crumbly in appearance and may be punctuated with keratin-filled pits. The lesions occur on the head, neck, trunk, and extremities, sparing the palms and soles.

> A flesh-colored, tan/brown/dark brown/black, well-marginated, "pasted on" appearance is distinctive in seborrheic keratoses.

Differential Diagnosis

Wart, actinic keratosis, lichenoid keratosis, and pigmented growths such as a *nevus, pigmented basal cell carcinoma,* or *malignant melanoma* may be confused with a seborrheic keratosis. The occurrence of multiple similar scaling growths with a greasy, well-marginated, "pasted on" appearance gives the observer the clue that these lesions are seborrheic keratoses. On occasion, a single thin seborrheic keratosis becomes inflamed resulting in a lichenoid keratosis. The superficial, exophytic, epidermal growth and keratotic surface of a seborrheic keratosis differentiate it from a nevus, a pigmented dermal growth with which it is often confused.

<table>
<tr><td>

DIFFERENTIAL DIAGNOSIS OF SEBORRHEIC KERATOSIS

- Wart
- Actinic keratosis
- Nevus
- Pigmented basal cell carcinoma
- Malignant melanoma
- Lichenoid keratosis

</td></tr>
</table>

Laboratory and Biopsy

If there is concern for a melanoma, then an excisional or deep shave biopsy confirms the clinical impression of seborrheic keratosis. This neoplasm is characterized by a uniform, well-demarcated, intraepidermal proliferation of small, benign squamous cells. Invaginations of the epidermis form small, keratin-filled pseudocysts (Fig. 5.8C).

> Deep shave or excisional biopsy is indicated for uncertain lesions.

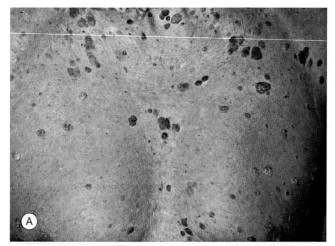

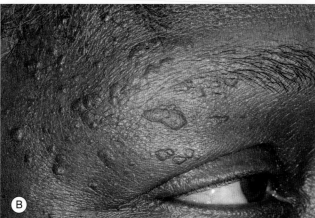

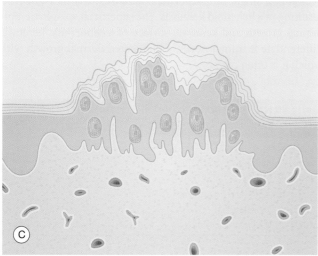

Fig. 5.8 Seborrheic keratosis. (A, B) Thick, corrugated, scaling, well-marginated, pasted on, brown, and tan plaques. (C) Epidermis—hyperkeratosis with thickened epidermis containing horny pseudocysts.

Therapy

No therapy is necessary for seborrheic keratoses unless they become irritated, are cosmetically unacceptable, or require confirmation that they are benign. Cryotherapy with liquid nitrogen is an efficient and effective means of removal. As an alternative, seborrheic keratoses can be anesthetized and curetted or shaved off. Caution should be used; vigorous treatment may result in scarring. Excisional surgery is seldom needed unless concern about malignancy exists.

THERAPY FOR SEBORRHEIC KERATOSIS
Initial
• None
• Cryotherapy with liquid nitrogen
Alternative
• Curettage
• Shave

Course and Complications

The tendency is to acquire more seborrheic keratoses with age (wisdom spots). Sometimes, seborrheic keratoses become irritated from rubbing, clothing, or excoriations. Occasionally, their typical morphologic appearance becomes obscured by inflammation, thus making a biopsy necessary for diagnosis.

The number of seborrheic keratoses increases with age.

Of note is the very rare *sign of Leser-Trélat*, the rapid increase in size and number of seborrheic keratoses accompanied by pruritus. The extremities and shoulders are the most frequent sites of involvement. This is a cutaneous sign of internal malignancy, usually adenocarcinoma involving the stomach, ovary, uterus, or breast.

SKIN TAG

KEY POINTS
1. Soft pedunculated papules
2. No therapy necessary

Definition

A skin tag (acrochordon) is a benign, fleshy tumor that is frequently acquired in adult life. It is characterized by a slightly hyperplastic epithelium covering a dermal connective tissue stalk. It appears as a pedunculated, flesh-colored growth.

Incidence

This benign tumor is common in adulthood. The incidence of patients coming into the authors' clinic specifically for skin tags is 0.5%, but as an incidental finding 50%–60% of patients older than 50 years have skin tags. A steady increase in frequency occurs from the second decade (11%) to the fifth decade (59%) of life, after which the number of individuals with skin tags remains stable.

History

Most patients ignore skin tags and accept their acquisition as a sign of aging. Some patients request their removal because of irritation or cosmetic appearance.

Physical Examination

A skin tag is a soft, tan- to flesh-colored, 1–10 mm, pedunculated, fleshy papule (Fig. 5.9A). It has a smooth or folded surface and frequently appears boggy or filiform. It is found on any skin surface, but has a predilection for the axilla, neck, inframammary region, inguinal region, and eyelids. When irritated or injured, it can appear as a necrotic, crusted papule that may not be clinically distinctive but causes concern regarding a malignancy.

Differential Diagnosis

Intradermal nevi may have a boggy, flesh-colored appearance, making them impossible to differentiate from skin tags other than by histologic examination. The acquisition of skin tags in later life would help to differentiate them historically from nevi. *Neurofibromas* can resemble skin tags, but on palpation a neurofibroma can be invaginated into what feels like a "buttonhole" defect in the dermis. Uncommonly, *basal or squamous cell carcinoma* may have the appearance of a skin tag.

DIFFERENTIAL DIAGNOSIS OF SKIN TAG

- Intradermal nevus
- Neurofibroma
- Rarely, basal or squamous cell carcinoma

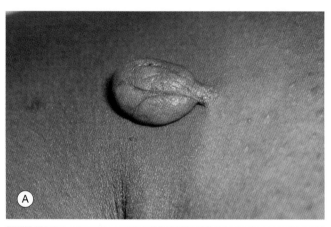

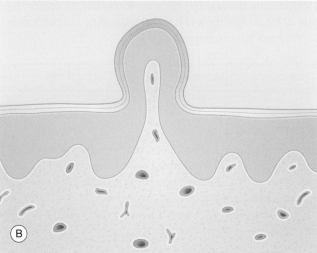

Fig. 5.9 Skin tag. (A) Soft, pedunculated, flesh-colored papule. (B) Epidermis—mildly thickened. Dermis—loose connective tissue stalk.

Laboratory and Biopsy

Skin tags are covered by a slightly hyperplastic epithelium consisting of hyperkeratosis, papillomatosis, and acanthosis. The underlying dermal connective tissue stalk is composed of loose collagen containing numerous capillaries (Fig. 5.9B). Typical multiple, 1- to 5-mm, flesh-colored, pedunculated skin tags need not be submitted for pathologic examination. Larger solitary and necrotic or crusted skin tags should be examined histologically.

> Large or necrotic skin tags should be sent to pathology.

Therapy

Skin tags need not be removed unless the patient requests it. The easiest means of removal of skin tags is by quickly snipping them with scissors. This usually requires no local anesthesia, and the crushing action of the scissors results in little bleeding. As an alternative, they may be frozen with liquid nitrogen.

THERAPY FOR SKIN TAGS

Initial
- None
- Snipping off with scissors

Alternative
- Cryotherapy with liquid nitrogen

Course and Complications

The number of skin tags increases with age. Tags normally are of little consequence and require no treatment. Concern has been expressed that skin tags may be a marker for the presence of colonic polyps in highly selected referral populations presenting for colonoscopy. In the primary care setting, no association exists between skin tags and colonic polyps.

SQUAMOUS CELL CARCINOMA

KEY POINTS

1. Malignancy of keratinocytes
2. Potential to metastasize

Definition

Squamous cell carcinoma is a malignant neoplasm of keratinocytes. It is locally invasive and has the potential to metastasize. It appears clinically as a scaling, patch, indurated plaque, or nodule that sometimes bleeds or ulcerates (Fig. 5.10). The etiology of squamous cell carcinoma includes UV radiation from sun exposure or tanning beds, chronic wounds or scars, chronic immunosuppression, and chemical carcinogens such as soot and arsenic.

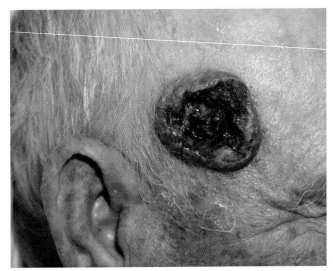

Fig. 5.10 **Squamous cell carcinoma**—ulcerated, crusted, red plaque.

Incidence

Squamous cell carcinoma is the second most common skin cancer, with nearly 2 million new cases diagnosed each year in the United States. The incidence of squamous cell carcinoma varies greatly with reference to ethnic group, geographic location, and occupation. It is most common in men aged over 60 years who have light skin and abundant sunlight exposure. Closer to the equator, the incidence increases. For example, squamous cell carcinoma is five times greater in New Orleans than in Chicago. In renal transplant patients, squamous cell carcinoma is 3.5 times more frequent than basal cell carcinoma, and more than 250 times more common than in the general population. Some 9 years after renal transplantation, patients have a more than 40% incidence of squamous cell carcinoma.

> Squamous cell carcinoma is the second most common skin cancer.

History

The patient's history of sunlight exposure in occupational and recreational activities is important in determining the risk of developing squamous cell carcinoma. A family history of skin cancer and a personal history of fair skin and sunburning are additional predisposing factors. The history of a chronic, non-healing, bleeding growth or ulcer should arouse suspicion of squamous cell carcinoma.

Physical Examination

Squamous cell carcinoma occurs most often in sun-exposed skin. It also develops on the mucous membranes and in sites of chronic injury, such as burn scars, irradiated sites, erosive discoid lupus erythematosus, and osteomyelitis sinuses. The occurrence of squamous cell carcinoma varies with anatomic location: head and neck, 81%; upper extremities, 16%; trunk, 1.5%; legs, 1.3%. The tumor nodule is hard, red to flesh colored, and has a smooth or verrucous surface. The central portion may

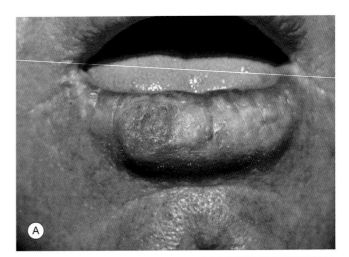

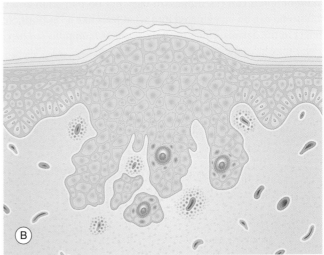

Fig. 5.11 **Squamous cell carcinoma**. (A) Slightly crusted, hyperkeratotic plaque on the lower lip. (B) Epidermis—hyperkeratosis, atypical keratinocytes. Dermis—invasive tumor, inflammation.

be hyperkeratotic, ulcerated, or crusted. Deep invasion results in fixation to underlying tissue. Squamous cell carcinoma of the lip involves the lower lip in 90% of cases and usually arises from a chronically damaged epithelium secondary to actinic exposure or smoking (Fig. 5.11). A chronic scaling red patch may be a squamous cell carcinoma.

> Most squamous cell carcinomas occur on the head, neck, and arms.

Differential Diagnosis

Squamous cell carcinoma can be differentiated clinically or by biopsy from a *keratoacanthoma (which may be a variant of a squamous cell carcinoma), hypertrophic actinic keratosis, wart, lichenoid keratosis, basal cell carcinoma,* and *seborrheic keratosis.* All persistent ulcers or crusted lesions must undergo biopsy to rule out squamous cell carcinoma.

> Chronic ulcers should undergo biopsy to exclude malignancy.

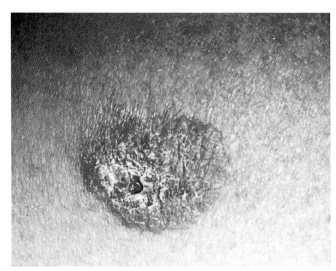

Fig. 5.12 Squamous cell carcinoma in situ—well-demarcated red, scaling, and slightly crusted patch.

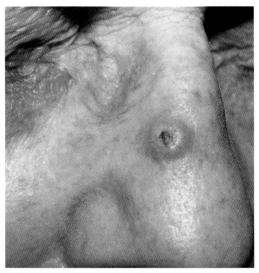

Fig. 5.13 Keratoacanthoma. Rapidly growing pink nodule with a crusted, hyperkeratotic central crater.

Squamous cell carcinoma in situ (*Bowen disease)* appears as an red, scaling, slightly crusted, well-marginated patch (Fig. 5.12). Squamous cell carcinoma in situ of the glans penis is referred to as erythroplasia of Queyrat; it appears as a red, velvety, moist patch.

Keratoacanthoma is a rapidly growing neoplasm of the epithelium that may be biologically benign but histologically resembles a squamous cell carcinoma and is thought by some to be a variant of squamous cell carcinoma. Keratoacanthoma is a round, flesh-colored nodule that characteristically grows rapidly (within 4–6 weeks) and has a central keratin-filled crater (Fig. 5.13). Keratoacanthomas may spontaneously involute within 6 months. However, because some may be difficult to differentiate from squamous cell carcinoma, excision or other destructive treatment is recommended.

Laboratory and Biopsy

Any lesion suspected of being squamous cell carcinoma should undergo biopsy. Squamous cell carcinoma consists of malignant

DIFFERENTIAL DIAGNOSIS OF SQUAMOUS CELL CARCINOMA

- Keratoacanthoma (squamous cell variant?)
- Hypertrophic actinic keratosis
- Wart
- Basal cell carcinoma
- Seborrheic keratosis
- Lichenoid keratosis

epidermal cells that invade the dermis (Fig. 5.11B). It is graded according to the degree of atypicality of the tumor cells, with grade 1 predominantly mature, whereas grades 2, 3, and 4 are less well-differentiated. Grade 4 tumors may be difficult to differentiate from malignant melanoma because their spindle-shape cells lack intercellular bridges.

The biopsy of squamous cell carcinoma in situ (*Bowen disease*) reveals a thickened epidermis consisting of atypical, poorly oriented, dysplastic cells that lie completely within the epidermis. *Keratoacanthoma* has a large, central, keratin-filled crater surrounded by well-differentiated epidermal cells that sometimes appear dysplastic, thus making it difficult to distinguish from a squamous cell carcinoma.

Therapy

Sun protective measures, such as the use of sunscreens, protective clothing, and avoiding midday UV light exposure, are important for the prevention of future squamous cell carcinomas. Nicotinamide 500 mg twice a day is also effective in reducing squamous cell carcinoma.

Excision is the treatment of choice, although a well-differentiated small squamous cell carcinoma occurring in actinically damaged skin may be effectively treated with curettage and electrodesiccation. These surgical techniques are reviewed in Chapter 4. Large or recurrent poorly differentiated tumors, as well as those occurring on the mucous membrane and in scars, should be treated by scalpel excision with narrow margins (3–5 mm) that are checked histologically to be free of tumor or by the Mohs technique.

Nonsurgical therapy, such as ionizing radiation, is useful in selected patients. Intralesional methotrexate or 5-flourouracil have been used in selective squamous cell carcinomas, especially keratoacanthomas.

The immune checkpoint inhibitors, cemiplimab and pembrolizumab, are both monoclonol antibody medications that bind the PD-1 and work by increasing the body's immune response to tumors. They are indicated for patients with locally advanced squamous cell carcinoma who are not candidates for curative surgery or radiation, and for metastatic cutaneous squamous cell carcinoma.

Course and Complications

The course of squamous cell carcinoma is variable. Those carcinomas most likely to metastasize are relatively large, poorly differentiated, invade more deeply including perineural and lymphovascular invasion, occur in damaged skin and mucous

THERAPY FOR SQUAMOUS CELL CARCINOMA

Prevention
- Sunscreen ≥SPF 30. Reapply after a couple of hours
- Broad-brimmed hat, long-sleeved shirt, and pants
- Avoidance of intense midday sun (from 10:00 a.m. to 2:00 p.m.)
- Nicotinamide 500 mg twice a day

Initial
- Excision
- Curettage and electrodesiccation
- Mohs micrographic surgery

Alternative
- Radiation
- Intralesional methotrexate or 5-flourouracil
- Immunotherapy, chemotherapy

membranes, and in an immunosuppressed patient. Some 2% of all squamous cell carcinomas of the skin metastasize. Those that arise in actinic keratoses are less aggressive, with a metastatic rate of 0.5%.

> Squamous cell carcinoma arising in actinic keratosis has a low metastatic potential.

Much higher rates of metastasis, up to 9%, occur in squamous cell carcinoma arising in chronic leg ulcers, burn scars, radiodermatitis, osteomyelitis sinuses, and the mucous membrane of the lips, glans penis, and vulva. When metastasis occurs, it is usually through the lymphatics to the regional lymph nodes. Prophylactic lymph node dissection is not done unless the patient has lymphadenopathy.

> High-risk features include large size (2 cm), depth (2 mm), perineural or lymphovascular invasion, ear or mucous membrane, recurrent tumor, immunosuppression, and poor differentiation.

Pathogenesis

Sir Percivall Pott in 1775 was the first to describe occupationally induced cancer and to relate cancer to an etiologic agent. He described the occurrence of squamous cell carcinoma of the scrotum in chimney sweeps and suggested that its cause was chronic soot exposure. In 1809, Lambe related squamous cell carcinoma to arsenic in drinking water. The relationship between UV radiation and squamous cell carcinoma was suggested in 1875 by Thiersch. Frieben in 1902 described the occurrence of squamous cell carcinoma after exposure to X-rays.

Experimentally, Yamagiwa and Ichikawa in 1915 were the first to produce squamous cell carcinoma in mice and rabbits after the topical application of coal tar. Several years later, in 1924, Block induced squamous cell carcinoma in rabbits after X-irradiation. Using mice repeatedly exposed to UV radiation, Findlay in 1928 was the first to produce UV radiation–induced carcinoma.

Human papillomavirus (HPV) has been implicated as the cause of cutaneous and cervical carcinoma. Patients with *epidermodysplasia verruciformis*, a rare genetic disorder, develop hundreds of flat warts, and those warts caused by specific types of HPV, particularly HPV-5 and -8, are prone to transform into squamous cell carcinoma. The finding of HPV-16 and -18 genomes in carcinoma of the cervix has provided strong circumstantial evidence for HPV carcinogenic potential.

All of these carcinogens—UV radiation, X-irradiation, coal tar, arsenic, and viruses—are active in the skin, initiating malignancy by altering cellular DNA, RNA, and proteins. In addition, UV radiation also alters the immune system, making the host more susceptible to these tumors. Chronic immunosuppression, as occurs in organ transplant recipients, is also associated with an increased frequency of squamous cell carcinoma, especially in sun-damaged skin.

WART

KEY POINTS
1. Caused by multiple papillomavirus types.
2. Vary in appearance.
3. Treatments are nonspecific and destructive.

Definition

Warts are benign neoplasms caused by infection of epidermal cells with papillomaviruses. The thickening of the epidermis with scaling and an upward extension of the dermal papillae containing prominent capillaries give them their "warty" or verrucous appearance.

> Warts are caused by papillomaviruses.

Incidence

Warts generally occur in healthy children and young adults. Genital HPV infection may be the most common sexually transmitted disease. Of sexually active adults, 1% are estimated to have genital warts, and a further 10%–20% have latent infection. For sexually active young college women, the incidence of infection is high: 43% prior to the advent of HPV vaccines. Some 5%–7% of patients seen by dermatologists present with warts.

History

Predisposing conditions make the occurrence of multiple warts more likely. Immunosuppressed patients, such as renal transplant recipients, are prone to the development of warts. Inquiry into the patient's occupation is important because butchers and meat cutters have a significantly higher incidence of common warts. Anogenital warts (condylomata acuminata) affect sexually active individuals, and their occurrence in children should raise suspicions of sexual abuse. However, most patients with warts do not have any significant predisposing conditions.

Physical Examination

The *common wart* (Fig. 5.14), or verruca vulgaris, is a flesh-colored firm papule or nodule that has a corrugated or hyperkeratotic surface. It interrupts the normal skin lines and is studded with black puncta, which represent thrombosed blood vessels. Common warts occur individually, in groups, or in a linear fashion from autoinoculation. The hands and fingers are the usual sites. Involvement around nails frequently results in extension underneath the nail plate. A filiform variant of verruca vulgaris occurs on the head and neck.

A *flat wart* has a subtle appearance (Fig. 5.15). It is a flesh-colored or reddish brown, slightly raised, flat-surfaced, 2- to 5-mm, well-marginated papule. On extremely close inspection (a hand magnifying lens may be needed), the surface appears finely verrucous. Multiple lesions commonly affect the hands and face. A linear arrangement of lesions is common.

A *plantar wart* may occur as a single, painful papule on the plantar aspect of the foot. It is often covered by a thick callus. When the callus is pared down with a scalpel, the underlying wart is visualized with interruption of skin lines and black puncta. Multiple plantar warts may coalesce (Fig. 5.16) in a mosaic configuration or remain discrete in a mother–daughter relationship, with a central large wart surrounded by multiple smaller warts.

> Common and plantar warts interrupt skin lines and have black puncta.

Venereal/anogenital warts (*condyloma acuminatum*) (Fig. 5.17) involve the rectum, perineal region, inguinal folds, external genitalia, and, occasionally, urethra and vagina. This wart is composed of a soft, moist papule and plaque that may be sessile or pedunculated. It has a verrucous surface that is often cauliflower-like. Soaking the genital area for 5 minutes with 3% to 5% acetic acid (white vinegar) causes warts to turn white. Subsequent use of

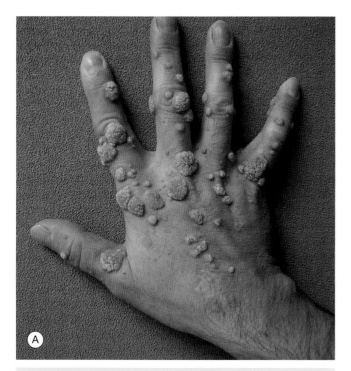

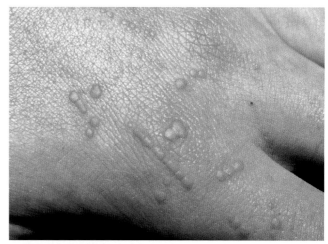

Fig. 5.15 **Flat warts**—pink flat papules in a linear arrangement, suggesting autoinoculation.

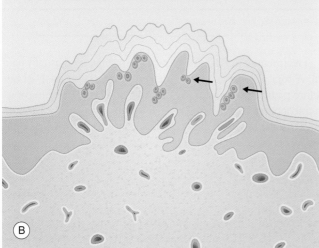

Fig. 5.14 **Wart**. (A) Scaling, verrucous papules/plaques with interrupted skin lines and black puncta. (B) Thickened epidermis, with overlying hyperkeratosis. Vacuolated keratinocytes are present in the granular cell layer (arrow).

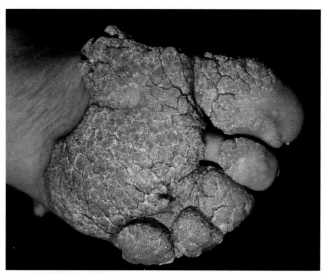

Fig. 5.16 **Plantar warts**—confluent verrucous plaque.

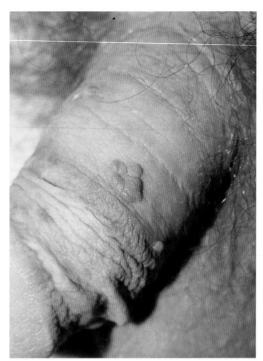

Fig. 5.17 Genital warts—verrucous, flesh-colored papules on the genitalia.

a hand magnifying lens or colposcopy enables better visualization of small genital warts (aceto-whitening). Although aceto-whitening increases the sensitivity of detection, it is not specific for HPV lesions and is not recommended for routine screening because over diagnosis of external genital warts may occur.

Differential Diagnosis

A common wart usually is easily recognized. When covered with thick scale, it may be confused with a *callus*, which on paring does not have interrupted skin lines. The diagnosis of *squamous cell carcinoma* should be entertained for a lesion that is resistant to treatment, is enlarging, and is crusted or ulcerated.

A flat wart on the face may be confused with a noninflammatory acne lesion, the "whitehead" or *comedo*. The tops of comedones are smooth and dome-shaped, whereas flat warts have roughened flat tops. When flat warts occur on the hand and forearm, *lichen planus* (see Chapter 11), an idiopathic inflammatory skin disease, is in the differential diagnosis. Lichen planus papules are red to purple; warts are flesh colored.

Plantar warts and *corns* are often confused because both are painful and have a thick, scaling surface. However, paring down the surface demonstrates the interruption of skin lines and black puncta characteristic of a plantar wart.

Genital warts may resemble the verrucous form of squamous cell carcinoma. Lesions that do not respond to treatment must undergo biopsy. *Secondary syphilis* of the anus and genitals (condyloma latum) is ruled out with a darkfield examination and serology. *Seborrheic keratoses* in the genital region also may resemble venereal warts.

Bowenoid papulosis is an uncommon disorder characterized by erythematous, sometimes pigmented, papules occurring in the genital region of sexually active young adults. Histologically,

bowenoid papulosis has the appearance of squamous cell carcinoma in situ. Its relationship with HPV infection has been confirmed by finding HPV DNA in bowenoid papulosis, especially HPV-16. Conservative surgical modalities or topical therapies should be used to treat bowenoid papulosis. Radical, mutilating procedures are unwarranted.

DIFFERENTIAL DIAGNOSIS OF WARTS
Common
• Callus
• Squamous cell carcinoma
Flat
• Comedo
• Lichen planus
Plantar
• Corn
Genital
• Squamous cell carcinoma
• Secondary syphilis
• Seborrheic keratosis
• Bowenoid papulosis

Laboratory and Biopsy

Warts are usually not biopsied unless a suspicion of carcinoma exists. When examined by biopsy, warts demonstrate a thickened epidermis (acanthosis) with overlying hyperkeratosis (Fig. 5.14B). Distinctive large keratinocytes (koilocytes) with small pyknotic nuclei surrounded by clear cytoplasm are found in the upper layers of the epidermis. Typing of HPV is based on DNA homology.

Therapy

Prevention of warts is better than treatment. A quadrivalent vaccine (Gardasil), preventing types 6 and 11 (which cause anogenital warts), and types 16 and 18 (responsible for >70% of cervical cancers), is highly effective for young males and females.

Prevention is better than treatment.

Treatment of warts is nonspecific, destructive, and usually painful. A topical local anesthetic applied under occlusion 1–2 hours before painful procedures may be beneficial when treating warts in uncooperative children. The goal is destruction of the keratinocytes that are infected with HPV. This may be accomplished with a variety of physical, chemical, or biologic modalities.

Avoid overzealous treatment, which produces scars.

The physical modalities include cryotherapy with liquid nitrogen, electrodesiccation and curettage, surgical excision, and laser therapy. Cryotherapy, the most common initial mode of treatment, uses either a cotton-tipped stick or a cryospray unit to apply the liquid nitrogen onto the verruca. A white ice ball develops at the site of freezing and should extend 1–2 mm beyond the margins of the wart. After the area has thawed, a second freezing results in greater destruction of the wart. Subsequent blister formation often occurs within 24 hours. After a couple of weeks, the blister dries, and the skin containing the wart peels off. Often, follow-up treatments every 4–8 weeks are necessary to eradicate any residual wart. Eradication generally requires at least two or three visits. The advantages of cryotherapy are that it is quick, does not require local anesthesia, and the discomfort from the freezing is tolerated well by most patients, except young children. Caution must be used with all the physical modalities, especially surgical excision, because of potential scarring. The scar may be cosmetically unacceptable, or it may be painful if on the plantar surface. Although laser surgery was initially thought to be superior to other surgical procedures in removing warts, this now appears not to be true.

Numerous chemotherapeutic agents are used to treat warts either in the office or at home. The initial treatments include salicylic acid at home or trichloroacetic acid in the office. Common warts may be treated with nonprescription 17% salicylic acid preparations applied daily with or without occlusion (duct tape). The wart is softened by soaking in water for 5 minutes before application; any loosened tissue is gently removed. Once the acid has been applied, the wart can be covered with adhesive tape. Cantharidin, a potent blistering agent derived from the blister beetle, is an alternative office treatment that is applied to common warts and covered with tape. After 24 hours, a blister forms beneath the wart. The blister roof dries and peels off, taking with it the wart. Occasionally, cantharidin or cryotherapy may result in the formation of a new wart in an annular configuration (ring) at the periphery of the blister.

> Tretinoin (Retin-A) is useful in the treatment of flat warts; its efficacy probably results from its irritant effect.

THERAPY FOR WARTS
Initial
- Cryotherapy with liquid nitrogen—all warts
- Salicylic acid plus occlusion with tape—common and plantar warts
- Cantharidin—especially for children
- Tretinoin 0.1% cream—flat warts
- Podophyllin 25%—genital warts
- Podofilox solution or gel—genital warts: twice daily for 3 days/week for 4 weeks
- Imiquimod cream—genital warts: once daily for 3 days/week for 16 weeks

Alternative
- Surgical excision, curettage, electrocautery
- Laser
- Interferon
- Bleomycin intralesionally
- 5-Fluorouracil
- Sinecatechins 15% ointment—genital warts: three times daily for 16 weeks
- Squaric acid

Plantar verrucae are treated with daily applications of a 40% salicylic acid plaster or 17% salicylic acid liquid under occlusion (duct tape).

Genital warts are commonly treated with 25% podophyllin resin (Podocon-25), which can be very toxic and is used only in the clinician's office. Within 4–6 hours after application, excess podophyllin should be washed off to prevent excessive local irritation. Caution must be used when applying podophyllin to extensive lesions because severe systemic reactions may result from absorption. The Centers for Disease Control and Prevention prefer cryotherapy over podophyllin for the treatment of genital warts. Podophyllin is a cytotoxic agent and has resulted in renal toxicity, polyneuritis, and shock. Podophyllin must never be used during pregnancy because of potential harmful effects on the fetus. Podofilox, a chemically pure ligand derived from podophyllin, is available as a 0.5% topical solution or gel (Condylox, podofilox) for patient self-treatment of external genital warts. Application is made twice daily for 3 consecutive days followed by a 4-day rest period. This cycle may be repeated up to four times. Sinecatechins 15% ointment (Veregen) is an alternative treatment. The sexual partners of infected individuals should be examined for the presence of genital warts. Female patients with genital warts should have periodic gynecologic examinations with Papanicolaou smears. Screening for other sexually transmitted diseases should be considered. Children greater than 4 years old with genital warts should be screened for sexual abuse. Genital warts in children under 4 years old are typically acquired from a nonsexual transmission.

> Podophyllin is toxic; do not apply to extensive lesions or use to treat pregnant women.

Recalcitrant warts have been treated with 5-fluorouracil topically, bleomycin intralesionally, and interferon topically, intralesionally, and systemically.

Biologic treatments have centered on the induction of immune responses. Imiquimod (Aldara) cream 5% applied topically induces the cytokines interferon-α, tumor necrosis factor-α, and interleukins-1, 6, and 8. It is indicated for the treatment of external genital and perianal warts, with three applications per week. Squaric acid dibutylester has been used to induce allergic contact dermatitis. Presumably, the wart is destroyed by the delayed hypersensitivity reaction that occurs at the site of application of the allergens.

Course and Complications
A total of 35% to 65% of warts resolve spontaneously within 2 years. Treatment results in cure rates of as high as 80%.

Of concern is the relationship between papillomavirus and carcinoma. Papillomavirus-associated cancers occur in humans, cattle, horses, and rabbits, and experimentally in rodents. In patients with the rare syndrome *epidermodysplasia verruciformis*, manifest by widespread refractory warts, who are infected with HPV-5 or HPV-8, sun-exposed flat warts progress into squamous cell carcinoma. Furthermore, HPV genomes have been demonstrated within the malignant squamous cells. The evidence for mucosal papillomaviruses (type 16, 18) causing cervical cancer is overwhelming. HPV infection of the cervix appears to represent a necessary but not sufficient condition for developing malignancy. Other possible cofactors, such as cigarette smoking, appear to be required for carcinogenesis. HPV typing, however, has not been proven to be beneficial in the diagnosis and management of external genital warts.

> Mucosal papillomavirus types 16 and 18 are the leading cause of cervical and anal carcinomas.

Pathogenesis

The contagious nature of warts was observed in ancient times. Jadassohn in the 1800s was the first to prove conclusively the infectious nature of warts. He ground up wart material and inoculated in the normal skin of volunteers. After an incubation period of 2–3 months, warts developed in the inoculation sites. In 1907 Ciuffo proved the viral nature of warts using ultrafiltration techniques.

The papillomavirus is a double-stranded DNA virus that infects and replicates in keratinizing cells in the epidermis. The HPV virion is an icosahedral particle composed of a viral genome surrounded by a proteinaceous capsid. Progeny HPV virions are assembled and become apparent in the upper layers of the epidermis, especially the stratum corneum and stratum granulosum. Viral genomes are found in lower layers of the epidermis and probably help to explain the chronicity and treatment failure of many warts. The presence of the wart virus stimulates epidermal proliferation, resulting in epidermal thickening and hyperkeratosis. Papillomaviruses have been subdivided into distinct types based on DNA homology. On this basis, more than 150 genotypes have been described. The clinical type of wart had been thought to be determined by local conditions at the site of infection. However, it now appears that different HPV types are responsible for the different clinical lesions—common, flat, plantar, and genital—because good correlation often exists between clinical presentation and HPV type.

The viral and host factors that influence persistence, regression, latency, and reactivation of warts are poorly understood. Serum antibodies to warts have been detected. More importantly, cell-mediated immunity appears to contribute to the regression of warts; in immunodeficient hosts (e.g., those with organ transplants or epidermodysplasia verruciformis), warts may reactivate or persist.

UNCOMMON EPIDERMAL GROWTHS

Birt–Hogg–Dube Syndrome

Birt–Hogg–Dube syndrome is an autosomal-dominant genodermatosis manifested by numerous 2- to 4-mm flesh-colored papules affecting the face (Fig. 5.18). These asymptomatic benign hair follicle hamartoma growths are fibrofolliculomas and trichodiscomas. The mouth and upper trunk are also affected with these growths and skin tags are always present in the axillae. These patients are at increased risk of developing renal tumors, including renal cell carcinoma, lung cysts, and spontaneous pneumothorax. The syndrome is caused by a mutation in the FLCN gene that encodes the protein, folliculin.

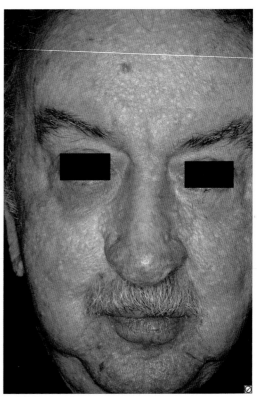

Fig. 5.18 Birt–Hogg–Dube syndrome—numerous flesh-colored to whitish papules scattered on the entire face.

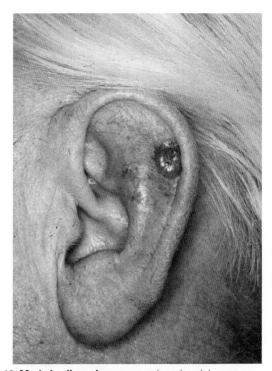

Fig. 5.19 Merkel cell carcinoma—pearly red nodule.

Merkel Cell Carcinoma

Merkel cell carcinoma is a rare malignant tumor that usually occurs as an asymptomatic, solitary nodule on the head and neck of elderly, fair-skinned patients (Fig. 5.19). The etiology

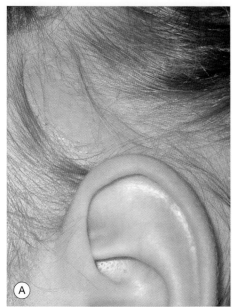

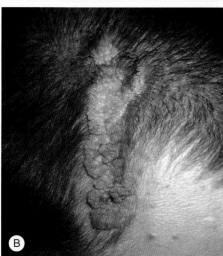

Fig. 5.20 **Nevus sebaceous**. (A) Smooth, yellow plaque with alopecia in a child. (B) Yellow-brown, verrucous, linear plaque with alopecia and a pink papule (syringocystadenoma papilliferum).

of this tumor appears to be the Merkel cell polyomavirus. Of great concern is its high rate of local recurrence, metastasis to regional lymph nodes and distant viscera, and mortality. The

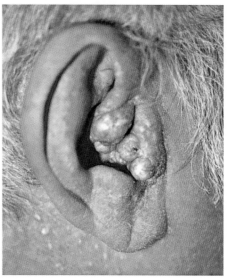

Fig. 5.21 **Trichoepithelioma**—flesh-colored and yellowish nodular plaque.

histologic appearance of the tumor can be confused with that of other primary and metastatic neoplasms of the skin. Treatment requires wide local excision, sentinel lymph node biopsy, and radiotherapy. Chemotherapy or immunotherapy is administered for disseminated disease.

Nevus Sebaceous

This hamartoma of the sebaceous glands and other cutaneous structures appears at birth as a thin yellowish plaque with alopecia. In adulthood, the plaque becomes verrucous, and both benign and malignant tumors may develop (Fig. 5.20). For this reason, excision is often recommended when the individual is a teen or young adult. Extensive nevus sebaceous may be associated with neurologic or skeletal abnormalities, as found in the epidermal nevus syndrome.

Trichoepithelioma

Trichoepithelioma is a benign tumor of the hair follicle. It usually appears on the face as solitary or multiple, firm, smooth, flesh-colored papules or nodules (Fig. 5.21). Multiple trichoepitheliomas may be inherited as an autosomal-dominant condition. Differentiation from basal cell carcinoma is important.

SELF-ASSESSMENT

Case 1—Pearly Nodule (Fig. 5.22)

What Is Your Differential Diagnosis?

This pearly nodule with telangiectasia and a central depression is characteristic of a nodular basal cell carcinoma. The surrounding skin is thickened and furrowed and has a yellowish hue typical of sun damage. Also to be considered in the differential diagnosis is a squamous cell carcinoma. The relatively recent onset of the lesion rules out a flesh-colored nevus, and its size and color make sebaceous hyperplasia (yellow) unlikely.

How Would You Treat It?

Excisional surgery was chosen to remove this tumor. Histologic examination confirmed the clinical diagnosis of basal cell carcinoma, and the margins of the excision were free of tumor.

What Precautions Should This Patient Take in the Future?

This patient should prevent further sun damage to the skin by wearing protective clothing, including a broad-brimmed hat and a long-sleeved shirt, when working outside. In addition, he should use a broad-spectrum sunscreen with an SPF of 30

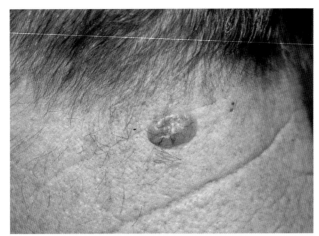

Fig. 5.22 This 55-year-old man was seen in the dermatology clinic because of a nodule on his neck. It had been present for the past year and was growing slowly. His occupation was farming. He had a history of tanning poorly and numerous sunburns. His previous medical and dermatologic history was otherwise negative.

or greater. He should be seen again in the clinic for yearly skin examinations because his chances of developing skin cancer in the future are high: 30% in the next 5 years.

> **IMPORTANT POINTS**
> 1. The recent acquisition of a pearly nodule may indicate a skin cancer.
> 2. Basal cell carcinoma is treatable and rarely metastasizes.
> 3. Precautions should be started to prevent excessive UV radiation exposure, because this is the most common etiologic agent of basal cell carcinoma.

Case 2—Ulcer Behind the Ear (Fig. 5.23)

What Is Your Differential Diagnosis of This Ulcer?

The differential diagnosis of an ulcer is extensive. Neither the history nor the physical examination gives us a clue to its origin. However, a negative medical history and normal general physical examination make a vascular, hematologic, neurologic, drug, connective tissue disease, or physical cause of this ulcer less likely. This leaves a neoplastic, infectious, or unknown origin.

What Would You Do Now?

The next step is a biopsy of the ulcer.

What Is the Best Treatment?

The biopsy revealed a basal cell carcinoma. Treatment was excision of the tumor with the Mohs technique, which conserves as much normal skin as possible and ensures the greatest potential for cure.

> **IMPORTANT POINTS**
> 1. Ulcers of unknown origin must be examined by biopsy to rule out neoplasm.
> 2. Appropriate therapy is dictated by correct identification of the cause.

Case 3—Lip Ulcer (Fig. 5.24)

How Would You Complete the Physical Examination?

Palpate the lesion and feel for local lymph nodes. This lesion felt firm and indurated. The patient's head and neck were examined for lymphadenopathy, but none was found.

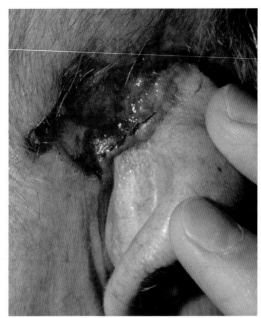

Fig. 5.23 This 60-year-old man had a 1-year history of a nonhealing ulcer. He had otherwise been in excellent health and had no previous history of ulcers. The general physical examination was normal. The skin examination revealed a fair-skinned white man with a 6-cm shallow ulcer behind his ear. The base of the ulcer was clean and the surrounding skin appeared normal. The patient had used a number of topical preparations and had been treated with systemic antibiotics without success.

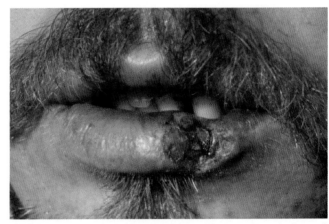

Fig. 5.24 This 33-year-old man presented with a lesion on the lower lip that started with a "cigarette burn" 1 year earlier. He remained a heavy smoker. On examination, you see a crusted and scaling ulcer.

What Is Your Most Likely Diagnosis?

For a chronic mucous membrane ulcer, squamous cell carcinoma is the favored diagnosis. The suspicion is heightened by the finding of induration.

How Would You Confirm It?

A biopsy is required. In this case, it confirmed the diagnosis of squamous cell carcinoma. The lesion was totally excised subsequently.

> **IMPORTANT POINTS**
> 1. Smoking is a risk factor for the development of mucous membrane squamous cell carcinoma.
> 2. Biopsy is required for all chronic ulcers, especially when these lesions are indurated.

CHAPTER CONTENTS

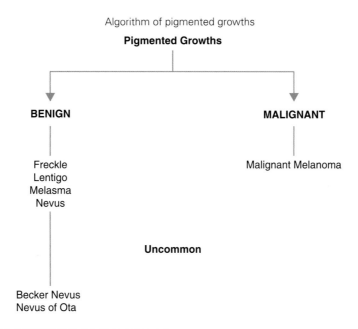

Algorithm of pigmented growths

Pigmented Growths

BENIGN — Freckle, Lentigo, Melasma, Nevus

MALIGNANT — Malignant Melanoma

Uncommon — Becker Nevus, Nevus of Ota

ABSTRACT

The skin has one pigment-forming cell: the melanocyte. Melanocytes are dendritic cells found in the basal layer of the epidermis. Nevus cells, a type of melanocyte, found in the basal layer of the epidermis as well as in the dermis, are arranged in nests and do not have dendritic processes. Melanocytes contain tyrosinase, the enzyme necessary for pigment (melanin) synthesis, and are thought to be derived from a progenitor cell in the neural crest.

KEY POINTS

1. Melanocytes produce melanin, the skin pigment.
2. When recognized early, malignant melanoma is curable.

Pigmented growths (Table 6.1) are the result of an increased number of melanocytes, nevus cells, or pigment deposition. The diagnosis of malignant melanoma is important because it can be recognized early, when it is curable.

FRECKLE

KEY POINTS

1. Sun-induced brown macules
2. Evidence of significant sun exposure and light complexion

Definition

A freckle (ephelis) is a brown macule found in sun-exposed areas of the skin (Fig. 6.1). The amount of melanin in the basal area of the epidermis is increased, with no increase in the number of melanocytes.

Incidence

Freckles are a common incidental finding during a skin examination and are rarely a reason, in and of themselves, for seeking medical attention.

TABLE 6.1 Pigmented Growths

	Frequency (%)[a]	History	Physical Examination	Differential Diagnosis	Laboratory Test (Biopsy)
Freckle		Appear before the age of 3 years	Tan macule, sun-exposed skin	Junctional nevus Lentigo Seborrheic keratosis	No
Lentigo	0.2	Acquired at any age	Brown macule	Junctional nevus Freckle Seborrheic keratosis	If uneven color
Melanoma	0.3	Recent acquisition Itches Bleeds Growing			Excision or deep shave biopsy
Superficial spreading			Irregular surface, border, color	Nevus Seborrheic keratosis Angioma Pigmented basal cell carcinoma	
Lentigo maligna			Irregular surface, border, color	Actinic lentigo Seborrheic keratosis	
Acral lentiginous melanoma			Irregular surface, border, color	Nevus Tinea nigra palmaris	
Nodular			Blue-black nodule	Blue nevus Pyogenic granuloma Angioma Dermatofibroma	
Melasma	0.2	Adults	Brown macules on face	Postinflammatory hyperpigmentation Freckle	No
Nevus	2.8	Not acquired past third decade	Flesh- or brown-colored macule or papule; smooth or verrucous surface	Melanoma Seborrheic keratosis Skin tag Neurofibroma Dermatofibroma Basal cell carcinoma Lentigo Freckle	If change

[a]Percentage of new dermatology patients with this diagnosis seen in the Hershey Medical Center Dermatology Clinic, Hershey, Pennsylvania.

History

Freckles usually appear before 3 years of age and darken after ultraviolet (UV) light exposure. The patient has a history of sunburning easily. Freckles can fade significantly in colder months.

Sunlight darkens freckles.

Physical Examination

The freckled individual typically has a fair complexion and reddish or sandy hair. Hundreds of freckles occur on sun-exposed skin. They are 1–6 mm in size, irregularly shaped, discrete brown macules.

Freckles occur only in sun-exposed areas.

Differential Diagnosis

Lentigo and *junctional nevus* can look like a freckle. *Actinic lentigo* does not darken with sun exposure and is acquired later in life. In contrast, freckles darken after sun exposure and are present from early childhood. *Lentigo simplex* is acquired in childhood, but the lentigines are not confined to sun-exposed skin. *Junctional nevi* and freckles are acquired in childhood. Darker pigmentation and lack of change after sunlight exposure favor a diagnosis of junctional nevus.

DIFFERENTIAL DIAGNOSIS OF FRECKLE

- Junctional nevus
- Actinic lentigo
- Lentigo simplex

Laboratory and Biopsy

Ordinarily, freckles do not require biopsy (Fig. 6.1B).

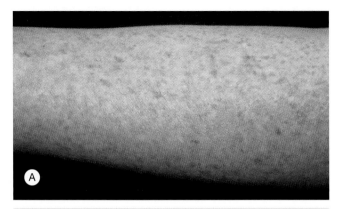

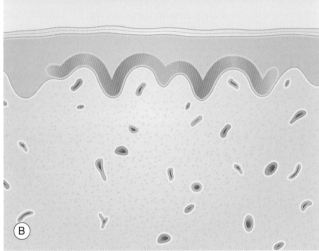

Fig. 6.1 **Freckles**. (A) Brown macules on sun-exposed skin of a youth. (B) Epidermis—melanin pigmentation in basal layer.

Therapy

> Freckles should be accepted as normal. Prevention by sunlight avoidance is effective but not practical.

THERAPY FOR FRECKLES

- None

Pathogenesis

UV radiation induces an increase in melanin pigment in the basal layer of the epidermis without an increase in melanocytes.

LENTIGO

KEY POINTS

1. Lentigo simplex occurs in childhood and is idiopathic.
2. Actinic lentigo occurs in adults and is sun-induced.

Definition

A lentigo (plural, lentigines) is a brown macule caused by an increased number of melanocytes. Two types are recognized: lentigo simplex lesions arise in childhood and are few in number,

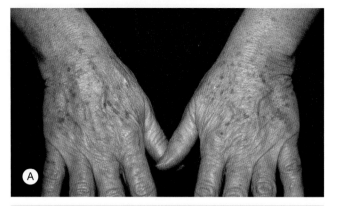

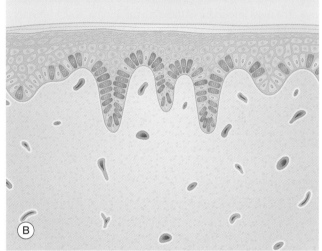

Fig. 6.2 **Actinic lentigo**. (A) Small brown macules in sun-exposed skin of a middle-aged person. (B) Epidermis—increased basal layer pigmentation resulting from an increase in melanocytes and melanin; rete ridges are elongated.

whereas actinic (solar) lentigines (Fig. 6.2) arise in middle age and are numerous in sun-exposed skin.

> Types of lentigo:
> 1. Simplex—few, congenital or in childhood
> 2. Actinic—many, sun-exposed skin, in middle age

Incidence

Lentigo simplex is uncommon. Actinic lentigines are found on more than 90% of whites patients after the age of 70 years, but seldom cause a patient to seek medical advice.

History

Lentigo simplex may be congenital or may arise in childhood. It has no relation to sun exposure. Conversely, actinic lentigo is acquired in middle age, does not fade, and occurs in sun-exposed skin. Patients often call actinic lentigo "liver spots."

Physical Examination

Lentigo is a uniform, tan, brown, or dark brown macule. Lentigo simplex is sharply marginated and occurs anywhere on the body and mucosae. These lesions are usually few in number.

Lentigo is a brown macule with uniform color.

Actinic or solar lentigo is a tan or brown macule, ranging in size from several millimeters to several centimeters, with distinct borders. The lesion occurs in sun-exposed areas of the body: particularly on the dorsum of the hands, neck, head, shoulders, upper trunk, and lower legs.

Differential Diagnosis

In childhood, the differential diagnosis of lentigo includes *junctional nevus* and *freckle*. In adults, *seborrheic keratosis* and *malignant melanoma in situ* (lentigo maligna) are included in the differential diagnosis. The most important of these is a melanoma, which appears as an irregularly colored (varying shades of brown and black), irregularly bordered macule, typically on sun-exposed regions of the body.

DIFFERENTIAL DIAGNOSIS OF LENTIGO

- Junctional nevus
- Freckle
- Seborrheic keratosis
- Malignant melanoma in situ

Laboratory and Biopsy

Biopsy is seldom indicated unless there is concern for a malignant melanoma. If biopsy is performed, the histologic picture is characterized by an increased number of melanocytes within the epidermis as well as increased pigmentation within the keratinocytes. The rete ridges may be normal or elongated (Fig. 6.2B).

Therapy

No therapeutic intervention is required, except for cosmetic purposes. For multiple actinic lentigines, tretinoin cream 0.1% (Retin-A) applied nightly is effective in lightening these photoaging spots. Irritation, however, is common, thus requiring less frequent application (every other night or every third night) or use of a less concentrated cream (0.025% or 0.05%). Preparations containing hydroquinone are generally ineffective. A combination product, 2% mequinol plus 0.01% tretinoin solution (Solage) applied twice daily, lightens these spots. Mild freezing with liquid nitrogen or laser destruction of these pigmented lesions is effective. Sunscreens with a sun protective factor (SPF) of 30 or greater should be used to prevent the development of more actinic lentigines.

THERAPY FOR ACTINIC LENTIGO

Prevention
- Sun protection

Initial
- Cryotherapy

Alternative
- Laser
- Tretinoin cream 0.1% daily or less frequently
- Mequinol 2% plus tretinoin 0.01% solution (Solage) twice daily

Course and Complications

Lentigo has no malignant potential. *Noonan syndrome with multiple lentigines*, a rare but distinctive syndrome, is characterized by hundreds of lentigines on the trunk, head, and extremities, including the palms and soles. It is dominantly inherited and formerly called *LEOPARD* syndrome (**L**entigines, **E**lectrocardiographic abnormalities, **O**cular hypertelorism, **P**ulmonary stenosis, **A**bnormal genitalia, **R**etarded growth and development, and **D**eafness).

1. Syndromes with numerous lentigines:
   - NOONAN (LEOPARD)
2. Peutz–Jeghers syndrome

Peutz–Jeghers syndrome is a dominantly inherited trait that is distinctive because of numerous lentigines occurring around the mouth and eyes as well as on the lips, oral mucosa, hands, and feet, in association with gastrointestinal polyps. Intussusception, hemorrhage, and malignancy are complications of these polyps.

MALIGNANT MELANOMA

KEY POINTS

1. Thin melanoma is curable.
2. Prognosis is best predicted by depth of invasion (Breslow thickness) in primary cutaneous melanoma.
3. Sentinel lymph node biopsy is prognostic, not therapeutic.

Definition

Malignant melanoma is a cancerous neoplasm of pigment-forming cells, melanocytes, and nevus cells. Clinically, its hallmarks are an irregularly shaped and colored macule, papule, or plaque. Four types of melanoma are recognized (Table 6.2): (1) superficial spreading, (2) lentigo maligna, (3) nodular, and (4) acral lentiginous.

Incidence

The occurrence of malignant melanoma is increasing faster than that of any other cancer in the United States, with increased sunlight exposure implicated as one factor. More than 100,000 new cases of melanoma are diagnosed yearly in the United States. The estimated lifetime risk of developing a malignant melanoma is approaching 1 in 38 for White population, 1 in 167 for Hispanic population, and 1 in a 1000 for Black population.

The incidence of malignant melanoma is increasing and related to UV light exposure.

History

An increase in the size of the lesion or a change in its color is noted by the most patients who have melanoma. Development of a new growth, bleeding, and itching are other symptoms that may accompany a melanoma. Occasionally, patients have a family history of malignant melanoma.

Physical Examination

Lentigo maligna melanoma, superficial spreading melanoma, and acral lentiginous melanoma are characterized by a horizontal growth phase that allows for clinical identification before deeper invasion and metastasis occur.

TABLE 6.2 Clinical Features of Melanoma

Type	Location	Median Age (Years)	Premetastatic	Frequency (%)[a]	Ethnicity
Lentigo maligna	Sun-exposed surfaces (head, neck)	70	5–15 years	10	White
Superficial spreading	All surfaces (back, legs)	47	1–7 years	27	White
Nodular	All surfaces	50	Months to 2 years	9	White
Acral lentiginous	Palms, soles, nail beds	61	Months to 8 years	1	Black, Asian

[a]Fifty-three percent of melanomas are unclassified.

1. Melanoma signs (ABCDs):
   - Asymmetry
2. Border irregularity—notched border
3. Color variegation—red, white, blue, black, dark brown
4. Diameter >6 mm

The ABCDs of identifying characteristics for these three types of melanoma are **A**symmetry, **B**order irregularity, **C**olor variegation, and **D**iameter greater than 6 mm. The suspicious lesion is red, white, black, dark brown, and blue; has a notched border; and may have a papule or nodule within it. However, in approximately 10% of melanomas, the ABCD rule does not apply. Therefore any pigmented lesion or "nevus" that looks significantly different from an individual's other nevi—the "*ugly duckling*" mole—should be viewed suspiciously and biopsied.

The "ugly duckling" mole should be biopsied.

Lentigo maligna melanoma (Fig. 6.3) occurs on sun-exposed skin, especially the head and neck. It is multicolored, with dark brown, black, red, white, and blue hues, and it is elevated in areas. It is preceded by lentigo maligna (in situ melanoma), which extends peripherally and is an unevenly pigmented, dark brown, and black macule. Lentigo maligna often reaches a diameter of 5–7 cm before showing signs of invasion. The change in size and darkening are insidious, occurring over a period of years.

The most common type of melanoma is the *superficial spreading melanoma* (Fig. 6.4). This lesion is irregular in color (red, white, black, dark brown, and blue), surface (macule, papule, or nodule), and border (notched), and may occur anywhere on the body. It is found most frequently on the chest and upper back in males, and on the upper back and lower legs in females. During the horizontal growth phase, the lesion is flat, extending to approximately 2.5 cm in diameter before invasion develops.

Nodular melanoma (Fig. 6.5) is a rapidly growing, blue-black, smooth or eroded nodule. It occurs anywhere on the body. It begins in the vertical growth phase, so is less likely to be diagnosed in a premetastatic stage.

Acral lentiginous melanoma (Fig. 6.6) occurs on the palms, soles, and distal portion of the toes or fingers. It is an irregular, enlarging, black growth similar to a lentigo maligna melanoma, but much rarer. The vertical growth phase in this type of melanoma can be deceptive, showing only a small degree of papular elevation associated with a deep invasion. Acral lentiginous melanomas have no relation to skin phenotype, occur at equal rates across ethnicities,

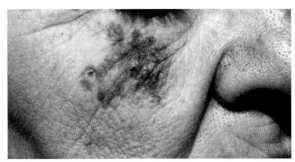

Fig. 6.3 Lentigo maligna melanoma—large, brown, black, irregularly shaped macule that typically occurs on the face of the elderly.

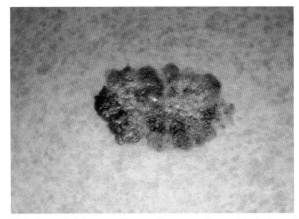

Fig. 6.4 Superficial spreading melanoma—brown-black, irregularly surfaced, and bordered plaque with a red papule.

and are not induced by UV exposure. However, they account for a higher percentage of melanoma diagnoses in darker-skinned patients, while making up less than 1% of melanomas in fair-skinned patients, who are more prone to sun-induced melanoma subtypes. Acral lentiginous melanomas are diagnosed and treated at later stages in Black patients, likely due to the lack of social campaigns aimed at raising awareness of melanoma in dark skin, coupled with the relative lack of efficacy of available immunotherapies, which are more effective in sun-induced melanomas.

Differential Diagnosis

Although the clinical criteria outlined above allow for the early diagnosis of malignant melanoma, other pigmented lesions must be considered before definitive therapy is undertaken. In one study, two-thirds of the pigmented lesions that were thought clinically to be malignant melanoma were not malignant by histopathologic criteria.

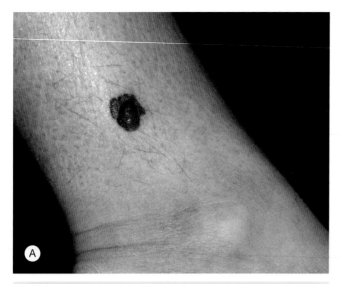

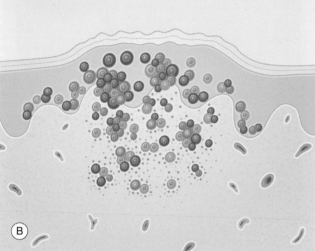

Fig. 6.5 (A) Nodular melanoma—blue-black nodule. (B) Epidermis—atypical pigmented melanoma cells. Dermis—variously sized nests of atypical melanoma cells, inflammation.

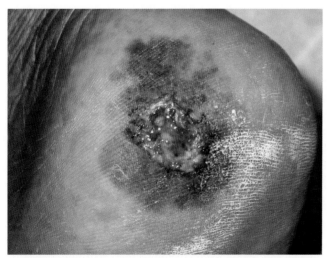

Fig. 6.6 Acral lentiginous melanoma on the sole of the foot—black, brown, and whitish, irregularly shaped and bordered plaque with an erosion.

The differential diagnosis of lentigo maligna melanoma includes *actinic lentigo* and *seborrheic keratosis*. The brown color of these latter lesions is a reassuring sign of their benignity.

Pigmented basal cell carcinoma, seborrheic keratosis, nevus, and *angioma* can look like superficial spreading malignant melanoma.

Nodular melanoma can resemble *pyogenic granuloma, angioma, blue nevus,* and *dermatofibroma.* A pyogenic granuloma is an easily bleeding nodule composed of numerous benign blood vessels. It often occurs after minor trauma and can be viewed as excessive granulation tissue.

Tinea nigra palmaris, a rare superficial fungal infection, and nevus should be considered in the differential diagnosis of acral lentiginous melanoma. Tinea nigra palmaris can easily be diagnosed with a potassium hydroxide scraping that reveals fungal hyphae.

DIFFERENTIAL DIAGNOSIS OF MALIGNANT MELANOMA

Lentigo Maligna
- Actinic lentigo
- Seborrheic keratosis

Superficial Spreading
- Pigmented basal cell carcinoma
- Seborrheic keratosis
- Angioma
- Nevus

Nodular
- Pyogenic granuloma
- Angioma
- Blue nevus
- Dermatofibroma

Acral Lentiginous
- Tinea nigra palmaris
- Nevus

Biopsy

All suspicious pigmented lesions must undergo biopsy, by excision with narrow 2- to 3-mm margins of normal skin or by deep shave biopsy. Definitive treatment by wide surgical excision should not be undertaken until confirmation of malignant melanoma has been made histologically. For extensive lesions, such as lentigo maligna melanoma, it is acceptable to perform an incisional biopsy before definitive therapy. The histologic features vary with the type of melanoma and require a skilled pathologist for interpretation (Fig. 6.5B).

Gene expression profiling is used in selected lesions for diagnosis (atypical nevus vs. melanoma) and prognosis (melanoma).

All suspicious pigmented lesions, especially the "ugly duckling" mole, that could be a melanoma should undergo excisional or deep shave biopsy.

Therapy

The survival of patients with malignant melanoma depends on early diagnosis, when surgical excision is often curative. The margin of normal skin excised around the melanoma increases with the depth of invasion or thickness: in situ, 0.5 cm margin; thickness less than 2 mm, 1-cm margin; thickness equal to or more than 2 mm, 2-cm margin.

> Cure of malignant melanoma rests in the hands of the surgeon, if the lesion is treated early enough.

Radiolymphatic *sentinel node* mapping and biopsy have been used for melanomas deeper than 0.8 mm in thickness in patients with clinically negative lymph nodes. A radioactive tracer is injected at the site of the primary melanoma before wider excision is performed. The first draining or sentinel lymph node can be identified by lymphoscintigraphy and examined by biopsy for the presence of metastatic melanoma. In this way, the surgeon can identify patients who may benefit from adjuvant immunotherapy. Prognostic information is also garnered.

> Sentinel lymph node biopsy is an appropriate staging procedure. Its survival benefit is controversial.

Once a malignant melanoma has metastasized, several therapeutic options are available and best managed by a medical oncologist familiar with these agents—immunotherapy, kinase inhibitors, chemotherapy, radiation, and oncolytic viruses. Radiation therapy is used for palliation of bone and brain metastasis, and when lentigo maligna is so large that surgical removal is technically difficult. Chemotherapy (dacarbazine) has a limited effect and its role is diminished.

Immunotherapeutic approaches for the treatment of disseminated or inoperable melanoma are preferred, especially the immune checkpoint inhibitors, which include cytotoxic T-lymphocyte–associated antigen 4 (CTLA-4) blocking antibody (ipilimumab) and programed death receptor-1 blocking antibody (nivolumab, pembrolizumab). Cytokines (interleukin-2) are less frequently used.

Targeted therapy or kinase inhibitors (vemurafenib, dabrafenib, trametinib, cobimetinib) and biologic agents (talimogene laherparepvec) have caused significant response rates. However, they are not usually long-lasting as a solo therapy. Known mutations (BRAF, Met, KIT, N-RAS, PTEN) provide therapeutic signaling pathway targets for the inhibition of melanoma growth.

THERAPY FOR MALIGNANT MELANOMA
Initial
- Wide excision with margins of normal skin based on thickness of melanoma: in situ 0.5 cm margin; thickness <2 mm, 1 cm margin; thickness equal to or >2 mm, 2 cm margin

Alternative—Metastatic or Inoperable
- Immunotherapy (immune checkpoint inhibitors)
- Kinase inhibitors (targeted therapies)
- Oncolytic viruses
- Chemotherapy
- Radiation

Course and Complications

Lentigo maligna melanoma, superficial spreading melanoma, and acral lentiginous melanoma initially have a horizontal growth phase manifested as a macular or slightly raised pigmented lesion. During the horizontal growth phase, malignant melanoma is curable. Nodular melanoma has only a vertical growth phase, which forebodes a worse prognosis.

> 1. Certain principles are important concerning malignant melanoma: a horizontal growth phase makes surgical cure possible for superficial melanoma
> 2. The prognosis is related to tumor thickness
> 3. Clinical criteria allow for an early diagnosis of malignant melanoma

Pathologist Wallace Clark and dermatopathologist Alexander Breslow correlated survival with tumor thickness. Clark and coworkers devised a system of microstaging melanoma based on the level of invasion in the dermis. The difficulty with this system is variability in differentiating between level 3 and level 4 melanomas. Breslow, using an ocular micrometer, measured tumor thickness from the stratum granulosum to the depth of invasion. These measurements are reproducible and are the preferred method of calculating tumor thickness and, thus, of predicting 5-year survival (Fig. 6.7).

> Guidelines for Recommended Follow-Up of Patients With Malignant Melanoma
> - New or changing mole?
> - Review of symptoms
> - Examine complete skin surface and lymph nodes
> - More extensive studies based on patient's symptoms and signs
> - Follow-up visit every 6 months for 2 years, and then annually

It is estimated that patients with melanoma have a 5% chance of developing a second one. Extensive laboratory tests such as brain, bone, liver, and spleen scans; magnetic resonance imaging; or positron emission tomography are not indicated unless the history or physical examination suggests possible metastasis to these organs.

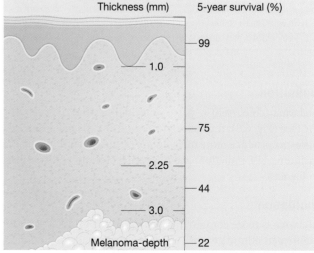

Fig. 6.7 Survival is related to the depth of invasion (thickness measured in millimeters).

Pathogenesis

The pathogenesis of malignant melanoma is unknown. However, sunlight (sunburn), indoor tanning, and heredity (*CDKN2A* and *CDK4* gene mutations) have been implicated as risk factors. Other risk factors for melanoma include a large number of small nevi, large nevi, and dysplastic nevi. The production of melanoma by UV radiation is suggested both epidemiologically and experimentally. The cause-and-effect relationship, however, is less well proven than with other skin cancers. Familial occurrence of malignant melanoma is rare but well established. The *familial atypical mole and melanoma syndrome* (*dysplastic nevus syndrome* or *B-K mole syndrome*) occurs in family members with numerous atypical-appearing, haphazardly colored, and bordered nevi (*atypical moles*) and who have one or several malignant melanomas.

> Familial atypical mole and melanoma syndrome should be suspected: 1—personal or family history of melanoma and 2—numerous (>50) atypical nevi.

Biopsy of these atypical moles reveals disordered melanocytic proliferation. These atypical moles are markers for an increased risk of developing malignant melanoma and, in some cases, precursors of melanoma. This syndrome occurs sporadically and in a familial pattern. Close clinical follow-up and biopsy of suspicious nevi are mandatory (see Nevus section, below, for guidelines). Genetic testing may be considered when three family members have melanoma; an individual has three melanomas; or three cancer events (melanoma or pancreatic cancer) occur in a family.

> Rule of 3s for familial melanoma genetic testing: three melanomas in a family, three melanomas in an individual, and three cancers (melanoma or pancreatic) in a family.

MELASMA

KEY POINTS
1. Brown macules on the face
2. Treat with 4% hydroquinone and sun protection

Definition

Melasma (chloasma) is patchy macular hyperpigmentation of the face (Fig. 6.8). It usually affects women. The melanocytes in melasma produce more melanin in response to multiple factors, including UV radiation, genetic predisposition, and hormonal influences.

Incidence

Melasma is more common in women and in those from darkly pigmented ethnic groups. The frequency of new patients presenting in the authors' clinic with the chief complaint of melasma is 0.2%, but it is a common incidental finding.

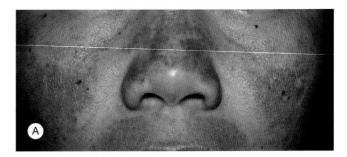

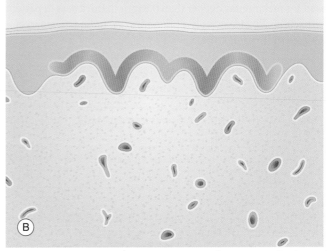

Fig. 6.8 Melasma. (A) Brown macules on the face—nose, cheeks, and lip. (B) Epidermis—melanin pigmentation in basal layer.

History

Displeasure with their self-image causes patients to seek medical attention. Adults acquire melasma most commonly in association with sunlight exposure, pregnancy (chloasma, the "mask of pregnancy"), and the use of oral contraceptive pills.

> Sunlight, pregnancy, and oral contraceptives exacerbate melasma.

Physical Examination

Brown macules of melasma occur symmetrically on the face. They are sharply delineated and involve the malar eminences, forehead, upper lip, and mandible. The brown pigmentation is often patchy within the macule, giving it a reticulated appearance.

Differential Diagnosis

Postinflammatory hyperpigmentation and *freckles* are pigmented macules. For the former, patients have a history of dermatitis. Freckles are smaller and more numerous and involve the trunk and extremities in addition to the face.

DIFFERENTIAL DIAGNOSIS OF MELASMA
- Postinflammatory hyperpigmentation
- Freckles

Laboratory and Biopsy

No laboratory tests are necessary.

Therapy

Hydroquinone, a bleaching agent, is most frequently used to treat melasma. A 2% concentration is available over the counter, whereas 4% hydroquinone cream or higher requires a prescription. It is applied twice daily to affected areas until lightening occurs, followed by reduction in use to a few times a week for maintenance. Sunscreens with an SPF of 30 or greater should be used prophylactically. If no lightening has occurred after several months, tretinoin cream 0.1% may be cautiously applied daily in addition to the use of hydroquinone and a sunscreen. In addition, a combination product containing fluocinolone, hydroquinone, and tretinoin (Tri-Luma) is effective. Less commonly used treatments include azelaic acid cream (Azelex) and chemical peels. Newer therapies include the use of tranexamic acid, topically or by mouth. The oral formulation, taken twice daily, requires patient screening as it can increase the risk of blood clots in patients at risk or with a history of thrombi.

THERAPY FOR MELASMA

Initial
- Hydroquinone cream 4% or higher, twice daily
- Sun protection—sunscreen SPF 30 or greater, hats, shade

Alternative
- Tretinoin cream 0.1% daily or less frequently
- Fluocinolone 0.01% plus hydroquinone 4% plus tretinoin 0.05% cream (Tri-Luma) twice daily
- Azelaic acid cream 20%
- Chemical peels
- Tranexamic acid

Course and Complications

Melasma fades postpartum, with sunlight protection, and with discontinuation of oral contraceptive pills. However, it may take months to years for normal skin color to return, and topical therapies take months to prove their effectiveness.

Pathogenesis

The melanocytes in the areas of involvement are increased in number as well as in activity, producing a greater number of melanosomes. Hormonal factors have been implicated because of the association with pregnancy and oral contraceptive pills, but melasma is infrequently found in menopausal women who receive estrogen replacement. Plasma measurements of β-melanocyte-stimulating hormone are normal.

NEVUS

KEY POINTS

1. Nevi generally have uniform color, surface, and border.
2. Changing or symptomatic nevi should be viewed with suspicion.
3. The "ugly duckling" mole should be biopsied.

Definition

A nevus (mole) is a benign neoplasm of pigment-forming cells, the nevus cell. Nevi are congenital or acquired. A junctional nevus is macular, with nevus cells confined to the base of the epidermis. Compound (Fig. 6.9) and intradermal nevi are papular, with nevus cells in the epidermis and dermis, and in the dermis only, respectively.

Types of nevi:
1. Junctional
2. Compound
3. Intradermal

Incidence

Nevi should be considered a normal skin finding. The average number of nevi per person is 2–11 for Black people and 15–40 for White people. In the authors' clinic, 3% of new patients are seen because of the concern about nevi that have become irritated, have changed in color or size, or are cosmetically unattractive.

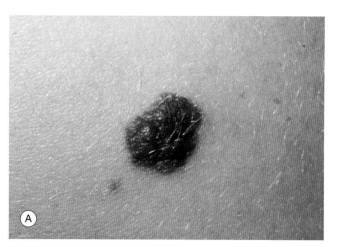

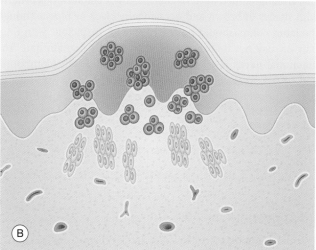

Fig. 6.9 Compound nevus. (A) Even bordered and surfaced, brown papule. (B) Epidermis—pigmented nevus cell nests in lower epidermis. Dermis—pigmented nests of round nevus cells in upper dermis; bundles of spindle-shaped nevus cells in lower dermis.

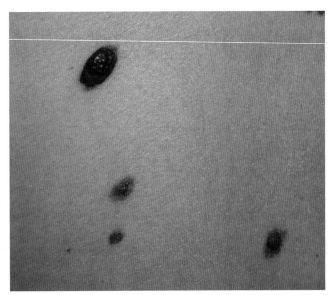

Fig. 6.10 Brown and tan nevi showing variation in appearance.

History

Most nevi are acquired after 6 months of age and before the age of 35 years. Thereafter, one sees a progressive decline in number, so that nevi are infrequent by age 80 years. Moles usually appear singularly, rarely in crops. It is common to have darkening in color, itching, and development of new nevi during pregnancy and adolescence. Otherwise, symptomatic nevi should be regarded suspiciously.

Physical Examination

Nevi vary greatly in appearance and coloration (Fig. 6.10). However, individuals tend to have similar appearing nevi that are generally uniform in color, surface, and border. The pigmented lesion that differs from other nevi—the *"ugly duckling"*—should be biopsied to rule out malignant melanoma. Nevi are flat or elevated, smooth or verrucoid, polypoid or sessile, and pigmented or flesh colored. Their coloration is orderly, with shades of brown and occasionally black or blue, although the latter colors should be regarded with suspicion. Skin lines may or may not be present. Nevi frequently contain hair. The junctional nevus is a light to dark brown macule. Compound and intradermal nevi are flesh-colored or brown, smooth- or rough-surfaced papules that occur in older children and adults.

> Uniform color, surface, and border are characteristics of nevi. The "ugly duckling" nevus, the one that looks different from the patient's other nevi, should be biopsied.

Differential Diagnosis

The most important task is to differentiate a nevus from a *malignant melanoma*. Regular brown color, surface, and border are characteristic features of a nevus that differentiate it from melanoma. A junctional nevus may appear similar to other pigmented macules, such as a *lentigo* or *freckle*. Compound and intradermal nevi, when flesh colored, can be confused with a

skin tag, *basal cell carcinoma*, and *neurofibroma*. The presence of telangiectasia and central depression, as well as a recent acquisition, in an adult, is characteristic of a nodular basal cell carcinoma. When pigmented, these nevi can resemble *seborrheic keratoses* and *dermatofibromas*. The presence of scale and a "pasted on" appearance is typical of seborrheic keratosis. Dermatofibromas are hard dermal papules that dimple when pinched, whereas nevi are soft.

DIFFERENTIAL DIAGNOSIS OF NEVUS

- Malignant melanoma
- Freckle
- Lentigo
- Skin tag
- Basal cell carcinoma
- Neurofibroma
- Seborrheic keratosis
- Dermatofibroma

The *Spitz nevus (benign juvenile melanoma)* is composed of spindle and epithelioid nevus cells. It is a smooth, round, slightly scaling, pink nodule that occurs most frequently in children. The most important aspect of dealing with this lesion is to recognize that it is a nevus and not a melanoma and to avoid extensive surgical intervention.

Special nevi:
1. Spitz
2. Blue
3. Dysplastic/atypical
4. Congenital

Blue nevi are small, steel-blue macules, papules, and nodules that usually begin early in life (Fig. 6.11). Their importance in diagnosis is their similar appearance to nodular melanoma. If any doubt exists, a biopsy should be performed.

The *dysplastic nevus*, or *atypical mole*, is both controversial and confusing (Fig. 6.12). Controversy exists regarding its propensity to develop into a malignant melanoma. The confusion stems from differing histologic criteria for diagnosis. Clinically, the atypical mole is more than 5 mm, is variegated in color with a pink background, and has an irregular, indistinct border. Atypical moles were initially recognized as markers for increased risk of melanoma in family members with inherited malignant melanoma, the *familial atypical mole and melanoma syndrome*, or *dysplastic nevus syndrome*. In these families, virtually all members with atypical moles developed a melanoma in their lifetime, whereas family members without atypical moles did not. Subsequently, investigators discovered that approximately 5% of the healthy white population in the United States has atypical moles. The risk of developing a melanoma in these individuals, many of whom have only one or a few atypical moles and no personal or familial history of melanoma, is unclear, but, for most, a melanoma never develops.

Congenital nevi (Fig. 6.13) are present at birth or shortly thereafter; they are usually elevated and have uniform, dark

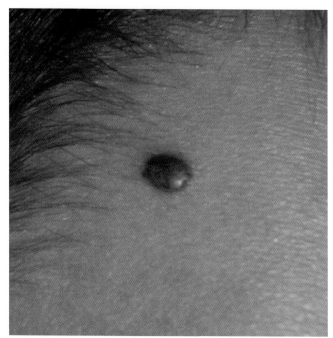

Fig. 6.11 Blue nevus.

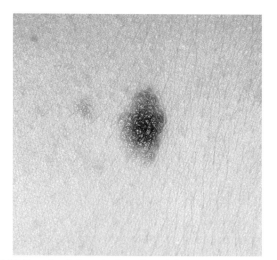

Fig. 6.12 **Dysplastic/atypical mole**—pink, tan, brown, irregularly shaped papule with an indistinct border.

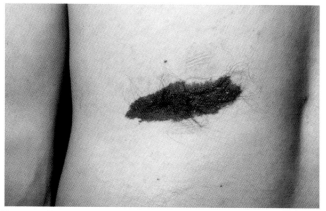

Fig. 6.13 **Congenital nevus**—black plaque containing dark hairs.

cell appearance, resembling fibroblasts. Immunohistochemical markers can be used to identify melanocytic lesions. Atypical moles histologically have (1) abnormal architecture of melanocytes within the epidermis; (2) a dermal fibrotic response; and (3) depending on the pathologist, variable cytologic atypia.

Therapy

The prophylactic removal of nevi is not required. Worrisome lesions are those that have changed in color, shape, or size; have been acquired in adulthood; bleed; or are itching. An excisional or deep shave biopsy with narrow margins (2–3 mm) is recommended for suspicious lesions. Clinically benign and cosmetically unsightly nevi may be removed by shaving off the lesion with a scalpel. However, a superficial shave biopsy leaves some residual nevus cells at the biopsy site that may become darkly pigmented.

> All nevi that are removed should be examined by a pathologist.

THERAPY FOR NEVUS

Initial
- Shave biopsy or deep shave excision for worrisome lesions

Alternative
- Elliptical excision

brown pigmentation with discrete borders. Of newborns, 1% have congenital nevi. Large congenital nevi (>20 cm across or covering 5% of body area) have a 6%–12% chance of developing into a malignant melanoma. Small congenital nevi have little to no increased risk of transformation into melanoma and therefore do not need to be removed prophylactically.

Laboratory and Biopsy

Nevus cells vary in morphology, depending on their location in the skin (Fig. 6.9B). They are arranged in nests in the basal layer of the epidermis and upper dermis. When they extend deeper, cord-like or sheet-like formations occur. In the upper dermis and epidermis, the individual cells are epithelioid in appearance with a cuboidal or oval shape, indistinct cytoplasm, and a round or oval nucleus, and are pigmented. In the middle dermis, nevus cells are smaller, do not contain pigment, and have a lymphoid appearance. In the lower dermis, they have a spindle

The management of *congenital nevi* is difficult when these lesions are large (diameter >20 cm or covering 5% of body area), and somewhat controversial when they are small. Large congenital nevi, such as the bathing-suit nevus, cover extensive areas of the trunk in a garment-like fashion and are generally associated with many satellite lesions. They are rare but have a significant potential for developing into malignant melanoma (6%–12%). The optimal treatment is excision of the lesions, although the technical difficulty of removing such wide areas of skin may preclude this therapy. At the least, patients should be followed carefully, with excision of nodules that develop within the nevus. Large congenital nevi covering the head and neck are sometimes associated with underlying meningeal melanosis, seizures, mental retardation, and development of meningeal malignant melanoma. For small congenital nevi, no excision is needed unless the lesion changes clinically.

The recommended advice to the healthy person with (multiple) atypical moles but no personal or familial history of malignant melanoma is patient education about sun exposure, self-examination, and yearly full skin examination by a physician.

> Guidelines for the Management and Follow-Up of Patients With Multiple Atypical Moles
> - Biopsy of at least two lesions to confirm diagnosis
> - Sun protection
> - Patient self-examination periodically
> - Screen blood relatives for atypical nevi and melanoma
> - Frequency of follow-up:
>   - Patients with no personal or family history of melanoma: yearly
>   - Patients with personal or family history of melanoma: every 6 months for 2 years, then yearly

Course and Complications

Approximately 50% of malignant melanomas have associated nevi. The relative risk of melanoma increases as the number of nevi increases; that is, persons with large numbers of nevi have a greater risk of melanoma than do persons with a few nevi. No evidence indicates that mild irritation or rubbing results in the transformation of a nevus into a melanoma.

Some nevi develop a surrounding depigmented zone and are referred to as *halo nevi* (Fig. 6.14). They occur singularly or multiply, usually on the trunk in teenagers. The development of a halo around the nevus is a harbinger of its disappearance. Both humoral and cellular immunities appear to be involved with the development of halo nevi, a process that results in the destruction of nevus cells. On rare occasions, a depigmented halo develops around a malignant melanoma. If the central lesion has a uniform brown color typical of a nevus, a biopsy is not necessary.

> Halo nevi are rarely a malignant melanoma.

Pathogenesis

Nevus cells are derived from the neural crest. Morphologically, one can recognize the nevus cell because it has no dendritic processes and groups together in nests within the epidermis and dermis.

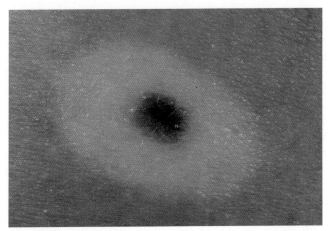

Fig. 6.14 Halo nevus. Red, tan-brown papule with surrounding white halo.

UNCOMMON PIGMENTED GROWTHS

Becker Nevus

Becker nevus (melanosis) is a brown patch with dark, coarse hairs that occurs on the upper trunk and arms (Fig. 6.15). It usually appears in teenage and young adult males. It has no malignant potential and treatment is for cosmetic appearance.

Nevus of Ota

Nevus of Ota (oculodermal melanocytosis) is a mottled or confluent brown, blue, gray macule of the face that usually affects female Asians (Fig. 6.16). Besides the skin, the eye can be involved with associated glaucoma. Onset occurs at birth, before 1 year of age, and at puberty. Malignant melanoma is a rare complication. Laser treatment can be cosmetically successful.

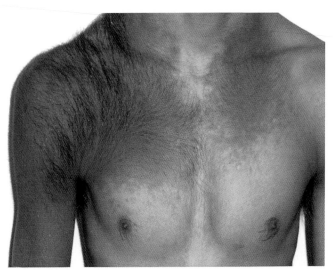

Fig. 6.15 Becker nevus.

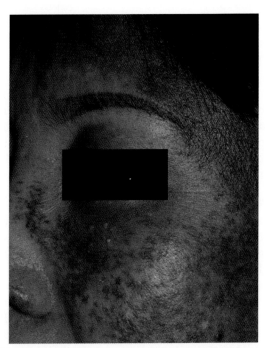

Fig. 6.16 Nevus of Ota.

SELF-ASSESSMENT

Case 1—Bleeding Growth (Fig. 6.17)

What Is Your Differential Diagnosis of This Lesion?

This 6-mm nodule has the blue-black color and eroded surface typical of a nodular malignant melanoma. The differential diagnosis includes blue nevus, nodular pyogenic granuloma, and hemangioma.

What Would You Do Now?

An excisional biopsy revealed histopathologic changes typical of a nodular melanoma invading to a depth of 3.7 mm. The remainder of the skin examination and a general physical examination were normal. A sentinel lymph node biopsy was free of tumor. A 2.0-cm margin of normal skin was excised around the biopsy scar.

How Would You Determine the Prognosis of This Patient?

The prognosis of malignant melanoma is related to tumor thickness. Because this is a thick melanoma, the patient's prognosis is poorer despite having negative sentinel lymph nodes.

IMPORTANT POINTS

1. All bleeding pigmented lesions should be examined by biopsy, not merely watched.
2. Patients with thick melanomas have a poor prognosis.
3. Most melanomas can be removed (and cured) when they are thin—if physicians and the public are alert to these diagnostic signs.

Case 2—Firm Nodule (Fig. 6.18)

What Is the Most Likely Diagnosis?

Malignancy must be suspected for all firm dermal nodules. A benign process would be particularly unlikely in this patient because of the size and firmness of the nodule.

What Should be Done Next?

All suspicious nodules must be examined by biopsy. Biopsy of this nodule was initially interpreted as undifferentiated metastatic malignancy, not further classifiable.

Do You See Any Other Skin Lesions of Note?

The patient was examined to search for the primary tumor. The physician noted on the patient's mid-thigh a small, darkly pigmented plaque with bluish color, irregular border, and white halo (arrow). Excision and histologic examination of this lesion revealed a primary malignant melanoma. Retrospective review of the original biopsy from the nodule showed it to be metastatic melanoma.

IMPORTANT POINTS

1. For firm nodules in the skin, malignancy must be suspected, and biopsy must be performed.
2. A complete skin examination is an important part of every physical examination. In this case, it revealed the source of the primary malignant disease—malignant melanoma.

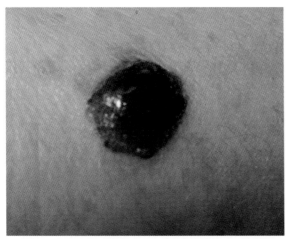

Fig. 6.17 This 29-year-old white woman was seen in the dermatology clinic because of a bleeding growth. It had been present for 6 months and had grown rapidly. Her medical history was otherwise unremarkable.

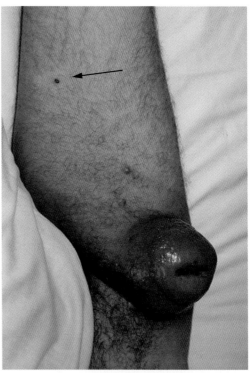

Fig. 6.18 This 50-year-old man sought medical attention because of the large nodule on his right hip. Otherwise, he felt well. On examination, the nodule felt extremely firm. A healing excision from a recent biopsy was present.

7

Dermal and Subcutaneous Growths

CHAPTER CONTENTS

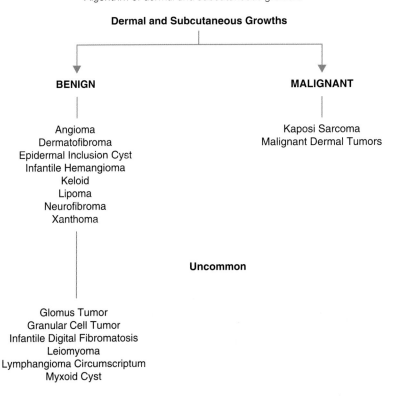

Algorithm of dermal and subcutaneous growths

Dermal and Subcutaneous Growths

BENIGN

Angioma
Dermatofibroma
Epidermal Inclusion Cyst
Infantile Hemangioma
Keloid
Lipoma
Neurofibroma
Xanthoma

MALIGNANT

Kaposi Sarcoma
Malignant Dermal Tumors

Uncommon

Glomus Tumor
Granular Cell Tumor
Infantile Digital Fibromatosis
Leiomyoma
Lymphangioma Circumscriptum
Myxoid Cyst

ABSTRACT

This chapter deals with nodular and cystic "lumps" in the skin (Table 7.1). With the exception of lipomas, the lesions are located in the dermis, often with no alteration in the overlying epidermis. For many patients, common lesions, such as epidermal inclusion cysts, small angiomas, dermatofibromas, and lipomas, are not troubling and are not brought to the attention of a physician. However, these lesions are often found during routine physical examinations, and it is important to be able to distinguish them from malignant dermal growths. The usual question asked by patients who present with a "lump" in the skin is: "Is it cancer?" This concern is appropriate and must always be addressed.

KEY POINTS

1. Biopsy nodules of uncertain origin
2. Suspect cancer for hard dermal nodules

TABLE 7.1 Dermal and Subcutaneous Growths

	Frequency[a]	Physical Examination	Differential Diagnosis[b]	Laboratory Test (Biopsy) Diagnostic But Usually Not Necessary	Diagnostic and Necessary
Angioma	100% in elderly	Bright red macule or papule	Petechiae Blue nevus Melanoma	Check mark like boxes below	
Dermatofibroma	0.2	Tan to brown, firm, flat to slightly elevated papule; "dimples" with lateral pressure	Nevus Melanoma Dermatofibrosarcoma protuberans (rare)	✓	
Epidermal inclusion (follicular) cyst	0.5	Flesh-colored, firm, but malleable nodule	Pilar cyst Lipoma Malignant dermal tumor	✓[c]	
Hemangioma	0.8	Red or purple (often blanchable) soft-to-firm macule, papule, or nodule	Vascular malformation Rapidly involuting congenital hemangioma Noninvoluting congenital hemangioma	✓	
Kaposi sarcoma	<0.1	Purple macules, plaques, or nodules	Bruise Angioma Bacillary angiomatosis		✓
Keloid	0.2	Flesh-colored to pink, firm, elevated scar	Hypertrophic scar Dermatofibrosarcoma protuberans (rare)	✓	
Lipoma	0.2	Flesh-colored, rubbery, subcutaneous nodule	Epidermal inclusion cyst Angiolipoma Malignant tumor	✓	
Neurofibroma	0.1	Flesh to brown, soft, and often compressible ("buttonhole" sign) papule or nodule	Skin tag Dermal nevus	✓	
Xanthoma	<0.1	Yellow papules and nodules Hard subcutaneous tendon nodules	Sebaceous gland hyperplasia Juvenile xanthogranuloma Rheumatoid nodules	✓	
Malignant dermal tumors	<0.1	Flesh, red, or purple, hard nodules	Any of the above		✓

[a]Percentage of new dermatology patients with this diagnosis seen in the Hershey Medical Center Dermatology Clinic, Hershey, Pennsylvania.
[b]A malignant tumor should be in the differential diagnosis for all dermal growths.
[c]Incision and drainage reveals cheesy, foul-smelling material.

Color and consistency are helpful distinguishing features.

Color and consistency are helpful in distinguishing clinical features. The color of the lesion sometimes reflects the nature of the proliferating elements. Vascular lesions, for example, have hues ranging from red to purple. Consistency often distinguishes a nodule from a cyst. A cyst is usually fluctuant or malleable. For nodules, a soft consistency lends reassurance that the lesion is benign, a firm consistency is of intermediate concern, and a hard consistency should lead to suspicion of a possible malignant process. Sometimes, the diagnosis can be made only with a biopsy. This is particularly important for firm to hard nodules in which the clinical diagnosis is uncertain and malignancy needs to be ruled out.

For any skin nodule of uncertain origin, a biopsy is indicated to rule out malignancy.

ANGIOMA

KEY POINTS

1. Very common in older adults
2. Typically cherry red color but can be dark red or purple

Definition

An angioma is a common benign vascular growth in older adults. It is also referred to as cherry angioma because of its bright red color (Fig. 7.1A).

Incidence

Angiomas are very common and increase in number as one ages. Virtually all elderly individuals have angiomas.

History

Angiomas are frequently an incidental finding on the skin examination. They are asymptomatic unless traumatized. Occasionally, the patient or physician is concerned that an angioma may be a melanoma if it is deep purple in color (Fig. 7.2).

Physical Examination

Angiomas are easily recognized by their smooth surface and red color. There may be a few to numerous angiomas occurring most commonly on the trunk but can be on the head and extremities. They vary from being pinpoint macules resembling petechiae to papules or small plaques. Angiomas usually are bright red but may be shades of deep red to purple.

Differential Diagnosis

An angioma is easily recognized most of the time. Petechiae are sometimes confused with numerous small flat angiomas. The occurrence on the trunk and the presence for years in a healthy individual makes angioma the diagnosis. When deep purple, a blue nevus or melanoma should be considered. Examination with the dermatoscope is very helpful in visualizing the vascular globules seen in an angioma. If uncertain, a biopsy should be performed.

DIFFERENTIAL DIAGNOSIS

- Petechiae
- Blue nevus
- Melanoma

Laboratory and Biopsy

The diagnosis of angioma is almost always made clinically. If in doubt, a biopsy reveals a well-demarcated collection of small blood vessels in the dermis (Fig. 7.1B).

Therapy

In most cases, no therapy is needed. If irritated or cosmetically unattractive to the patient, they can be shaved off, electrodesiccated, or lasered.

THERAPY FOR ANGIOMA

- None
- Shave biopsy
- Electrodesiccation
- Laser

Course and Complications

The number of angiomas increases with age. They are usually of no concern other than for their cosmetic appearance. They

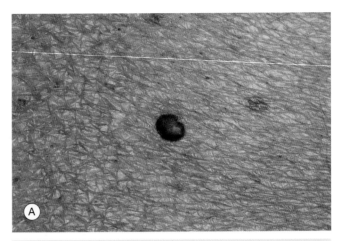

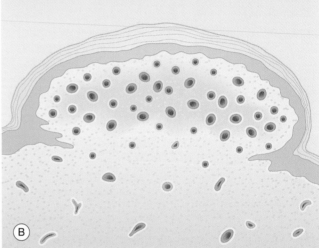

Fig. 7.1 **Angioma**. (A) Bright red pinpoint macules and papules. (B) Epidermis—normal. Dermis—well-demarcated collection of blood vessels.

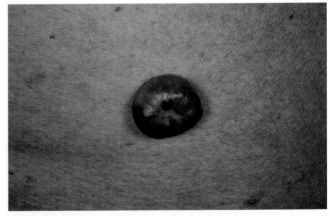

Fig. 7.2 **Angioma**. Red/purple vascular papule.

are chronic and not associated with complications other than bleeding if traumatized.

DERMATOFIBROMA

KEY POINTS

1. Dermal fibrotic papule or small nodule
2. Chronic, asymptomatic, and stable

Definition

A dermatofibroma is an area of focal dermal fibrosis, often accompanied by overlying epidermal thickening and hyperpigmentation. It appears clinically as a brown papule or small nodule, often more indurated than elevated. The origin is unknown; however, it is probably a response to trauma.

Incidence

Dermatofibromas are common and are often found incidentally during cutaneous examinations. Occasionally, they cause a patient to seek medical advice. They are seen most often in young adults.

History

Dermatofibromas usually are asymptomatic. The patient's concern, if any, is over the possibility of malignancy.

Physical Examination

Typical dermatofibromas are approximately 5 mm in size and are slightly elevated. They vary in color from light tan to dark brown. The fibrotic nature of the lesion is best appreciated by palpation, which reveals a firm consistency. A helpful diagnostic test is the "dimple sign," in which pinching results in central dimpling (Fig. 7.3A). Most dermatofibromas exhibit this sign; it is rarely seen with any other skin lesion. Dermatofibromas may occur anywhere, but the thighs and legs are the most common locations. One or several lesions may be present.

> The "dimple sign" is characteristic of dermatofibroma.

Differential Diagnosis

With its brown color, a dermatofibroma may be confused with a *nevus*. Nevi, however, are usually softer and do not exhibit the dimple sign. Darker dermatofibromas may raise a clinical suspicion of *melanoma*. Dermatofibromas are usually purely brown (a benign color), whereas a nodular melanoma usually has shades of dark gray or blue. If any doubt exists, however, a biopsy should be performed.

> Enlarging or atypically colored lesions should undergo a biopsy to rule out malignancy.

Dermatofibrosarcoma protuberans is a low-grade malignant fibrous tumor that grows slowly but persistently, and rarely metastasizes. It is a rare tumor and is distinguished clinically from a dermatofibroma by its larger size, irregular shape, and continued growth.

Laboratory and Biopsy

The diagnosis is usually made clinically. If any doubt exists, a biopsy should be performed to rule out malignancy. The histologic picture is diagnostic and shows a focal proliferation of densely packed collagen bands that are twisting and intertwining

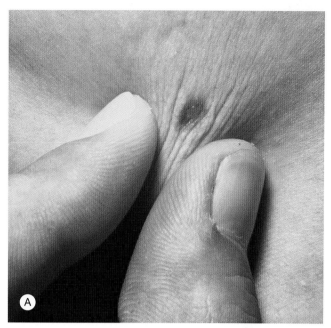

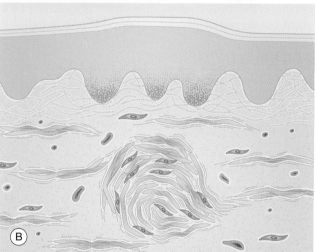

Fig. 7.3 Dermatofibroma. (A) Firm, reddish papule with "dimple sign." (B) Epidermis—slightly thickened and hyperpigmented. Dermis—nodular aggregate of fibroblasts and densely packed collagen.

DIFFERENTIAL DIAGNOSIS OF DERMATOFIBROMA

- Nevus
- Melanoma
- Dermatofibrosarcoma protuberans

(Fig. 7.3B). Fibroblasts are interspersed and increased in number. Increased pigmentation of the slightly thickened overlying epidermis accounts for the frequently brown color of these lesions.

Therapy

Therapy is usually not indicated. If desired, a simple excision is sufficient for removal and histologic examination.

Course and Complications

Dermatofibromas are chronic and usually stable in size. They are not associated with any complications.

Pathogenesis

Although the origin is unknown, trauma (e.g., an insect bite) may be an initiating factor for some of these lesions. The proliferation of fibroblasts and subsequent fibrosis may represent an exuberant healing response to injury. However, most patients do not recollect a history of trauma in the area.

Two other lesions are considered within the spectrum of a dermatofibroma. A *histiocytoma* (an aggregate of histiocytes in a focal area within the dermis) probably represents an early phase in the formation of a dermatofibroma. A *sclerosing hemangioma*, as the name suggests, shows more of a vascular component, but the end result is that of dermal fibrosis as well.

EPIDERMAL INCLUSION CYST

KEY POINTS
1. Central pore and cheesy, foul-smelling discharge is diagnostic.
2. Origin is from the hair follicle.

Definition

An epidermal inclusion cyst (Fig. 7.4A) is derived from the upper portion (infundibulum) of the epithelial lining of a hair follicle and is located in the middle and lower dermis. It is also called an *epidermoid cyst*. Clinically, it appears as a flesh-colored, firm, but often malleable, solitary nodule in the skin with a central punctum.

Incidence

These lesions are common but usually are not brought to the attention of a physician, so the exact incidence is not known. They may occur at any age.

History

Epidermal inclusion cysts are usually asymptomatic, slow growing, and most frequently are found incidentally by either the patient or the examining physician. Occasionally, they are the primary complaint in a patient concerned about the possibility of malignancy. Another reason for medical attention is rupture of the cyst or secondary infection, either of which produces inflammation, pain, and drainage of foul-smelling material.

Physical Examination

Characteristically, the lesion is a flesh-colored, dome-shaped nodule that feels firm (but not hard). On palpation, it often feels slightly malleable, a finding that suggests the contents are semisolid. This is a helpful diagnostic aid, as is the finding of a *central*

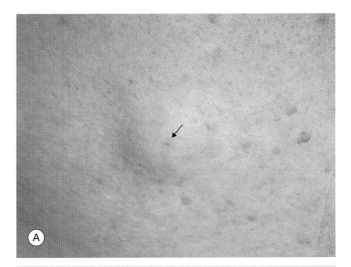

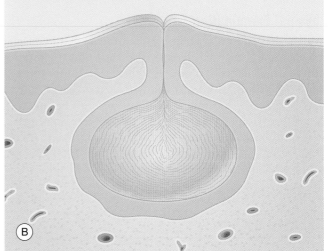

Fig. 7.4 Epidermal inclusion cyst. (A) Flesh-colored, firm nodule with central pore (*arrow*). (B) Epidermis—invaginates into dermis. Dermis—keratin-filled, epidermal-lined cyst.

pore, which represents the opening of the follicle from which the cyst originated. Lesions range in size from 0.5 to 5 cm. They may be located anywhere but occur most frequently on the head and trunk. If the central pore is open, the diagnosis is sometimes confirmed by squeezing the lesion and expressing some of the whitish, cheesy, foul-smelling material that is trapped within. This material represents macerated keratin.

A central pore is the characteristic of an epidermal inclusion cyst.

Differential Diagnosis

Pilar (trichilemmal) *cysts* arise from the middle third (isthmus) of the follicular canal. They occur most frequently on the scalp, where they are the most common type of cyst. In other locations, they are less common than epidermal inclusion cysts, but the two may be indistinguishable clinically, and histologically, some cysts may have elements of both. The difference is not critical: both are benign. A *lipoma* is usually deeper than an epidermal inclusion cyst, and although a lipoma may feel rubbery, it is usually not malleable. When the diagnosis is uncertain, particularly if the lesion feels firm, a *malignant tumor* must be considered.

> ## DIFFERENTIAL DIAGNOSIS OF EPIDERMAL INCLUSION CYST
> - Pilar cyst
> - Lipoma
> - Malignant tumor

Laboratory and Biopsy

Usually, the diagnosis can be made clinically. If desired, confirmation can be obtained by incising and draining the lesion, which reveals the cheesy, foul-smelling, keratinous contents. A biopsy is equally confirmatory but usually not necessary (Fig. 7.4B).

Therapy

Frequently, no therapy is requested or needed. If removal is desired, the entire cyst should be excised with its lining to prevent recurrence. This is accomplished by incising the skin overlying the cyst without disrupting the cyst wall and then bluntly dissecting the entire cyst along with its wall. If the cyst breaks, a curette can be used to remove the remaining contents and cyst wall. Elliptical excision is usually required for the removal of cysts that have previously ruptured and scarred.

> To prevent recurrence, the entire cyst, with its lining, should be removed.

> ## THERAPY FOR EPIDERMAL CYSTS
> - None
> - Incision and drainage
> - Excision

Course and Complications

Untreated, most epidermal inclusion cysts reach a stable size, often in the range of 1–3 cm, rarely larger.

Complications are rare and usually limited to occasional rupture or infection. Rupture or infection results in redness and tenderness of the cyst and, on examination, increased fluctuance. If this occurs, the lesion should be treated as an abscess with incision and drainage, and occasionally oral antibiotics.

Multiple epidermal inclusion cysts are a feature of *Gardner syndrome*, an uncommon, autosomal dominant, heritable disorder manifested by multiple epidermal cysts, fibromas, osteomas, and intestinal polyps. The intestinal polyps often undergo malignant degeneration.

Pathogenesis

Epidermal inclusion cysts arise from the upper portion (infundibulum) of a hair follicle. The epidermal lining of the cyst is identical to that of the surface epidermis and produces keratin, which, having no place to shed, accumulates and forms the cystic mass.

INFANTILE HEMANGIOMA

> ### KEY POINTS
> 1. Benign vascular tumor in infancy
> 2. Superficial and subcutaneous involvement
> 3. Although most regress spontaneously, treat early if esthetic or functional impairment anticipated

Definition

An infantile hemangioma (Fig. 7.5A) is a benign proliferation of blood vessels in the dermis and subcutis. The vascularity imparts a red, blue, or purple color to these lesions, depending on the size and depth of the proliferative vessels.

Incidence

Infantile hemangiomas are the most common soft tissue tumor of infancy, occurring more frequently in females, premature, and white infants. They are likely to be brought to the attention of a physician because of their rapid growth or cosmetic concerns.

History

Most arise in the first few weeks of infancy. Infantile hemangiomas are usually asymptomatic, except when they ulcerate, or cause local obstruction—fortunately an uncommon occurrence.

Physical Examination

Superficial infantile hemangiomas have a bright red color, whereas the deeper subcutaneous forms have a bluish hue. Mixed infantile hemangiomas are bright red, dome-shaped nodules.

> Types of infantile hemangioma:
> 1. Superficial (strawberry)
> 2. Subcutaneous (cavernous)
> 3. Mixed

Differential Diagnosis

> The diagnosis of infantile hemangioma is usually made clinically, without difficulty.

In contrast, vascular malformations (port-wine stain, lymphangioma circumscriptum, venous malformation) are generally present at birth and do not regress spontaneously. Rapidly involuting congenital hemangioma (RICH) is present at birth, rapidly involutes by 1–2 years, and is GLUT1 (glucose transporter isoform 1) negative on biopsy, in contrast to infantile hemangiomas, which are GLUT1 positive. Noninvoluting congenital hemangioma (NICH), which is present at birth, has superficial telangiectasia, gradually enlarges as one ages, is GLUT1 negative, and usually requires surgery.

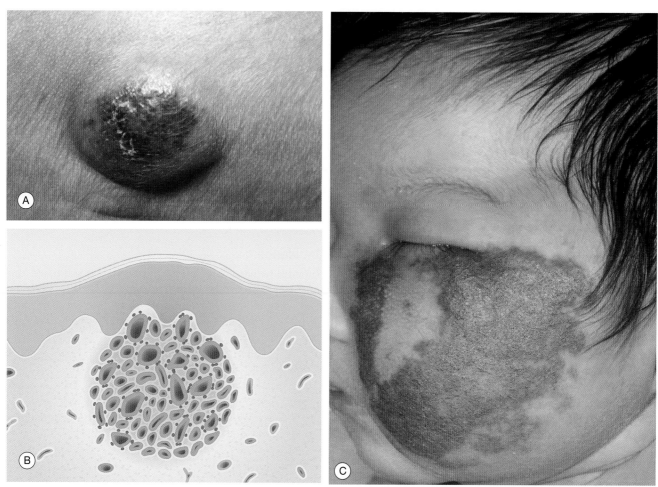

Fig. 7.5 Infantile hemangioma. (A) Reddish, blue, soft nodule. (B) Dermis—Focal proliferation of blood vessels and endothelial cells. (C) Rapidly growing hemangioma that requires systemic treatment to prevent serious complications.

DIFFERENTIAL DIAGNOSIS OF HEMANGIOMA
• Vascular malformation • RICH • NICH

Laboratory and Biopsy

A biopsy, if done, reveals a marked increase in the number of blood vessels, many of which are dilated (Fig. 7.5B). An infantile hemangioma has GLUT1-positive staining.

Therapy

Observation is the most appropriate therapy for many infantile hemangiomas. Although these lesions grow over the first year of life (and during this time, the parents will need repeated reassurance), they usually involute spontaneously over the ensuing years with a good cosmetic result. For ulcerating, large, head and neck or groin infantile hemangiomas, therapeutic intervention may be necessary as vision, respiration, or a good cosmetic result may be compromised.

Early treatment may prevent serious complications.

Therapeutic options include systemic propranolol as the first line of therapy, topical timolol, intralesional and potent topical steroids, pulsed-dye laser, and surgical excision.

THERAPY FOR INFANTILE HEMANGIOMAS
Initial • None • Topical timolol 0.5% or high-potency topical steroids **Alternative** • Propranolol: 1–3 mg/kg daily divided twice daily • Steroids: 3–5 mg/kg daily • Laser • Surgery

Course and Complications

Infantile hemangiomas often increase in size over the first year but then subside spontaneously, so that by the age of 5 years, 50% are involuted, and by the age of 9 years, 90% are involuted.

Some 20% have residual changes, including scarring and fibro-fatty tissue. Depending on their location, large subcutaneous or mixed infantile hemangiomas (Fig. 7.5C) may cause functional compromise of neighboring and underlying structures (e.g., the eye, ear, or oral pharynx). Hemangiomas occasionally ulcerate, become painful, and may be further complicated by infection.

> Most infantile hemangiomas involute spontaneously during childhood.

In infants with numerous hemangiomas (*diffuse neonatal hemangiomatosis*), internal organ involvement should be suspected; this rare syndrome occasionally leads to death from high-output cardiac failure or compromise of an affected vital organ (liver, spleen, intestine).

Pathogenesis

Although the pathomechanism of infantile hemangiomas is unknown, a localized proliferation of endothelial cells and the supporting stroma, resulting in a cellular mass containing increased vascular channels, suggests the importance of angiogenic growth factors.

KAPOSI SARCOMA

KEY POINTS

1. Malignant vascular tumor
2. Human herpesvirus-8 may be pathogenetic
3. Sign of AIDS, test for HIV

Definition

Kaposi sarcoma is a malignant tumor derived from endothelial cells. It is manifest by multiple vascular tumors that usually occur first in the skin, where they appear as purple macules, plaques, or nodules (Fig. 7.6A). It is associated with human herpesvirus-8.

Incidence

The disease occurs in three settings.

> Types of Kaposi sarcoma: classic, lymphadenopathic, and AIDS-associated.

Classic Kaposi sarcoma is a chronic cutaneous disorder that occurs primarily in elderly men, usually those of Eastern European, Mediterranean, and Middle Eastern descent. This is the type described by Moritz Kaposi in 1872. It remains an uncommon disorder with an annual incidence in the United States of approximately 0.05 per 100,000 population. It affects men 10–15 times more often than women and occurs most often in people older than 50 years.

An aggressive *lymphadenopathic* form occurs primarily in equatorial Africa, where it accounts for approximately 9% of all cancers. This type mainly affects young men and is rapidly fatal.

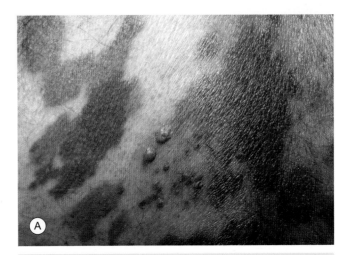

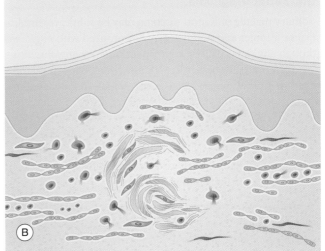

Fig. 7.6 **Kaposi sarcoma**. (A) Purple macules and papules. (B) Dermis—strands and clusters of spindle cells, hemorrhage, and blood-filled vascular slits.

AIDS-associated Kaposi sarcoma, which was first noted in 1979, represents the most common neoplasm associated with AIDS. Kaposi sarcoma occurs most commonly in LGBTQ+ males with AIDS, in whom it disseminates and is frequently fatal without HIV treatment. In the United States, the incidence of AIDS-associated Kaposi sarcoma has decreased dramatically because of potent antiretroviral therapy (ART).

History

The skin lesions in Kaposi sarcoma are usually asymptomatic, so patients seek advice because of the concern over appearance or uncertainty about the nature of newly appearing skin lesions. In some patients, Kaposi sarcoma may be an incidental physical finding. In this setting, it often is the first sign of AIDS, so the physician should obtain a blood test for HIV. Kaposi sarcoma can also develop in patients receiving immunosuppressive therapy for organ transplantation and other diseases.

> Test for HIV in patients newly diagnosed with Kaposi sarcoma.

Physical Examination

Lesions of Kaposi sarcoma may appear as macules, papules, dermal plaques, and nodules. However, in all forms, the lesions are characteristically *purple*. In the classic type of Kaposi sarcoma, multiple lesions are usually located on the lower legs, where they may be accompanied by edema. In AIDS-associated Kaposi sarcoma, lesions may occur anywhere on the skin and range in number from one to innumerable. Lymphadenopathy is also frequently present in patients with AIDS. Kaposi sarcoma may also involve the mucous membranes. When examining the mouth, one should also look for oral hairy leukoplakia (see Chapter 22) as another sign of AIDS. Additional skin manifestations of AIDS are listed in Chapter 23.

Differential Diagnosis

A solitary macule of Kaposi sarcoma may be subtle, resembling a *bruise*. Papules and nodules may be confused with *angiomas*, although angiomas usually are redder. *Bacillary angiomatosis* is a condition that also occurs in patients with AIDS. It is manifest by red or purple papules that may resemble Kaposi sarcoma. Biopsy of bacillary angiomatosis, however, shows a benign process, and a Warthin–Starry stain reveals clusters of *Bartonella* bacteria, the same microorganisms that cause cat-scratch disease. Distinguishing bacillary angiomatosis from Kaposi sarcoma is important because bacillary angiomatosis is benign and responds to erythromycin therapy.

DIFFERENTIAL DIAGNOSIS OF KAPOSI SARCOMA
- Bruise
- Angioma
- Bacillary angiomatosis

Laboratory and Biopsy

The diagnosis of Kaposi sarcoma is confirmed with a biopsy that shows a proliferation in the dermis of spindle cells arranged in strands and small nodular aggregates (Fig. 7.6B). The spindle cells also attempt to form small blood vessels, resulting in slit-like spaces filled with red blood cells. Hemorrhage is common; lymphocytes and histiocytes may also be present. As mentioned above, patients suspected to have AIDS-associated Kaposi sarcoma should have an HIV serologic test.

Therapy

Early classic Kaposi sarcoma may require no therapy or only occasional excision of a papule or nodule. With more advanced cutaneous disease, local radiation therapy is highly effective. Patients with disseminated disease are treated with one or more chemotherapeutic agents.

AIDS-associated Kaposi sarcoma has been treated with combined ART and then local radiation therapy, intralesional interferon-α, or intralesional chemotherapy (e.g., vinblastine). Disseminated disease is treated with a combination of zidovudine and systemic interferon-α, or with systemic chemotherapy

THERAPY FOR KAPOSI SARCOMA
Initial—Local
- Radiation therapy
- Excision

Alternative
- Interferon-α (intralesional or systemic)
- Chemotherapy (intralesional or systemic)

using agents such as pegylated liposomal doxorubicin, paclitaxel, vincristine, vinblastine, bleomycin, and etoposide, either alone or in combination.

Course and Complications

Classic Kaposi sarcoma progresses slowly, and because it affects primarily elderly patients, many die from other causes. In the United States, the average survival time for patients with classic Kaposi sarcoma has been reported to be 8–13 years, but much longer times have been noted, and spontaneous remissions have occurred. Patients have an increased frequency of second malignant diseases, especially lymphoma and leukemia.

Lymphadenopathic Kaposi sarcoma disseminates rapidly to internal organs and results in early death. AIDS-associated Kaposi sarcoma also disseminates early in its course, but some patients respond to therapy, and many die from other causes, such as opportunistic infections.

Pathogenesis

Kaposi sarcoma is a malignant disease in which endothelial cells proliferate to form tumors. Multiple tumors apparently result from a multifocal rather than a metastatic process. Immunosuppression may play a permissive role because, in the United States, the disease occurs most frequently in patients who are immunosuppressed by drugs or AIDS. The findings of Kaposi sarcoma in several homosexual patients who are HIV-negative, and the epidemic occurrences of lymphadenopathic Kaposi sarcoma in Africa, also suggest an etiologic role for an infectious, transmissible organism. In this regard, human herpesvirus-8 has now been detected in all forms of Kaposi sarcoma and so is strongly implicated in the pathogenetic process.

KELOID

KEY POINTS
1. Exuberant scar tissue
2. Treat cautiously because of high recurrence rate

Definition

A keloid represents excessive proliferation of collagen (scar tissue) after trauma to the skin (Fig. 7.7A). Clinically, a keloid appears as an elevated, firm, protuberant nodule or plaque.

Keloids occur most often in young Black population.

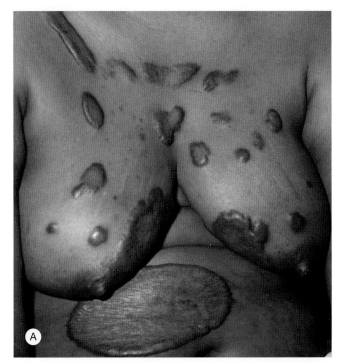

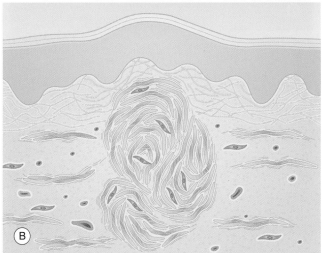

Fig. 7.7 **Keloid**. (A) Multiple hyperpigmented, smooth, firm, protuberant nodules and plaques. (B) Dermis—highly compacted whorls of collagen.

Incidence

Keloids are relatively common. The incidence is highest in people aged 10–30 years. Black people are particularly prone to keloids; in African descendent populations, the prevalence is approximately 6%.

History

The trauma responsible for inducing the keloid is almost always remembered by the patient. Often, the trauma is obvious, such as ear piercing, surgical incisions, or other wounds. Keloids develop over weeks to months after the trauma. New and actively growing keloids often itch, whereas stable, long-standing ones are asymptomatic.

Physical Examination

A keloid looks like an overgrown scar—which is what it is. It is protuberant and firm and usually conforms roughly to a pattern of the original trauma, although it is more extensive. Keloids are often pink or dark brown and have an irregular border with claw-like extensions. They may occur anywhere, but they are more common on the earlobes (secondary to ear piercing), shoulders, upper chest, and back.

Differential Diagnosis

The difference between a keloid and a *hypertrophic scar* is mainly quantitative, with a keloid expanding beyond the limits of the original trauma.

A *dermatofibrosarcoma protuberans* is a rare, malignant, fibrous tumor that clinically may look like a keloid, but the patient usually has no history of trauma, and the lesion continues to enlarge. If malignancy is suspected, a biopsy should be performed.

DIFFERENTIAL DIAGNOSIS OF KELOID

- Hypertrophic scar
- Dermatofibrosarcoma protuberans

Laboratory and Biopsy

The diagnosis can usually be made on clinical grounds. If doubt remains, a biopsy can be performed for confirmation. The histologic examination shows whorls and nodules of highly compacted hyalinized bands of collagen (Fig. 7.7B). Fibroblasts may be increased in number but not markedly so in mature keloids. Mast cells are prominent, and release of their histamine content may be the cause of the often associated pruritus. The overlying epidermis may be atrophic.

Therapy

Surgical removal alone, although tempting, is contraindicated because it is often followed by a recurrence that is larger than the original lesion. Repeated intralesional injections of steroids (triamcinolone; Kenalog-40) at monthly intervals may cause keloids to flatten, which is a goal desired by some patients. Keloids can also be injected with a mixture of steroids and 5-fluorouracil and must be injected superficially to avoid ulceration. Light cryotherapy can also be used prior to injections to aid in pain control and softening of the scar tissue. Surgery may be used if it is combined with another modality such as intralesional steroids or low-dose radiotherapy. Pressure dressings are also helpful when applied after surgery or injections. Silicone (Silastic) gel dressings applied daily for 2 months have been shown to help flatten hypertrophic scars by mechanisms that are unknown.

Surgical excision should never be used alone in treating keloids.

THERAPY FOR KELOIDS
- None
- Intralesional steroids: Kenalog-40
- Compression
- Surgery with intralesional steroids

Course and Complications

Untreated, the usual course of a keloid is that of gradual enlargement to a steady-state size. Keloids are much less likely to regress than are hypertrophic scars, but in either case, the time course for regression (if it occurs at all) is measured in years. The major complication is cosmetic disfigurement, which may be profound.

Pathogenesis

Increased fibroblast activity, initiated by tissue injury, results in a marked increase in collagen synthesis. Dermal ground substance (primarily the chondroitin 4-sulfate component) is also increased; investigators have suggested that this change may inhibit collagen degradation. Collagen production may also be affected by imbalance in, or altered fibroblastic responsiveness to, tissue cytokines. For example, collagen synthesis by fibroblasts is stimulated by transforming growth factor-β and is inhibited by interferon.

LIPOMA

KEY POINTS
1. Benign subcutaneous fat tumor
2. Slow growing or stable
3. Biopsy rapidly growing tumors and if uncertain of the diagnosis

Definition

A lipoma represents a benign tumor of subcutaneous fat (Fig. 7.8A). Clinically, it is a rubbery nodule that appears only slightly elevated above the skin's surface but is easily palpable deep in the skin. The origin is unknown.

Incidence

Most lipomas are never brought to a physician's attention. When they are, it is because of the patient's concern that the lesion may be malignant. They are most common in midlife.

History

Lipomas are usually asymptomatic. They may grow slowly, but most patients are not aware of any change in size.

Physical Examination

A typical lipoma is flesh colored and imparts a slight elevation to the normal-appearing overlying skin. It feels rubbery but not hard and is usually freely movable. Lipomas range in size from 1 to 10 cm, rarely larger. They may occur anywhere but are found most often on the trunk, neck, and upper extremities.

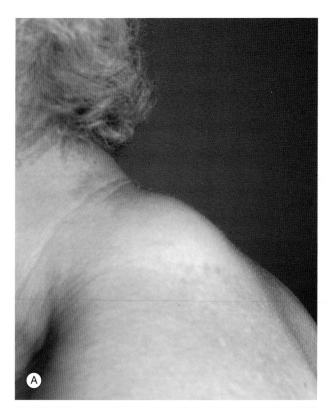

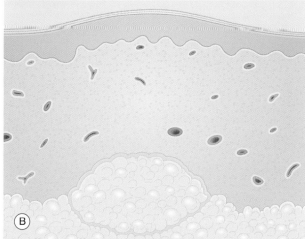

Fig. 7.8 Lipoma. (A) Deep, movable, flesh-colored, rubbery nodule. (B) Dermis—impinged on by encapsulated tumor of normal-appearing fat cells.

Lipoma is a stable or slow-growing, movable, rubbery, subcutaneous nodule.

Differential Diagnosis

A lipoma usually is deeper, more freely movable, and more rubbery than an *epidermal inclusion cyst*.

Angiolipomas are uncommon tumors that are often painful and sometimes locally invasive. Histologically, they have a prominent vascular component.

Metastatic *malignant tumors* of the skin can be deep but usually are firm (if not hard) and also involve the dermis, so the skin cannot be freely moved over them. A lipoma may also be mistaken for a soft tissue sarcoma, which is harder.

DIFFERENTIAL DIAGNOSIS OF LIPOMA

- Epidermal inclusion cyst
- Angiolipoma
- Malignant tumor

Laboratory and Biopsy

The diagnosis can usually be made clinically. When any doubt exists, particularly if a malignant tumor is even remotely suspected, a biopsy should be performed. One needs to be sure to extend the biopsy deep enough to sample the tumor. A deep elliptical excision is preferred. Histologically, a lipoma is an encapsulated collection of normal fat cells (Fig. 7.8B).

Therapy

Therapy is usually not required.

THERAPY FOR LIPOMA

- None
- Excision

Course and Complications

Lipomas found incidentally by the physician are usually reported by the patient to have been present without change in size for a number of years. For lesions recently detected or those that appear to be growing, a biopsy should be considered to confirm the diagnosis. These lesions have no complications.

NEUROFIBROMA

KEY POINTS

1. Soft, "buttonhole," papule or nodule
2. Think of neurofibromatosis type 1 if there is more than one neurofibroma

Definition

A neurofibroma represents a focal proliferation of neural tissue within the dermis (Fig. 7.9A). Clinically, neurofibromas may appear in two ways: (1) most often, as soft, protruding papules and nodules and (2) less often, as deep, firm, subcutaneous nodules. Multiple neurofibromas are a cutaneous expression of *neurofibromatosis 1 (von Recklinghausen disease)*, a dominantly inherited neurocutaneous disorder with prominent skin, skeletal, and nervous system abnormalities. *Neurofibromatosis 2* is characterized primarily by bilateral acoustic neuromas and usually lacks the cutaneous findings of neurofibromatosis 1.

Incidence

Solitary neurofibromas are infrequent and inconsequential. Neurofibromatosis 1 is one of the more common genetic disorders, with an estimated birth incidence of 1 in 3000.

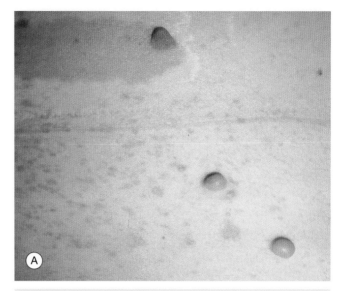

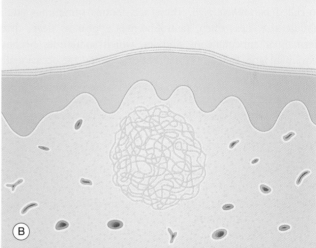

Fig. 7.9 **Neurofibroma**. (A) Multiple soft papules that invaginate into skin with pressure (buttonhole). Note the associated café-au-lait macule. (B) Dermis—circumscribed collection of loosely packed neural fibers.

A solitary neurofibroma is inconsequential; multiple ones are a sign of neurofibromatosis.

History

In neurofibromatosis 1, the onset of skin tumors usually occurs in late childhood, with more rapid growth occurring in adolescence and pregnancy. Inheritance is determined by an autosomal dominant mechanism, but the expressivity is variable. A family history is important and should be followed by a cutaneous examination of both parents. However, spontaneous mutations are common and account for approximately 50% of patients with neurofibromatosis 1. Patients with neurofibromatosis may have signs and symptoms relating to other organ involvement, most often the skeletal and central nervous systems.

Physical Examination

A typical neurofibroma appears as a soft, flesh-colored, protruding papule or nodule that characteristically, on compression, can be invaginated into what feels like a defect in the skin. This is the

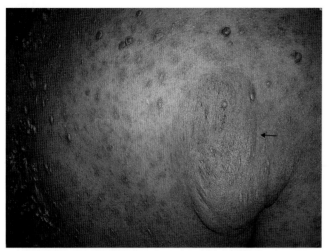

Fig. 7.10 Neurofibromatosis 1. Numerous soft papules (neurofibromas) and a large soft plaque (plexiform neurofibroma—*arrow*).

so-called *buttonhole sign*. These soft lesions sometimes attain nodule size. Less often, neurofibromas appear as deep, firm, dermal, or subcutaneous nodules, which sometimes become extremely large (plexiform neurofibromas) and are occasionally tender (Fig. 7.10).

> The "buttonhole" sign, a soft papule/nodule that can be invaginated into an apparent defect in the skin is characteristic of neurofibroma.

Neurofibromas in neurofibromatosis 1 are multiple, occasionally numbering in the thousands in a given patient. In the extreme case, particularly when combined with bony abnormalities, the condition can be remarkably disfiguring.

DIAGNOSTIC CRITERIA FOR NEUROFIBROMATOSIS TYPE 1

Two or more of the following:
1. Six or more *café-au-lait macules*—≥5 mm in prepubertal individuals and ≥15 mm in postpubertal individuals
2. Two or more *neurofibromas* of any type or one plexiform neurofibroma
3. Axillary or inguinal *freckling*
4. Optic nerve *glioma*
5. Two or more *Lisch nodules* (iris hamartomas)
6. Distinctive *osseous lesions* such as sphenoid wing dysplasia or long bone cortex thinning/dysplasia
7. A *first-degree relative* with neurofibromatosis 1

Café-au-lait spots, which are light brown macules, are present early in life—99% by the age of 1 year. Six or more *café-au-lait macules* 5 mm or larger in prepubertal individuals and 15 mm or larger in postpubertal individuals are diagnostic. Axillary and inguinal freckling is another characteristic sign. Ophthalmologic evaluation is extremely helpful because iris hamartomas (*Lisch nodules*) are found in 70% of affected individuals by the age of 10 years.

> Ophthalmologic examination for Lisch nodules is useful in diagnosing neurofibromatosis 1.

Differential Diagnosis

Skin tags are also soft but more superficial; they are narrower at the base (pedunculated) and lack the buttonhole sign.

A *dermal nevus* can appear as a soft, flesh-colored papule in the skin that clinically is similar to a small neurofibroma. Sometimes, only a biopsy can differentiate the two with certainty. Biopsies are done more often for solitary neurofibromas than for multiple neurofibromas, in which the diagnosis is more clinically evident.

DIFFERENTIAL DIAGNOSIS OF NEUROFIBROMA

- Skin tag
- Dermal nevus

Laboratory and Biopsy

The diagnosis of neurofibromatosis can usually be made clinically. Magnetic resonance imaging is helpful in detecting brain hamartomas in children affected with neurofibromatosis 1 and in revealing acoustic neuromas in patients with neurofibromatosis 2. For solitary neurofibromas or when histologic confirmation is needed for neurofibromatosis, a biopsy specimen provides the diagnosis. The histologic picture shows a well-circumscribed collection of fine, wavy fibers loosely packed in the dermis (Fig. 7.9B). Special stains for nerve fibers are positive.

Therapy

Individual lesions can be removed surgically, but if excision is incomplete, recurrence is common. No known medical therapy is available to treat, prevent, or retard the progression of either the cutaneous features or the systemic disease in neurofibromatosis 1. Patients who are diagnosed with neurofibromatosis 1 should have genetic counseling.

THERAPY FOR NEUROFIBROMA

- None
- Excision

Course and Complications

Solitary neurofibromas are of little consequence. They are usually asymptomatic, have no complications, and are stable. In neurofibromatosis 1, the cutaneous condition is usually progressive. Lesions continue to form and grow, sometimes to the point of resulting in marked cosmetic disfigurement. With the variable expressivity of the disease, some patients are affected only mildly. Deep nodular lesions (plexiform neurofibromas) can rarely degenerate into malignant neurofibrosarcoma. Clinical clues that this is occurring include lesion enlargement and the development of tenderness. In most patients, the skin lesions remain histologically benign, although, as mentioned, they can become a source of cosmetic disfigurement and social stigmatization. Systemic complications of neurofibromatosis are potentially numerous and include the following: central nervous system involvement with tumors, mental retardation, and seizures; skeletal abnormalities, including kyphoscoliosis, pseudarthrosis, and localized gigantism; and endocrine disorders such as precocious puberty and pheochromocytoma. Patients with neurofibromatosis and hypertension should be screened for pheochromocytoma.

Pathogenesis

Neurofibromatosis 1 is caused by an abnormal gene, *NF-1*, on chromosome 17, transmitted in an autosomal dominant manner in half of the affected individuals. The other half have spontaneous mutations. The gene encodes for a protein named *neurofibromin*, which appears to possess tumor-suppressing activity. Accordingly, inherited abnormalities of this gene may lead to tumor development (e.g., neurofibromas and possibly other tumors found in patients with neurofibromatosis 1). Genetic testing for *NF-1* mutations is complex, and a negative test does not exclude the diagnosis.

XANTHOMA

KEY POINTS

1. Composed of lipid-laden histiocytes
2. Skin sign of hyperlipidemia

Definition

A xanthoma represents a focal collection of lipid-laden histiocytes in the dermis or tendons. Clinically, xanthomas located in the dermis appear as yellowish (*xanthous*, Greek for yellow) papules, plaques, and nodules. Tendon xanthomas are deep, flesh-colored, hard nodules located within peripheral tendons. Xanthomas usually are a manifestation of a hyperlipoproteinemic state.

Xanthomas are yellow tumors in the skin.

Incidence

Flat xanthomas on the eyelids (xanthelasmas) are the most frequently encountered xanthomas but are still not very common. Other xanthomas are even less common, both as a presenting complaint in a dermatology clinic and as an incidental finding in the general population. Familial hypertriglyceridemia and familial hypercholesterolemia are both inherited as autosomal dominant traits, each at a frequency of 1 in 500 of the general population. Patients who are homozygous for the disease are obviously much fewer in number but are more severely affected and more likely to have xanthomas.

History

In patients with one of the inherited hyperlipoproteinemias, a positive family history may be elicited. In addition, the patient may have systemic signs and symptoms that accompany the cutaneous xanthomas, including a history of coronary artery disease and diabetes. Patients with eruptive xanthomas have markedly raised triglyceride levels that usually result from a familial metabolic abnormality combined with a secondary factor such as alcohol, obesity, glucose intolerance, hyperinsulinemia, and drugs, including estrogens, corticosteroids, and isotretinoin. Eruptive xanthomas appear relatively quickly in several weeks and correspondingly disappear rapidly after reduction of serum triglyceride levels.

Physical Examination

Several types of xanthoma have been characterized. In all, except the tendon type, the yellow color of the lesion provides the clue to its lipid nature. The most common types are described below.

Xanthoma type	Raised plasma lipid levels
Xanthelasma	Often none
Eruptive	Triglycerides
Tendon	Cholesterol
Tuberous	Both or either of the above

Xanthelasmas are yellowish plaques on the eyelids. This is the only type that is not invariably accompanied by an increase in either plasma cholesterol or triglyceride concentration.

Eruptive xanthomas (Fig. 7.11A) are reddish-yellowish papules and plaques that occur in patients with markedly raised triglyceride levels. They occur most frequently on extensor surfaces but may appear anywhere.

Tendon xanthomas (Fig. 7.12) are stony hard nodules occurring on tendons, most often the Achilles tendon and the extensor tendons of the fingers. Because of their depth, the yellow color cannot be appreciated clinically. Tendon xanthomas are usually associated with severe hypercholesterolemia.

Tuberous xanthomas are "potato-like" papules and nodules, which are yellowish and most often found on the elbows and buttocks. Tuberous xanthomas are associated with increased serum triglyceride or cholesterol levels.

Differential Diagnosis

Sebaceous glands, lipid deposits, and granulomas are the major causes of the yellow color in skin papules. The lesions of *sebaceous gland hyperplasia* usually occur on the face as small superficial papules, often with a central umbilication.

The yellowish/orange papules and plaques of *juvenile xanthogranuloma* also contain lipid, which is responsible for their color (Fig. 7.13). As the name suggests, these lesions occur in childhood and usually involute spontaneously. Extracutaneous involvement is rare. However, multiple juvenile xanthogranulomas in children younger than 2 years of age are more likely to have eye involvement and should be referred to an ophthalmologist to rule out hyphema (hemorrhage) and glaucoma. Histologically, they have a distinctive appearance. They are not associated with raised plasma lipid levels.

Both *rheumatoid nodules* and *tendon xanthomas* are subcutaneous, but only tendon xanthomas are affixed to the tendon structures.

DIFFERENTIAL DIAGNOSIS OF XANTHOMA

- Sebaceous gland hyperplasia
- Juvenile xanthogranuloma
- Rheumatoid nodule

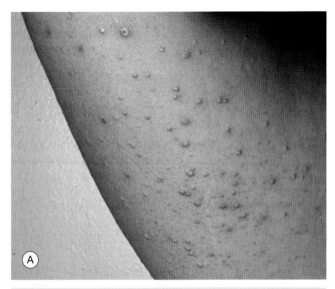

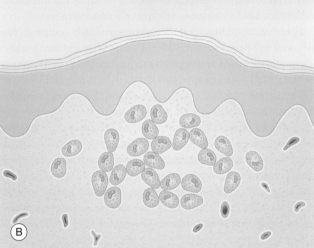

Fig. 7.11 **Eruptive xanthomas**. (A) Multiple yellowish-pink papules. (B) Dermis—dense infiltrate of lipid-laden histiocytes.

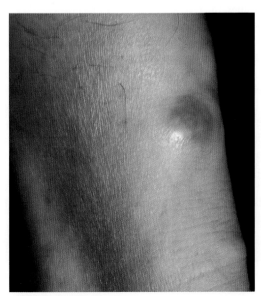

Fig. 7.12 **Tendon xanthoma**—hard, pinkish, flesh-colored nodule on the Achilles tendon.

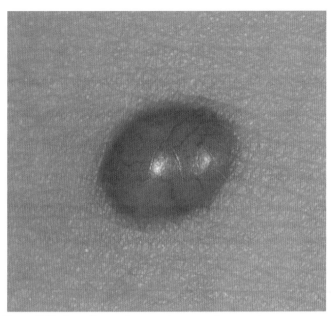

Figure 7.13 **Juvenile xanthogranuloma**—yellow papule.

Laboratory and Biopsy

The diagnosis is usually made clinically. All patients with xanthomas should have a screening for fasting lipid profile. In patients with xanthelasma, results are normal in approximately 50%. For the other types of xanthoma, lipid abnormalities are to be expected. The biopsy reveals an infiltrate of numerous lipid-laden histiocytes (Fig. 7.11B).

Therapy

Therapy is aimed at lowering the abnormal lipid levels with diet and, for patients with markedly increased lipid levels, medications. Xanthelasma lesions may be removed surgically for cosmetic reasons.

THERAPY FOR XANTHOMA
Initial
- Diet
- Medications—statins, bile-acid binding resins, fibrates, nicotinic acid

Alternative
- Surgery

Course and Complications

Eruptive xanthomas involute spontaneously after lowering of the serum triglyceride concentration. The other types of xanthoma are more persistent but may slowly regress if the lipid levels are lowered. The cutaneous lesions usually have no complications, but the lipid abnormality may be associated with significant systemic complications such as premature myocardial infarction in patients with raised cholesterol levels and pancreatitis in patients with markedly increased levels of serum triglycerides.

Eruptive xanthomas usually resolve when triglyceride levels are lowered; other xanthomas are more persistent.

Pathogenesis

Xanthomas represent accumulations of lipid-laden histiocytes. The lipid is thought to be extracted from plasma, although some evidence suggests that intracellular lipid synthesis may also be operative in some instances.

Patients with *familial hypertriglyceridemia* have increased endogenous hepatic production of very low-density lipoproteins (VLDLs), which are particles with a high triglyceride content. In these patients, VLDL production is further increased with high carbohydrate or alcohol ingestion, obesity, or diabetes, so triglyceride levels of more than 2000 mg/mL may be attained. Triglyceride deposits are polar and thereby more susceptible to intracellular lysosomal hydrolases; hence, eruptive xanthomas quickly resolve when the triglyceride level is lowered.

Patients with *familial hypercholesterolemia* have high levels of circulating low-density lipoproteins (LDLs), which are particles with a high cholesterol content. In these patients, the gene affected is the one that controls the synthesis of LDL cell surface receptors. As a result, LDL cannot be adequately removed from the plasma by cellular uptake. In addition, the cells perceive an intracellular deficiency of LDL and hence are stimulated to produce more LDL, a process resulting in even higher serum levels. Individuals who are heterozygous for this disease have plasma LDL levels that are two to three times the normal level and develop tendon xanthomas and premature atherosclerotic cardiovascular disease in midlife. Homozygotic patients have plasma LDL levels that are six to eight times normal levels, with cholesterol levels of greater than 800 mg/dL, and they develop symptomatic coronary artery disease before the age of 20 years. The nonpolar cholesterol esters are more resistant to degradation and therefore persist in both skin (tendon xanthomas) and blood vessels (atherosclerosis).

MALIGNANT DERMAL TUMORS

KEY POINTS

1. Rule out cancer for hard dermal nodules.
2. Although uncommon, skin metastases may be the first sign of internal cancer.

Definition

These tumors result from the deposition or proliferation of malignant cells in the dermis. They usually manifest clinically as hard nodules in the skin (Fig. 7.14A).

Incidence

Malignant dermal tumors can be primary or metastatic. Kaposi sarcoma, as discussed above, is an example of a primary (albeit multifocal) malignant tumor derived from endothelial cells in the skin. Tumors from other endogenous elements such as collagen (dermatofibrosarcoma protuberans), neural tissue (neurofibrosarcoma), vascular tissue (angiosarcoma), appendageal structures (sweat gland and sebaceous gland carcinomas), and subcutaneous fat (liposarcoma) are all extremely rare and are not discussed except with the usual admonition that, for undiagnosed nodules in the skin, a skin biopsy is necessary.

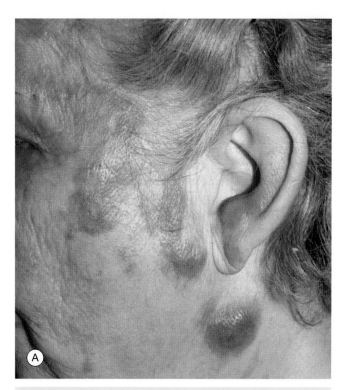

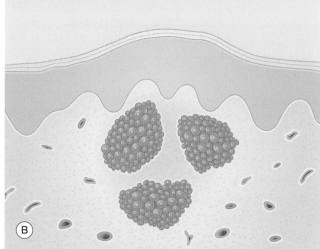

Fig. 7.14 Metastatic lymphoma. (A) Hard, red- to plum-colored nodules. (B) Dermis—dense aggregates of malignant cells.

Malignant tumors from endogenous dermal elements are rare. Metastatic tumors are more common.

The more common cause of malignant dermal tumors is metastatic disease. The authors performed a tumor registry survey of 4020 patients with metastatic carcinoma and found that 420 (10%) had cutaneous metastases. The incidence of metastatic nodules in the skin depends on the type of malignancy. For example, skin involvement is relatively common in acute myelomonocytic leukemia (occurring in 10%–20% of cases) but uncommon in acute lymphocytic leukemia. Moreover, skin nodules are common in metastatic breast carcinoma but extremely rare in prostatic carcinoma. Table 7.2 lists the tumor types that were found most likely to metastasize to skin.

Cutaneous metastases occasionally serve as the *first sign* of an internal malignancy. In a retrospective survey of 7316 patients with cancer, 59 (0.8%) patients presented with either direct extension (22 patients), local (20 patients), or distant (17 patients) metastases as the first manifestation of cancer. Most had breast cancer.

History

In patients with a known history of internal malignant disease, one should be particularly suspicious of a possible malignant origin of any new skin nodule. The nodules are usually asymptomatic, but the patient may have other signs and symptoms of malignancy, including weight loss, lymphadenopathy, or symptoms related to the location of the primary tumor.

Physical Examination

Malignant tumors in the dermis are characteristically hard or at least extremely firm. They vary in color from flesh tones to pink, red, and purple. Skin nodules of lymphoma and myeloma are frequently plum colored. Large nodules sometimes ulcerate. Lymphadenopathy or hepatosplenomegaly may also be present in patients with metastatic disease.

TABLE 7.2 **Frequency of Skin Metastases From Internal Malignancies**	
	Frequency (%)
Malignancy	
Leukemia	
Acute myelomonocytic	10–20
Chronic lymphocytic	5–10
Acute lymphocytic	Rare
Lymphoma (not including mycosis fungoides)	
Non-Hodgkin	3–20
Hodgkin	0.5
Multiple myeloma	4
Metastatic carcinoma	10
Type of Carcinoma Responsible for Skin Metastases	
Women	
Breast	73
Melanoma	11
Ovary	3
Oral cavity	2
Lung	2
Men	
Melanoma	34
Lung	12
Large intestine	12
Oral cavity	10

> Malignant tumors are hard dermal nodules.

Differential Diagnosis

A malignant tumor in the skin may be confused with any of the benign dermal growths. As is emphasized repeatedly, if any doubt exists, a biopsy is required.

DIFFERENTIAL DIAGNOSIS OF MALIGNANT DERMAL TUMORS
- Any dermal growth

Laboratory and Biopsy

The biopsy is diagnostic, showing an infiltrate of malignant cells, often in nodular aggregates (Fig. 7.14B). Occasionally, the histologic features are tumor specific, that is, the likely primary source is suggested by the histologic appearance of the skin involvement. Special histochemical or immunostains for cellular components (e.g., keratin) or tumor markers (e.g., carcinoembryonic antigen) may be helpful.

Therapy

For a primary malignant process in the skin, the preferred therapy is surgical excision. Therapy of metastatic disease is that of the primary tumor. The effect of systemic therapy can often be evaluated by measuring the metastatic skin lesion, an easily assessable marker. Troublesome skin metastases are sometimes also treated with palliative radiation or surgery.

THERAPY FOR MALIGNANT DERMAL TUMORS
- Excision for primary tumors
- Chemotherapy, immunotherapy, and so on, for metastases
- Palliative surgery or radiotherapy for metastases

Course and Complications

For metastatic disease, the course is similar to that of the primary process. For many diseases, the development of skin metastasis indicates a particularly poor prognosis. Acute myelomonocytic leukemia is an example.

The skin nodules of metastatic disease may ulcerate and become secondarily infected. This condition can lead to sepsis and death. The major complications, however, do not usually result from the skin but from the systemic disease.

Pathogenesis

Spread to the skin from an internal malignant disease usually occurs by a hematogenous route. Some tumors may also reach the skin via lymphatic pathways. Once lodged in the skin, the malignant cells proliferate in a three-dimensional fashion, clinically expressed as a nodule. The reason some tumors have a greater propensity for the skin than others is not known.

UNCOMMON DERMAL AND SUBCUTANEOUS GROWTHS

Glomus Tumor

Glomus tumor (glomangioma) is a benign growth of vascular smooth muscle which produces solitary or multiple flesh-colored to dusky blue nodules. Solitary glomus tumor is frequently extremely tender, occurring on the arms, fingers (subungual), and elsewhere. Multiple glomangiomas (Fig. 7.15) are usually nontender and may be inherited as an autosomal dominant trait.

Granular Cell Tumor

Granular cell tumors usually present in dark-skinned, middle-aged women, and are benign in the great majority of cases. It is found in the skin and the tongue, most frequently as a solitary, asymptomatic nodule (Fig. 7.16). The biopsy reveals large polyhedral cells with a characteristic granular cytoplasm.

Infantile Digital Fibromatosis

This is a rare benign tumor of myofibroblasts that occurs at birth or usually by the age of 1 year. The biopsy reveals spindle-shaped cells with characteristic eosinophilic inclusion bodies. These asymptomatic nodules affect the fingers and toes (Fig. 7.17). Surgical excision is usually unsuccessful because of a high recurrence rate.

Leiomyoma

Cutaneous leiomyoma is a benign smooth muscle tumor that is characteristically painful. It can be solitary or grouped (Fig. 7.18). An autosomal dominant familial form (hereditary leiomyomatosis and renal cell carcinoma) of multiple leiomyoma is associated with uterine leiomyomas and renal cell cancer. This is caused by a germline mutation in the gene encoding fumarate hydratase.

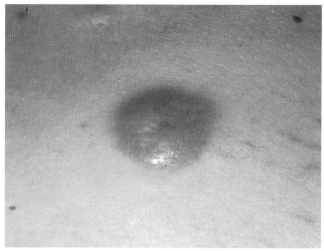

Fig. 7.16 Granular cell tumor—reddish-yellow, firm nodule.

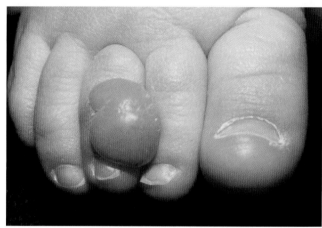

Fig. 7.17 Infantile digital fibromatosis—firm, red, smooth nodule.

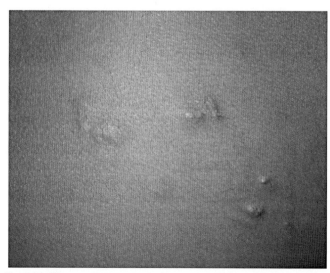

Fig. 7.15 Glomus tumor—dusky blue nontender papules and nodules.

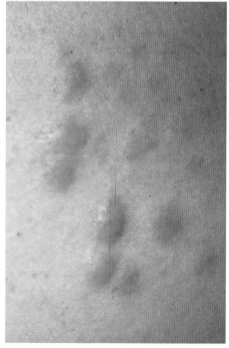

Fig. 7.18 Leiomyoma—grouped, pink, tender papules.

Lymphangioma Circumscriptum

This uncommon benign lymphatic tumor usually arises in infancy or early childhood. It is characterized by irregularly grouped, vesicle-like papules that are likened to frogspawn (Fig. 7.19). Trauma can result in weeping clear, colorless lymph. They also may be colored purple if filled with blood. These superficial lymphangiomas are frequently connected to deeper lymphatic cisterns, which makes treatment more difficult.

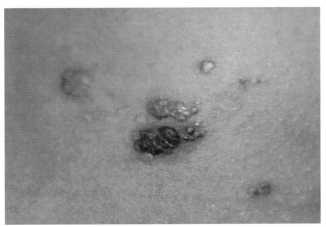

Fig. 7.19 Lymphangioma circumscriptum—irregularly grouped, translucent, and red papules.

Myxoid Cyst

Myxoid, or digital mucous, cyst occurs as a solitary, opalescent, or flesh-colored nodule. It is found over the distal interphalangeal joint or proximal nail fold, where it can cause a characteristic nail plate groove (Fig. 7.20). Puncture of the cyst results in a clear, viscous, sticky drainage. Connection with the underlying joint space makes treatment disappointing, unless careful excision is accomplished.

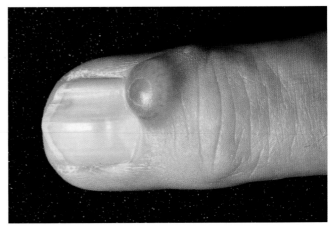

Fig. 7.20 Myxoid cyst—opalescent nodule of the proximal nail fold producing a characteristic groove of the nail plate.

SELF-ASSESSMENT

Case 1—Nodule on the Lower Leg (Fig. 7.21)

What Is Your Differential Diagnosis?

The first concern is whether this nodule represents a malignancy. If the patient was immunosuppressed or had a history of trauma, then an infectious or physical etiology could be considered.

What Diagnostic Workup Would You Do Now?

A skin biopsy is the next logical step. It revealed a dense dermal, hyperchromatic, lymphoid infiltrate of CD-20, BCL-2, and BCL-6-positive B cells. Further workup revealed a normal complete blood count and metabolic profile. A positron emission tomography/computed tomography whole-body scan showed enlarged lymph nodes in the neck.

What Is Your Diagnosis and How Would You Treat This?

The diagnosis is B-cell lymphoma, leg type. This lymphoma occurs in the elderly and has an overall 60% survival at 5 years. Treatment depends on the extent of the disease and can be local radiation, chemotherapy, and rituximab alone or in combination.

IMPORTANT POINTS

1. Consider a malignant neoplasm as the cause of nodules, especially if they are firm, dermal, and eroded.
2. A skin biopsy is an important diagnostic tool.

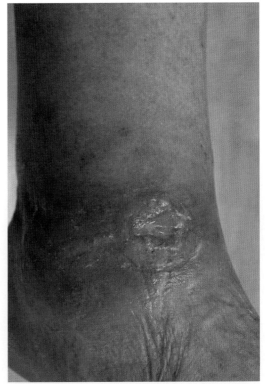

Fig. 7.21 This 81-year-old man developed this painless, pink, ulcerated nodule on his lower leg a couple of months ago. He otherwise felt healthy and the general physical examination was normal.

8

Eczematous Rashes

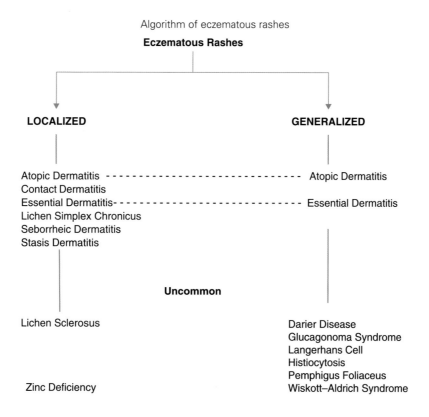

Algorithm of eczematous rashes

Eczematous Rashes

LOCALIZED

GENERALIZED

Atopic Dermatitis - Atopic Dermatitis
Contact Dermatitis
Essential Dermatitis - Essential Dermatitis
Lichen Simplex Chronicus
Seborrheic Dermatitis
Stasis Dermatitis

Uncommon

Lichen Sclerosus

Darier Disease
Glucagonoma Syndrome
Langerhans Cell
Histiocytosis
Pemphigus Foliaceus
Wiskott–Aldrich Syndrome

Zinc Deficiency

ABSTRACT

The term *eczema* is derived from the Greek word that means "to boil out or over." It is a convenient "wastebasket" for many undiagnosed rashes but is best applied to epidermal eruptions that are characterized histologically by intercellular edema, called *spongiosis* (Table 8.1). *Eczema* and *dermatitis* are synonyms. Acute dermatitis has a marked amount of spongiosis causing vesiculation. Subacute dermatitis has less spongiosis, resulting in "juicy papules." Chronic dermatitis involves

TABLE 8.1   Eczematous Eruptions

	Frequency[a]	History	Physical Examination	Differential Diagnosis	Laboratory Test
Atopic dermatitis	2.6	Allergic rhinitis Asthma	Vesicles, juicy papules—infants Lichenified plaques—adults and older children Head, neck, antecubital and popliteal fossa	Contact dermatitis Scabies Immunodeficiency syndromes Langerhans cell histiocytosis	IgE
Contact dermatitis	2.8	Irritant: contact precedes rash by hours to days Allergic: contact precedes rash by 1–4 days	Vesicles, juicy papules, lichenified plaques Sharp margins Geometric or linear configuration Conforms to area of contact	Eczematous dermatitis Fungal infection Cellulitis	Patch test
Essential dermatitis	11.4	Pruritus	Acute: vesicles, weeping, crusted patches Subacute: juicy papules Chronic: lichenified, scaling plaques	Contact dermatitis Atopic dermatitis Seborrheic dermatitis Fungal, viral, or bacterial infection Psoriasis Drug rash Dermatitis herpetiformis	–
Lichen simplex chronicus	0.8	Rash subsequent to pruritus	Lichenified plaque within reach of fingers	Contact dermatitis	–
Seborrheic dermatitis	3.7	Dandruff	Scaling papules and patches Scalp, eyebrows, nose, sternum	Atopic dermatitis Psoriasis Fungal infection Langerhans cell histiocytosis Lupus erythematosus Rosacea Perioral dermatitis	–
Stasis dermatitis	0.4	Varicose veins Leg swelling Thrombophlebitis	Juicy papules Lichenified plaques Brown pigmentation Lower legs	Cellulitis Contact dermatitis Fungal or bacterial infection	–

[a]Percentage of new dermatology patients with this diagnosis seen in the Hershey Medical Center Dermatology Clinic, Hershey, Pennsylvania.

a markedly thickened epidermis (*lichenification*) with only slight spongiosis.

KEY POINTS
1. Appearance varies from blisters to scaling, lichenified plaques.
2. Itching is prominent.
3. Distribution can be localized or generalized.

Types of dermatitis:
1. Acute—vesicles
2. Subacute—juicy papules
3. Chronic—lichenification

The hallmarks of dermatitis are marked pruritus, indistinct borders (except for contact dermatitis), and epidermal changes characterized by vesicles, juicy papules, or lichenification. Dermatitis may be localized or diffuse; it may be idiopathic or may have a specific cause. Contact allergy is the best understood cause of an eczematous reaction and potentially the most

correctable. For any eczematous rash, the first question to be asked is "Could it be contact dermatitis?"

If it does not itch, reconsider the diagnosis of dermatitis.

ATOPIC DERMATITIS

KEY POINTS
1. Itching is prominent.
2. The antecubital and popliteal fossae are typically affected.
3. Chronic waxing and waning course.

Definition

Atopic dermatitis is a chronic, relapsing, intensely pruritic, inflammatory condition of the skin that is associated with a personal or family history of atopic disease (e.g., asthma, allergic

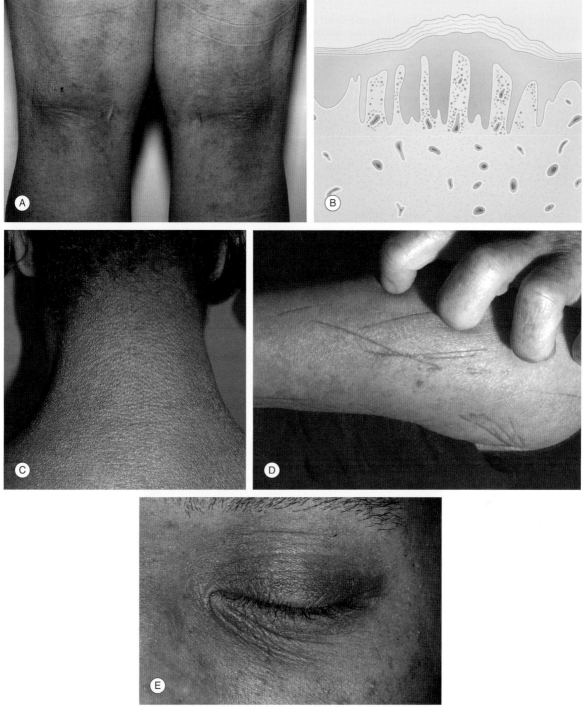

Fig. 8.1 **Atopic dermatitis**. (A) Hyperpigmented, pink, lichenified plaques affecting the popliteal fossae. (B) Epidermis—thickened, hyperkeratosis. Dermis—perivascular inflammation. (C) Hyperpigmented, licheni-fied plaque involving the whole neck. (D) Severe scratching, excoriations, and erythroderma. (E) Pink licheni-fied patch affecting the eyelids.

rhinitis, or atopic dermatitis). The cause of atopic dermatitis is thought to be altered skin barrier and immune dysfunction. Patients appear to have a genetic predisposition that can be exacerbated by numerous factors, including food allergy, skin infections, irritating clothes or chemicals, change in climate, and emotions. Lichenification is the clinical hallmark of chronic atopic dermatitis (Fig. 8.1).

Incidence

Atopic dermatitis is predominantly a disease of childhood, with 17% of children and 6% of adults affected. It usually starts after 2 months of age, and by 5 years of age, 90% of the patients who will develop atopic dermatitis have manifested the disease. It is uncommon for adults to develop atopic dermatitis without a history of childhood eczema.

History

A history of allergic respiratory disease is found in one-third of patients with atopic dermatitis and in two-thirds of their family members. Pruritus (Fig. 8.1D) is the most distressing and prominent symptom.

DIAGNOSTIC CRITERIA FOR ATOPIC DERMATITIS

- Pruritus
- Typical morphology and distribution
- Flexural lichenification in adults and older children
- Facial and extensor papulovesicles in infancy
- Chronic—relapsing course
- Personal or family history of atopic disease
- Lichenification is the clinical hallmark of chronic atopic dermatitis

Physical Examination

The morphology and distribution of atopic dermatitis are age-dependent (Fig. 8.2). Infantile atopic dermatitis is characterized by acute-to-subacute eczema with papules, vesicles, oozing, and crusting. It is distributed over the head, diaper area, and extensor surfaces of the extremities. In children and adults, eruption is a chronic dermatitis with lichenification and scaling. The distribution includes the neck, face, upper chest, and, characteristically, antecubital and popliteal fossae (Fig. 8.1).

> Atopic dermatitis in infants is papular or vesicular; in children and adults, it is lichenified, especially affecting the antecubital and popliteal fossae.

Individuals with atopic dermatitis have a characteristic expression. The face has mild-to-moderate erythema, perioral pallor, and infraorbital folds (Dennie–Morgan lines) associated with dermatitis and hyperpigmentation. The skin generally is dry and may have generalized fine, whitish scaling. The palms often have increased linear markings.

Differential Diagnosis

The differential diagnosis of atopic dermatitis includes other eczematous eruptions and *scabies*. The history of other family members with pruritus and a thorough skin examination that reveals burrows, particularly on the hands, are indicative of scabies. Infants with *Langerhans cell histiocytosis* and immunodeficiency syndromes such as *Wiskott–Aldrich syndrome, ataxia–telangiectasia,* and *Swiss-type agammaglobulinemia* have dermatitis that resembles atopic dermatitis, but these conditions are rare, and infants have systemic symptoms that distinguish their conditions from atopic dermatitis.

DIFFERENTIAL DIAGNOSIS OF ATOPIC DERMATITIS

- Contact dermatitis
- Scabies
- Langerhans cell histiocytosis
- Wiskott–Aldrich syndrome
- Ataxia–telangiectasia
- Swiss-type agammaglobulinemia

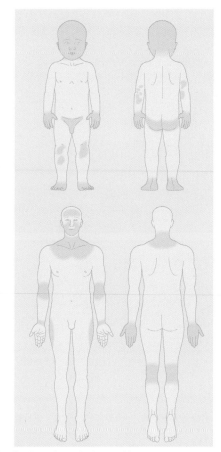

Fig. 8.2 Distribution of atopic dermatitis.

Laboratory and Biopsy

The diagnosis of atopic dermatitis is made clinically. Skin biopsy (rarely required) reveals an eczematous change that is not specific for atopic dermatitis (Fig. 8.1B). Serum immunoglobulin E (IgE) concentration is frequently raised but usually is not necessary to make the diagnosis.

Therapy

The treatment of atopic dermatitis is the same as for other eczematous eruptions and includes topical steroids, topical macrolide immunosuppressants (tacrolimus, pimecrolimus), and systemic antihistamines. However, the use of antihistamines to reduce pruritus is largely unproven. Only sedating antihistamines may be effective for itching that interferes with sleep. Treatment should be given in appropriate strength and frequency to reduce inflammation and itching significantly. A common error is undertreatment. Occasionally, a short course of systemic steroids (prednisone) is necessary to bring the disease under control. Wet dressings (plain water) and dilute bleach baths are helpful in treating acute atopic dermatitis. Avoiding environmental factors that induce itching, such as woolen clothes, emotional stress, and uncomfortable climatic conditions, is important. Moisturizers reduce dry skin and itching. Ultraviolet radiation B (UVB) or psoralen plus ultraviolet radiation A (PUVA) phototherapy can be used as a treatment. Systemic immunosuppressants including cyclosporine (Neoral), azathioprine (Imuran), mycophenolate mofetil (CellCept), and methotrexate are older medications that can help reduce steroid dependence. Immunosuppressing Janus kinase (JAK) inhibitors are now used for treating atopic dermatitis, and include ruxolitinib (Opzelura), upadacitinib (Rinvoq), and abrocitinib (Cibinqo), all of which also help to reduce steroid dependence. There are also excellent alternatives to chronic systemic steroids called immuno*modulators*, such as dupilumab (Dupixent) or tralokinumab (Adbry), both of which inhibit interleukin (IL)-4/IL-13 and require no laboratory monitoring. Immunosuppressants may be considered if satisfactory control is not achieved with initial treatment and the patient does not respond to dupilumab or tralokinumab.

> To be successful, treatment must eliminate pruritus.

In some children, food allergy can cause atopic dermatitis. Skin testing or radioallergosorbent tests may help to identify foods that are responsible. Positive tests must be confirmed with controlled food challenges and elimination diets. Eggs, peanuts, milk, and wheat appear to be the most frequently offending foods. Investigators have suggested that atopic dermatitis can be prevented by avoiding cow's milk, wheat, and eggs for the first 6 months of life. However, this approach is controversial and not generally recommended. Patients with atopic dermatitis have a higher frequency of immediate skin test reactivity in general, but hyposensitization is rarely of value in atopic dermatitis.

THERAPY FOR ATOPIC DERMATITIS (ALSO SEE THERAPY FOR ESSENTIAL DERMATITIS)

Initial
- Moisturizers
- Avoidance of irritants—woolen clothes, harsh soaps, uncomfortable climate
- Steroids, topical macrolide immunosuppressants, crisaborole ointment
- Antihistamines, baths, compresses, and antibiotics
- Avoidance of food allergens (eggs, peanuts, milk, wheat) in selected patients

Alternative
- Ultraviolet light—UVB, PUVA
- Immunomodulators—dupilumab, tralokinumab
- Immunosuppressants—cyclosporine, azathioprine, mycophenolate mofetil, methotrexate, JAK inhibitors
- Support group—National Eczema Association for Science and Education, www.nationaleczema.org

Course and Complications

Atopic dermatitis is a chronic disease punctuated by repeated acute flare-ups followed by longer periods of slow resolution. The cause of these flare-ups is frequently unknown—a feature that adds to the frustration of this disease. Most children (90%) outgrow their disease during adolescence, although some continue to have localized forms of atopic dermatitis as adults such as chronic hand or foot dermatitis, patches of lichen simplex chronicus, or eyelid dermatitis. Longitudinal studies suggest an "atopic march," in which over half of infants and children with atopic dermatitis will progress to develop allergic rhinitis and asthma.

Atopic dermatitis is frequently complicated by skin infections. Atopic skin has a higher rate of colonization with *Staphylococcus aureus*. The most serious cutaneous infection is *eczema herpeticum*, also known as Kaposi varicelliform eruption. This disseminated vesiculopustular eruption is caused by herpes simplex virus. Patients with this infection are acutely ill and may die, so it is imperative to start systemic antiviral therapy as soon as possible. *Hyper-IgE syndrome* refers to a syndrome of atopic dermatitis characterized by recurrent pyoderma (skin infections), raised serum IgE levels, and decreased chemotaxis of mononuclear cells.

> Bacterial and viral skin infections are common in atopic dermatitis.

Pathogenesis

Atopic dermatitis is a multifactorial cutaneous inflammatory disease caused, in part, by gene polymorphisms affecting the innate and adaptive immune response and epidermal barrier function. A disrupted skin barrier (filaggrin gene mutation) and disturbed immunologic response (Th2 + Th1 cytokines and IgE) have been implicated in the etiology of atopic dermatitis. The epidermal barrier defect results in dry skin and penetration of irritants, microbes, and antigens. The immunologic changes are most notable and frequent in patients with severe atopic dermatitis. These changes include increased serum IgE levels, defective cell-mediated immunity, decreased chemotaxis of mononuclear cells, increased T-lymphocyte activation with the production of T-helper Th1 and Th2 cytokines, and hyperstimulatory Langerhans cells. The increased IgE concentration is thought to reflect decreased numbers of T-suppressor cells and uninhibited production of IgE. Depressed cell-mediated immunity is manifested by an increased susceptibility to cutaneous viral and bacterial infections. In addition, responses to in vitro tests of cell-mediated immunity such as lymphocyte blastogenesis to mitogens and antigens are blunted. There are also low levels of antimicrobial peptides in lesional skin resulting in dysbiosis with increased susceptibility to pathogens such as *S. aureus*, herpes simplex virus, and vaccinia virus.

> Disruption of the skin barrier and immune dysfunction contribute to the development of atopic dermatitis.

CONTACT DERMATITIS

KEY POINTS
1. Irritant or allergic etiology
2. Distribution conforms to areas of contact
3. Avoidance of the contactant results in cure

Definition

Contact dermatitis (Fig. 8.3) is an inflammatory reaction of the skin precipitated by an exogenous chemical. The two types of contact dermatitis are irritant and allergic. *Irritant contact dermatitis* is produced by a substance that has a direct toxic effect on the skin. *Allergic contact dermatitis* triggers an immunologic reaction that causes tissue inflammation. Examples of irritants include acids, alkalis, solvents, and detergents. Innumerable chemicals cause allergic contact dermatitis, including metals, plants, medicines, cosmetics, and rubber compounds. Clinical appearance can range from acute (vesicles) to chronic (lichenification) eczematous reactions.

Types of contact dermatitis:
1. Irritant
2. Allergic

Incidence

Contact dermatitis is a frequent problem that most people experience during their lifetime, whether it is irritant diaper dermatitis or allergic poison ivy or oak dermatitis. A significant cause of occupational illness (excluding injury) is caused by contact dermatitis, resulting in impairment and time lost from work. In occupational contact dermatitis, irritant is usually more common than an allergic etiology.

History

One should first determine whether the contact dermatitis is an allergic or an irritant phenomenon. Skin damage is usually evident within several hours of contact with a strong irritant. Weaker irritants, however, may require multiple applications days before the development of dermatitis. Allergic contact dermatitis usually appears 24–48 hours after exposure, before the development of clinical disease. Occasionally, the dermatitis may develop as soon as 8–12 hours after contact or may be delayed as long as 4–7 days. The history of a precipitating contactant may be either obvious or obscure. Detailed history of occupation, hygienic habits, and hobbies is frequently necessary to find the contactant.

Causes of allergic contact dermatitis:
1. Poison ivy or oak
2. Cosmetics/personal care products
3. Nickel
4. Rubber compounds
5. Topical medications

Poison ivy or *oak* is a frequent cause of allergic contact dermatitis in the summer (Fig. 8.4). The sensitizing allergens are pentadecylcatechol and heptadecylcatechol chemicals located in the sap (urushiol) of the plant. Another familiar member of this family of poisonous plants is poison *sumac*. Less frequently recognized family members are cashew, mango, and lacquer trees. Sensitization to poison ivy results in sensitivity

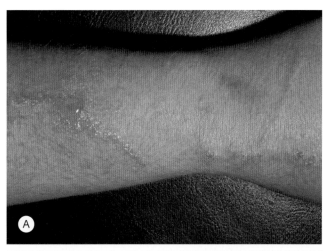
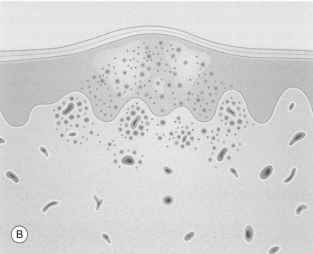

Fig. 8.3 Allergic contact dermatitis from poison ivy. (A) Linear, red papules and weeping vesicles. (B) Epidermis—vesicles, spongiosis. Dermis—perivascular inflammation.

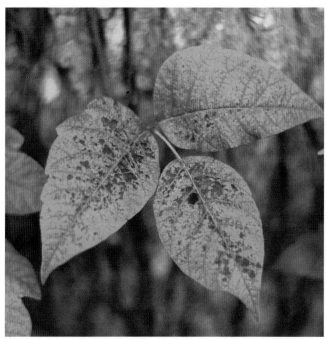

Fig. 8.4 Poison ivy plant with characteristic three leaves.

to the other poisonous plants in this family. The characteristic eruption resulting from contact with poison ivy or oak is manifested by linear streaks of papules and vesicles along with cellulitic appearing plaques and patches. Contact with the smoke of burning plants can result in confluent severe dermatitis of the exposed skin.

> Streaks of vesicles are characteristic of contact dermatitis to poison ivy or oak.

Cosmetics (personal care products) contain fragrances and preservatives that cause allergic contact dermatitis, particularly affecting the faces of those who frequently use makeup and moisturizers. *Paraphenylenediamine (PPD)* is a dye found in permanent hair coloring. Sensitization to PPD occurs in hairdressers and in clients who have their hair colored. Sometimes present in henna tattoos, PPD has caused severe blistering eruptions. When completely oxidized, as in the dye on a fur coat, PPD is not allergenic.

Nickel sensitivity is most often seen as a result of wearing "cheap" jewelry, commonly earrings. It is found in many metal alloys (Fig. 8.5). One cannot be certain that the commonly advertised "hypoallergenic" earrings are nickel-free. Although stainless steel contains nickel, it is bound so tightly that it usually does not allow an allergic reaction to occur.

Rubber compounds are ubiquitous. Shoes and gloves are the most common sources of allergic contact dermatitis caused by these chemicals. An eczematous reaction limited to the feet or hands is typical of shoe and glove dermatitis, respectively. The most frequent rubber allergens are *mercaptobenzothiazole* and *thiuram*.

In sleuthing the causes of contact dermatitis, one must not overlook the possibility of a *topical medication* perpetuating or exacerbating a preexisting dermatitis. *Neomycin* and *bacitracin*, found in topical antibiotic preparations, cause allergic contact dermatitis when these agents are used to treat cuts and abrasions, chronic ulcers, and surgical wounds.

Physical Examination

Contact dermatitis may be acute or chronic. The configuration of the lesions depends on the nature of the exposure, which may result in patches or plaques with angular corners, geometric outlines, and sharp margins. Poison ivy or oak characteristically causes linear streaks of papulovesicles.

The location of the dermatitis is helpful in predicting the causative irritant or allergen. The head and neck are frequent sites of contact dermatitis from fragrances and preservatives found in cosmetics. Hair dyes, permanent wave solutions, and shampoos produce dermatitis on the scalp. Eczema of the eyelids is caused by eye cosmetics or allergens that have been transferred from the hands, such as nail polish. Photoallergic contact dermatitis from sunscreens is produced by a photoreaction between sunlight and an allergen in exposed areas of the skin, such as the head, neck, V-shaped area of the chest, and arms. The hands are the most common area of contact dermatitis from industrial chemicals, particularly an irritant reaction from detergents, petroleum products, and solvents. Dermatitis of the feet is produced by allergens in shoes, such as rubber chemicals and leather tanning agents. The groin and buttocks in infants are frequently affected by *diaper dermatitis* (Fig. 8.6). This condition is an irritant contact dermatitis from moisture and feces. Diaper dermatitis is often complicated by secondary infection with bacteria and yeast.

> The location of the dermatitis often provides a clue to the nature of the contactant.

Differential Diagnosis

Morphologically, contact dermatitis is identical to other *eczematous eruptions* and may complicate atopic or stasis dermatitis if the patient becomes sensitized to the topical preparation used to treat these dermatoses. Other causes of eczematous-appearing dermatoses that may need to be ruled out include superficial *fungal*

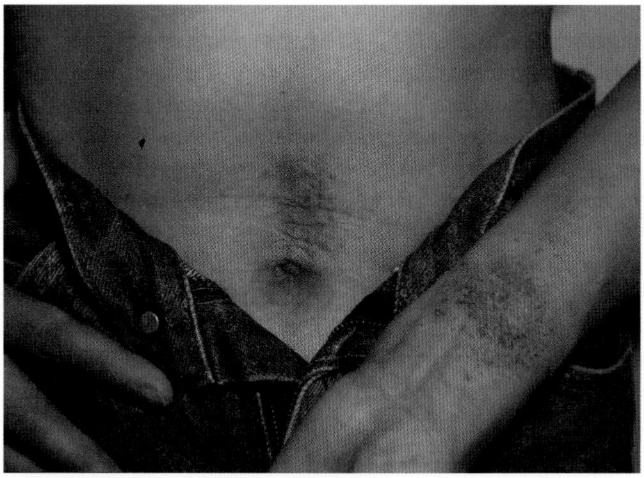

Fig. 8.5 Allergic contact dermatitis from nickel-containing snap and watch band—red, scaling and slightly crusted, lichenified plaques.

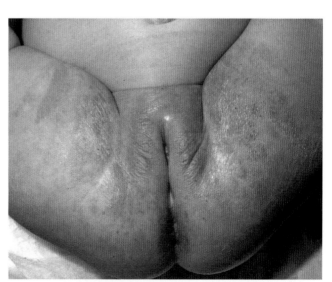

Fig. 8.6 Irritant contact dermatitis (diaper dermatitis)—red patches.

infections and *bacterial cellulitis*. In bacterial cellulitis, the skin is painful (rather than pruritic), and the patient is often febrile.

> For any dermatitis, ask "Could it be contact dermatitis?"

DIFFERENTIAL DIAGNOSIS OF CONTACT DERMATITIS

- Any eczematous eruption
- Superficial fungal infection
- Cellulitis

Laboratory and Biopsy

No standard testing method is available for diagnosing irritant contact dermatitis. For allergic contact dermatitis, the causative agent can be identified by patch tests, but these tests must be properly performed and interpreted (see Chapter 3). Patch testing is done with a screening patch test series. This series is composed of medications, fragrances, preservatives, metals, rubber compounds, botanicals, and miscellaneous other chemicals. Individual chemicals and special trays (e.g., allergens found in plants) supplement the screening series. The chemicals are applied to patches that are taped on the back of the test subject. After 48 hours, the patches are removed and the test site is examined for an eczematous reaction that is graded according to a standard interpretation key: a + 1 reaction indicates palpable erythema; a + 2 reaction indicates papules and vesicles; and a + 3 reaction indicates bullae. A further delayed reading 1–2 days after patch removal is mandatory. Although the patch testing procedure is simple, its interpretation is often difficult. A positive patch test must be relevant to the eruption to be meaningful (Fig. 8.7). Unknown chemicals and potential irritants must be patch tested cautiously and are best left to trained personnel who have experience in patch testing.

> Patch tests help in identifying the responsible allergen or allergens.

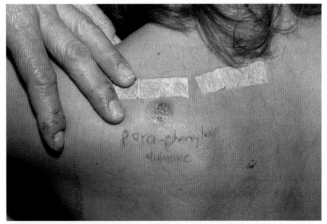

Fig. 8.7 Positive patch test to paraphenylenediamine. This was relevant to this hairdresser's hand dermatitis caused by permanent hair coloring.

Biopsy (Fig. 8.1B) of contact dermatitis cannot differentiate between irritant and allergic causes. Contact dermatitis also cannot be differentiated histologically from other causes of eczematous eruptions such as atopic or seborrheic dermatitis.

Therapy

Prevention of contact dermatitis is the most logical, but often the most difficult, solution. Avoidance of an irritant or allergen may require a change in lifestyle or occupation. Sometimes, protective clothing is curative. Allergens that have a high sensitizing potential are best used in closed systems in which workers have virtually no contact with the offending chemicals. Protective or barrier creams are of questionable benefit. Sometimes, the offending material can be substituted with another, less toxic or allergenic, chemical. Predictive testing for contact irritancy or sensitivity is a standard procedure before introducing new cosmetics or chemicals.

Acute, severe, generalized contact dermatitis is treated with a short course of systemic steroids: 40–60 mg prednisone daily for a *minimum* of 7 days and then tapered over the next 7–14 days or 1 mL triamcinolone suspension (Kenalog-40) intramuscularly. Astringent dressings (Domeboro) or soothing baths (Aveeno) reduce weeping and itching. Milder dermatitis responds to topical steroids (see Table 4.1) or to macrolide immunosuppressants (Protopic or Elidel). Systemic antihistamines such as 10–25 mg hydroxyzine (Atarax), 25–50 mg diphenhydramine (Benadryl) four times daily, or cetirizine (Zyrtec) 10 mg twice a day are helpful for pruritus.

THERAPY FOR CONTACT DERMATITIS

Preventative
- Avoidance of irritant or allergen
- Protective clothing—gloves and so on

Initial
- Steroids, antihistamines, baths, and compresses (see Therapy for Essential Dermatitis)

Course and Complications

Acute allergic contact dermatitis subsides within 3–4 weeks. If the patient has repeated exposure to the contactant, chronic dermatitis will develop. With the breakdown of the epidermal barrier, secondary bacterial infection may complicate contact dermatitis. Although contact dermatitis may start locally, generalized hypersensitivity of the skin can occur, with resultant generalized dermatitis autosensitization.

Pathogenesis

Irritant contact dermatitis is a nonspecific inflammatory reaction resulting from toxic injury of the skin. Allergic contact dermatitis is a cell-mediated, delayed type IV immunologic reaction. It is divided into a sensitization phase and an elicitation phase. The sensitization phase occurs when a chemical (hapten) is applied to the skin of a nonsensitized individual. This chemical in itself is unable to induce an allergic reaction because of its small molecular size, which is usually less than 500 Da. It must combine with an epidermal protein thought to be on the surface of the Langerhans cell (epidermal macrophage). After the formation of the hapten–protein complex, the Langerhans cell presents the allergen to T lymphocytes in the lymph node, where effector, memory, and suppressor lymphocytes are produced. The period of sensitization requires approximately 7–10 days. The elicitation phase occurs in sensitized individuals 1–2 days after reexposure to the antigen. After presentation of the antigen by Langerhans cells to memory T cells in the skin, effector T cells produce lymphokines, which recruit other inflammatory cells and produce allergic contact dermatitis. The dermatitis usually appears clinically 1–2 days after the elicitation exposure. The reaction is thought ultimately to be extinguished by suppressor T cells.

> Allergic contact dermatitis is a cell-mediated, delayed type IV immunologic reaction.

ESSENTIAL DERMATITIS

KEY POINTS
1. Idiopathic etiology.
2. Diagnosis of exclusion.
3. Treatment is symptomatic: suppress inflammation and itching.

Definition

Essential (nonspecific) dermatitis is an epidermal eruption that may be acute (Fig. 8.8) or chronic (Fig. 8.9) and localized or generalized. It is a diagnosis that is made by exclusion when an underlying cause such as an allergen or irritant cannot be found, and its distribution is not typical of defined eczematous eruptions such as atopic or seborrheic dermatitis.

Incidence

Essential dermatitis is one of the eruptions most frequently seen by the clinician. The authors' patients had this diagnosis in about 11% of them.

History

Itching is the chief complaint prompting patients to seek medical attention. It is often severe enough to interfere with normal daily activities and to interrupt sleep. The itching may be episodic or constant. The patient frequently has a history of "sensitive skin" that is intolerant to topical preparations such as moisturizers, soaps, and detergents and to irritating fabrics such as wool.

Physical Examination

The varied appearance of essential dermatitis occurs because of its evolution from an acute to a chronic process. Acutely, intercellular edema leads to vesiculation. Chronically, lichenification occurs. The polymorphism is manifest by vesicles, juicy papules, patches, and plaques. Secondary changes include oozing, crusting, scaling, and fissuring. Characteristic of essential dermatitis is the indistinct border between normal and abnormal skin.

Depending on the morphology and location, various types of dermatitis have been classified. *Dyshidrotic eczema* is characterized by deep-seated vesicles (which resemble the pearls

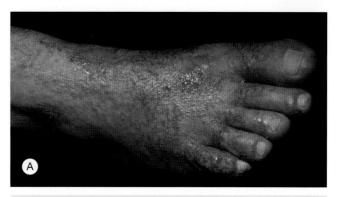

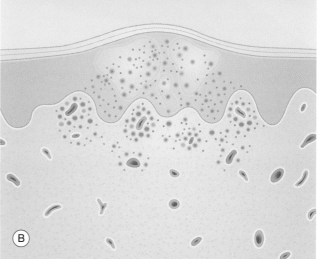

Fig. 8.8 Acute essential dermatitis. (A) Red, weeping, vesicles. (B) Epidermis—vesicles, spongiosis. Dermis—perivascular inflammation.

in tapioca pudding) involving the hands (palms), feet (soles), and sides of the digits. It occurs bilaterally and symmetrically. *Autosensitization* or *id eruption* is a generalized subacute dermatitis that follows a localized acute dermatitis, usually of the feet or hands. It is thought to be a hypersensitivity reaction to a substance produced by the acute dermatitis. *Xerotic eczema* (Fig. 8.10) is the result of low humidity and dry skin. It occurs in the winter and is manifest by dry, fissured skin of the trunk and extremities. It particularly affects the elderly and the lower legs of all age groups. *Nummular eczema* is characterized by oval, weeping patches with crusted papulovesicles (Fig. 8.11). It occurs on the trunk and extremities.

> Types of idiopathic eczema:
> 1. Dyshidrotic—hands and feet
> 2. Autosensitization—generalized
> 3. Xerotic—dry skin
> 4. Nummular—oval patches

Differential Diagnosis

The differential diagnosis of an acute vesiculopapular essential dermatitis includes, first, *contact dermatitis*. Also to be considered are infectious processes by a *dermatophyte*, *herpes simplex virus*, *varicella-zoster virus*, or *bacterium*, as in impetigo. The

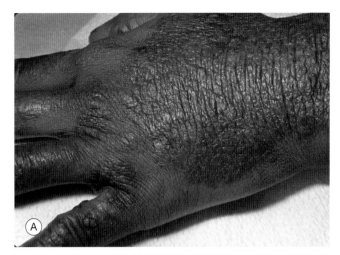

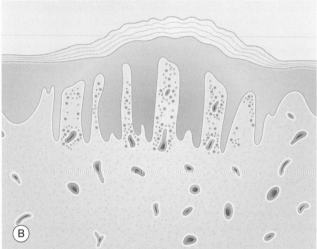

Fig. 8.9 Chronic essential dermatitis. (A) Hyperpigmented-brown, lichenified plaque. (B) Epidermis—thickened, hyperkeratosis. Dermis—perivascular inflammation.

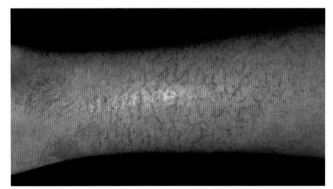

Fig. 8.10 Xerotic (dry skin) eczema—Pink, scaling, fissured, reticulated patch.

appearance of rectangular or linear areas of dermatitis would lead one to suspect contact dermatitis. Removal of the top of the vesicle or scales from the edge of the patch for potassium hydroxide (KOH) examination reveals the typical hyphae of a fungal infection. Scraping the base of the vesicle for a Tzanck preparation reveals the multinucleated giant cells of herpesvirus, which clinically appear as grouped vesicles on an erythematous

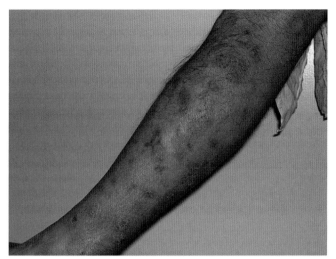

Fig. 8.11 Nummular eczema—Dusky pink oval scaling, slightly crusted patches.

base. Impetigo can be ruled out by Gram staining or culture of the yellow crusts typical of this infectious process.

The differential diagnosis of chronic essential dermatitis includes chronic *contact dermatitis, psoriasis, drug eruption, fungal infection, dermatitis herpetiformis, and mycosis fungoides.* The history and patch tests differentiate chronic nonspecific dermatitis from contact dermatitis. Clinically, psoriasis is usually easy to distinguish by its sharply demarcated, silvery, scaling plaques that affect but are not limited to the scalp, elbows, and knees. In any nonspecific dermatitis, one should consider drugs as the cause. Discontinuation of medication with subsequent clearing is the only reliable way to rule out a drug eruption. Fungal infections of the skin can mimic dermatitis, especially if lesions are treated with topical steroids. Any scaling patch, particularly if it has an annular inflammatory border, should be scraped and the scale examined for fungal hyphae (KOH preparation). Dermatitis herpetiformis (see Chapter 10) should be considered for any eczematous-appearing eruption involving the extensor elbows, knees, and low back (Fig. 8.12). A biopsy for routine and immunofluorescent staining will be diagnostic. Mycosis fungoides can be ruled out by a biopsy too. However, it may take multiple biopsies over time to confirm essential dermatitis vs. mycosis fungoides.

DIFFERENTIAL DIAGNOSIS OF ESSENTIAL DERMATITIS

Acute
- Contact dermatitis
- Dermatophyte infection
- Herpes simplex virus
- Herpes varicella-zoster
- Impetigo

Chronic
- Contact dermatitis
- Psoriasis
- Drug eruption
- Dermatophyte
- Dermatitis herpetiformi
- Mycosis fungoides

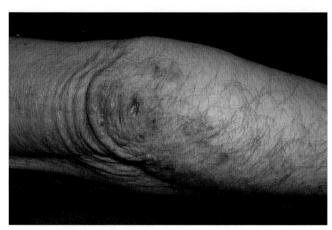

Fig. 8.12 **Dermatitis herpetiformis**—Red, slightly scaling, and excoriated patch.

Biopsy

The histologic hallmark of dermatitis is intercellular edema of the epidermis leading to widening of intercellular spaces with a sponge-like appearance of the epidermis (spongiosis). When the process is acute and severe, it results in intraepidermal vesicle formation (Fig. 8.8B). When it is chronic, the epidermis becomes hyperkeratotic and thickened (acanthotic) (Fig. 8.9B). The dermis is characterized by a lymphocytic infiltrate.

> Spongiosis is the histologic hallmark of dermatitis.

Therapy

Corticosteroids are the cornerstone of dermatitis treatment. They may be applied topically, injected intralesionally, or administered systemically. Steroid creams are used for acute papulovesicular eczema, whereas ointments are better for chronic lichenified dermatitis. However, patient preference of a cream versus an ointment is more important. Therapy with topical steroids such as hydrocortisone 1%, triamcinolone 0.1%, fluocinonide 0.05%, and clobetasol 0.05% is discussed in detail in Chapter 4. Alternatives to topical steroids are the macrolide immunosuppressants, tacrolimus and pimecrolimus. These nonsteroidal topicals have the advantage of not causing skin atrophy and, when used near the eyes, not causing glaucoma or cataracts. Thick, hyperkeratotic plaques that are unresponsive to topical steroids may be injected with intralesional triamcinolone suspension 10 mg/mL. This should be done cautiously because skin atrophy may occur. Severe, widespread acute or subacute dermatitis is treated most effectively with prednisone, but long-term use must be avoided if possible. In adults, prednisone, starting at a dosage of 40–60 mg daily and tapered over 2–4 weeks, is usually effective. Topical steroids may be added during the tapering period for recurrence of small areas of dermatitis. An alternative to prednisone is triamcinolone suspension at a dose of 40 mg intramuscularly, which has an effect for 3–6 weeks. Again, long-term administration should be avoided.

> Avoid the use of long-term systemic steroids because of systemic side-effects.

Astringent dressings (Domeboro) applied for 15 minutes twice daily are helpful in treating acute weeping dermatitis. For widespread dermatitis, baths have a soothing effect on the skin by reducing inflammation and oozing and by removing crust and scaling. Colloidal oatmeal or tar solution may be added to the bath water. Patients should soak in the bath for 15–20 minutes once or twice daily and then apply a topical steroid to the dermatitis *immediately* after towel drying.

Itching is a prominent component of dermatitis and must be reduced to prevent scratching. Antihistamines, such as hydroxyzine, cetirizine, or diphenhydramine, can be used, particularly at bedtime. However, the use of antihistamines to reduce pruritus is largely unproven. Only sedating antihistamines may be effective for itching that interferes with sleep. The nonsedating antihistamines, unfortunately, are not effective in reducing pruritus. An alternative oral antipruritic is gabapentin.

Secondary bacterial infections with *S. aureus* often complicate dermatitis, in which case a course of dicloxacillin or cephalexin for 7 days is indicated. Penicillin is *not* prescribed because *S. aureus* is usually resistant to this antibiotic. For methicillin-resistant *S. aureus*, trimethoprim–sulfamethoxazole or doxycycline are the preferred choices. Nasal and skin disinfection with Polysporin ointment and bleach baths, respectively, can be implemented. Impetiginized eczema has yellow crusting, purulent weeping, and pustules.

UV light can decrease inflammation and itching. Tanning in a salon or more intense light in a dermatologist's office with narrow-band UVB (nUVB) two to three times a week can be quite helpful.

Immunomodulants, dupilumab (Dupixent) or tralokinumab (Adbry), are safe and effective, particularly if there is a history suggestive of sensitive skin/atopic dermatitis.

Systemic immunosuppressants such as mycophenolate mofetil, azathioprine, cyclosporine, methotrexate, and JAK inhibitors can be considered as steroid-sparing agents.

THERAPY FOR ESSENTIAL DERMATITIS

Initial

Topical Steroids—Cream, Ointment, Solution, Lotion, Foam

- Hydrocortisone 1% (lowest potency)
- Triamcinolone 0.1% (medium potency)
- Fluocinonide 0.05% (high potency)
- Clobetasol 0.05% (super potent)

Antihistamines

- Hydroxyzine: 10–25 mg q.i.d.; syrup, 10 mg/5 mL—2 mg/kg daily in four divided doses
- Diphenhydramine: 25–50 mg q.i.d.; elixir, 12.5 mg/5 mL—5 mg/kg daily in four divided doses
- Cetirizine: 10 mg daily or b.i.d.

Alternative

Intralesional Steroid

- Triamcinolone suspension 10 mg/mL

Systemic Steroid

- Prednisone: 1 mg/kg or 40–60 mg daily in adults tapered over 2–3 weeks
- Triamcinolone suspension 40 mg/mL: 1 mL IM

Macrolide Immunosuppressants
- Tacrolimus ointment 0.03% and 0.1%
- Pimecrolimus cream 1%

Baths and Compresses
- Oatmeal
- Tar
- Aluminum acetate
- Bleach: ¼–½ cup of bleach in ½ tub of water

Antibiotics if Secondary Infection
- Dicloxacillin: 500 mg b.i.d.
- Erythromycin: 500 mg b.i.d.
- Cephalexin: 500 mg b.i.d.; suspension, 250 mg/5 mL—25–50 mg/kg daily in divided doses
- Trimethoprim–sulfamethoxazole DS b.i.d., suspension, 1 mL/kg/d b.i.d.
- Doxycycline 100 mg b.i.d.
- Polysporin ointment

Antipruritic
- Gabapentin: 100–300 mg q.h.s. and t.i.d. as necessary

UV light
- Tanning salon
- nUVB

Systemic Immunomodulators
- Dupilumab, tralokinumab

Systemic Immunosuppressants
- Mycophenolate mofetil, azathioprine, cyclosporine, methotrexate, JAK inhibitors

Pathogenesis

The cause of essential dermatitis is unknown. Scratching results in histamine release, which causes more itching, more dermatitis, and a chronic, self-perpetuating eruption.

LICHEN SIMPLEX CHRONICUS (CHRONIC DERMATITIS)

KEY POINTS

1. Localized chronic dermatitis from scratching.
2. Goal is to break itch–scratch–itch cycle.
3. Occluded topical steroids may help.

Definition

Lichen simplex chronicus (also called "neurodermatitis") is a chronic eczematous eruption of the skin that is the result of scratching (Fig. 8.13). Pruritus precedes the scratching and may be precipitated by frustration, depression, and stress. The scratching then causes the lichenification and further itching, resulting in an "itch–scratch–itch" cycle that perpetuates the process.

Incidence

Of all new patients seen in the authors' clinic, 0.8% have presented with lichen simplex chronicus.

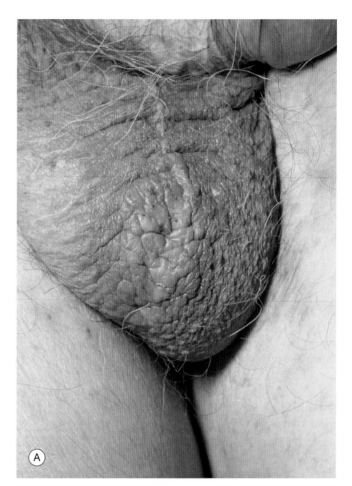

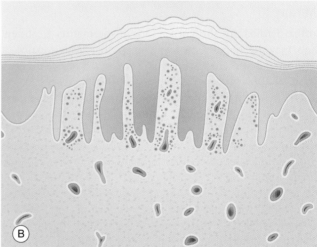

Fig. 8.13 **Lichen simplex chronicus**. (A) Lichenified, pink plaque. (B) Epidermis—thickened. Dermis—perivascular inflammation.

History

Some patients with lichen simplex chronicus have a history of emotional or psychiatric conditions. However, for most, it is simply a nervous habit. Preceding the eruption, the patient has a pruritic area of skin that is scratched, producing a plaque of chronic dermatitis.

Itching typically precedes the rash of lichen simplex chronicus.

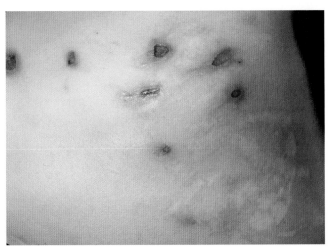

Fig. 8.14 Habitual (neurotic) excoriations—linear white scars and red, dug-out excoriations.

Physical Examination

The patient may appear anxious and may talk with pressured speech. There may be little insight into the cause of the eruption. The lichenified plaque always occurs within reach of scratching fingers.

Differential Diagnosis

The diagnosis of lichen simplex chronicus is usually obvious in patients who have a localized itching plaque of chronic dermatitis. *Chronic contact dermatitis* should be considered from a topical medicine used to treat the symptoms. Several more serious "psychodermatoses" are habitual (neurotic) excoriations, factitious dermatitis, and delusions of parasitosis.

> Types of "psychodermatoses":
> 1. Lichen simplex chronicus
> 2. Habitual (neurotic) excoriations
> 3. Factitious dermatitis
> 4. Delusions of parasitosis

Habitual (neurotic) excoriations (Fig. 8.14) are characterized by linear, "dug-out" lesions that typically spare the upper midback, where scratching fingers cannot reach. This condition appears to be more common in women and can start in teenage years.

Factitial dermatitis is a self-inflicted injury of the skin that presents as a bizarre eruption (often ulcerated) with linear and geometric outlines. The patient's history is vague and unclear. The diagnosis is made when the clinician has a high index of suspicion in a patient who has apparent secondary gain from perpetuating the condition.

Delusions of parasitosis occur in disturbed or anxious, often eccentric individuals. This disorder begins as intractable pruritus with a crawling sensation in the skin. The patients are convinced that they are harboring parasites and usually bring "specimens" to prove infestation. These bits of material or skin must be examined to rule out a true infestation and to assure the patient of your interest in the problem. More than half of these patients have no visible skin lesions. Those with active lesions have excoriated, crusted papules secondary to picking. Illicit drug addiction should also be ruled out.

> ### DIFFERENTIAL DIAGNOSIS OF LICHEN SIMPLEX CHRONICUS
> - Chronic contact dermatitis

Laboratory and Biopsy

The biopsy in lichen simplex chronicus is nonspecific, showing only chronic dermatitis (Fig. 8.13B).

Therapy

Treatment may be difficult, particularly if the patient has poor insight concerning the nature and cause of the eruption. Topical steroids under occlusion, which protect the area from scratching fingers, and intralesional triamcinolone suspension 10 mg/mL are helpful. Antipsychotics and antidepressants have a role in treating underlying emotional difficulties if such conditions are present.

> ### THERAPY FOR LICHEN SIMPLEX CHRONICUS
> **Initial**
> - Steroids
>   - Topical under occlusion
>   - Intralesional—triamcinolone suspension: 10 mg/mL
> - Emotional support
>
> **Alternative**
> - Antipsychotics and antidepressants

Course and Complications

Lichen simplex chronicus is a chronic, waxing, and waning problem that accompanies the mood changes of the patient.

SEBORRHEIC DERMATITIS

> ### KEY POINTS
> 1. Face and scalp most commonly involved
> 2. Treat with antiyeast and antiinflammatory agents
> 3. Check HIV status in severe cases

Definition

Seborrheic dermatitis is a chronic, superficial, inflammatory process affecting the hairy regions of the body, especially the scalp, eyebrows, and face (Fig. 8.15). Its cause is thought to be an inflammatory reaction to the *Malassezia* yeast (formerly *Pityrosporum ovale*). Dandruff is scaling of the scalp without inflammation.

> *Malassezia yeast* may contribute to the cause of seborrheic dermatitis.

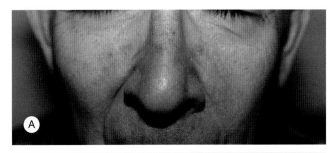

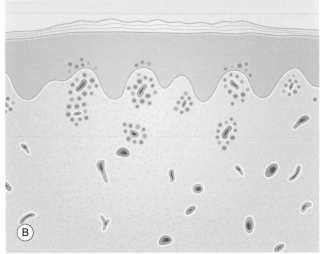

Fig. 8.15 Seborrheic dermatitis. (A) Pink, slightly scaling patches. (B) Epidermis—hyperkeratosis. Dermis—perivascular inflammation.

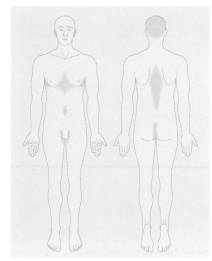

Fig. 8.16 Distribution of seborrheic dermatitis.

Incidence

Seborrheic dermatitis is a common problem affecting 3%–5% of the healthy population and may be higher in African Americans, although it is thought to be an underreported condition and true incidence is likely much higher.

History

The occurrence of seborrheic dermatitis parallels the increased sebaceous gland activity occurring in infancy and after puberty. It has a waxing and waning course with a variable amount of pruritus. It has been associated with Parkinson disease and AIDS, especially when it comes on abruptly. Approximately one-third of patients with AIDS and AIDS-related complex have seborrheic dermatitis. In Black patients, especially in the United States, seborrheic dermatitis is often normalized because it is so common.

Physical Examination

Seborrheic dermatitis has a predilection for the hairy regions of the skin, where sebaceous glands are numerous (Fig. 8.16). These regions are the scalp, eyebrows, eyelids, nasolabial creases, ears, chest, intertriginous areas, axilla, groin, buttocks, and inframammary folds. The rash is bilateral and symmetrically distributed. In its mildest form, dandruff, one sees fine, white scale without erythema. The patches and plaques of seborrheic dermatitis are characterized by indistinct margins, mild-to-moderate erythema, and yellowish, greasy scaling. It is uncommon for hair loss to result from seborrheic dermatitis; however,

it can happen more frequently in the Black community due to various hair styling and washing practices.

Differential Diagnosis

The differential diagnosis of seborrheic dermatitis includes atopic dermatitis, psoriasis, tinea capitis, Langerhans cell histiocytosis, lupus erythematosus, rosacea, and perioral dermatitis. The distinction between *seborrheic dermatitis* and *atopic dermatitis* in infancy is often difficult; so, many clinicians use the term "infantile eczema." When the dermatitis involves solely the diaper area and axillae, a diagnosis of seborrheic dermatitis is favored. Lesions on the forearms and shins favor the diagnosis of atopic dermatitis. *Psoriasis* may also enter into the differential diagnosis. Psoriasis limited to the scalp may be impossible to differentiate from seborrheic dermatitis. Involvement of nails, knees, and elbows favors the diagnosis of psoriasis. *Tinea capitis* should be considered in the differential diagnosis of seborrheic dermatitis, especially when the usual antiseborrheic agents have failed, when the patient has hair loss, and when the patient is Black and living in an underserved area. *Otitis externa* is not usually caused by a fungal infection but rather is a manifestation of seborrheic dermatitis. *Langerhans cell histiocytosis*, an uncommon Langerhans cell neoplasm, may appear as a seborrheic dermatitis-like eruption. The occurrence of petechiae and the failure of standard therapy should make one suspect this is cancer and obtain a skin biopsy. Facial involvement with seborrheic dermatitis may mimic lupus erythematosus or rosacea. *Lupus erythematosus* lacks yellowish, greasy scales and generally does not involve the eyebrows, as does seborrheic dermatitis. If in doubt, the history, physical examination, laboratory tests, and skin biopsy will rule out lupus. *Rosacea* has inflammatory papules and pustules not seen in seborrheic dermatitis. *Perioral dermatitis* is a hybrid of acneiform papules and pustules plus eczematous patches surrounding the mouth and nares. When the dermatitis predominates, topical steroids are often prescribed, which cause steroid addiction to suppress the acneiform eruption that will flare badly when the steroid is discontinued.

Seborrheic dermatitis is the most common cause of a "butterfly" rash.

- Atopic dermatitis
- Psoriasis
- Tinea capitis
- Langerhans cell histiocytosis
- Lupus erythematosus
- Rosacea
- Perioral dermatitis

Laboratory and Biopsy

Seborrheic dermatitis is usually not examined by biopsy unless concern exists about the possibility of another disease such as Langerhans cell histiocytosis. The histopathologic changes in seborrheic dermatitis are those of dermatitis and therefore are nondiagnostic with reference to other eczematous conditions (Fig. 8.15B).

Therapy

Nonprescription antiseborrheic shampoos containing zinc pyrithione, selenium sulfide, or ketoconazole are the mainstay of treatment. The shampoo must be rubbed into the scalp and be allowed to sit for 3–5 minutes before rinsing, followed by the patient's normal washing routine. Patients with inflammatory seborrheic dermatitis that has not responded to shampoos benefit from a topical steroid in a vehicle of the patient's choice. High-potency steroids should be used sparingly, particularly on the face. Tacrolimus ointment 0.1% or pimecrolimus 1% cream can be used as steroid-sparing agents.

> High-potency topical steroids should be avoided in prolonged treatment of seborrheic dermatitis, especially on the face and intertriginous skin.

THERAPY FOR SEBORRHEIC DERMATITIS

Initial
- Shampoos—one, two, or three times per week to start, then once every 2–4 weeks for maintenance
  - Zinc pyrithione 1%
  - Selenium sulfide 1% or 2.5%
  - Ketoconazole 1% or 2%
- Hydrocortisone cream 1% or 2.5% b.i.d. as needed

Alternative
- Tacrolimus ointment 0.1% or pimecrolimus cream

Course and Complications

In infants, seborrheic dermatitis can be expected to remit after 6–8 months. In adults, the course is chronic and unpredictable. However, it is usually easily controlled with shampoos and topical hydrocortisone preparations. Rarely, it can cause widespread exfoliative dermatitis. In infants, the association of a seborrhea-like dermatitis with failure to thrive and diarrhea is called *Leiner disease*.

Pathogenesis

The pathogenesis of seborrheic dermatitis is thought to be an inflammatory reaction to the resident skin *Malassezia* yeast. This lipophilic yeast is normally found on the seborrheic regions of skin, and proliferation is believed to play a role in this disease. The most effective antiseborrheic shampoos have antifungal activity against these yeast organisms.

STASIS DERMATITIS

KEY POINTS
1. Eczematous patches or plaques overlying lower leg edema
2. Chronic and itchy
3. Treat venous hypertension with compression stockings

Definition

Stasis dermatitis is an eczematous eruption of the lower legs secondary to peripheral venous disease (Fig. 8.17). Venous incompetence causes increased hydrostatic pressure and capillary damage with extravasation of red blood cells and serum. In some patients, this condition causes an inflammatory eczematous process.

Incidence

Stasis dermatitis is a disease of adults, predominantly of middle and older age.

History

Patients have a history of a chronic, pruritic eruption of the lower legs preceded by edema and swelling. Patients with stasis dermatitis have often had thrombophlebitis.

Physical Examination

Varicose veins are often prominent, as is pitting edema of the lower leg. The peripheral pulses are intact. The involved skin has brownish hyperpigmentation, dull erythema, petechiae, thickened skin, scaling, or weeping. Any portion of the lower leg may be affected, but the predominant site is above the medial malleolus.

> Characteristics of stasis dermatitis:
> 1. Edema
> 2. Brown pigmentation
> 3. Petechiae
> 4. Subacute and chronic dermatitis

Differential Diagnosis

Contact dermatitis, superficial fungal infection, and *bacterial cellulitis* must be considered in the differential diagnosis of stasis dermatitis. The history of application of a topical preparation to the skin and KOH testing will help to differentiate the first two conditions from stasis dermatitis. Gram staining and bacterial culture from bacterial cellulitis may be helpful but are often negative. An acute onset with fever particularly favors bacterial cellulitis.

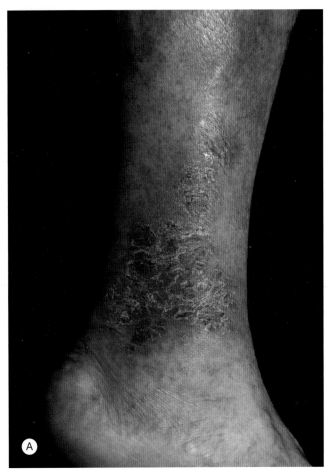

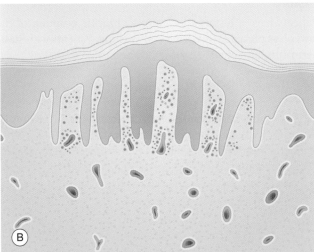

Fig. 8.17 Stasis dermatitis. (A) Dusky red, scaling, crusted, plaque. (B) Epidermis—hyperkeratosis, thickened. Dermis—perivascular inflammation.

DIFFERENTIAL DIAGNOSIS OF STASIS DERMATITIS

- Contact dermatitis
- Superficial fungal infection
- Bacterial cellulitis

Laboratory and Biopsy

The diagnosis of stasis dermatitis is usually made clinically. The biopsy shows a subacute or chronic dermatitis with hemosiderin, fibrosis, and dilated capillaries in the dermis (Fig. 8.17B). Vascular laboratory studies may be used to assess for peripheral vascular disease (see Chapter 19).

Therapy

The cornerstone of stasis dermatitis management is the prevention of venous stasis and edema. This is done by the use of compression stockings while the patient is ambulatory. Standing should be restricted, and patients who are obese should be placed on a weight reduction program. If this approach fails, bed rest with elevation of the legs is required. The dermatitis skin is treated with topical steroids and wet compresses (Domeboro), if oozing or crusting is present.

THERAPY FOR STASIS DERMATITIS

Initial
- Support stocking (knee high, 20–30 mm Hg pressure)
- Leg elevation
- Topical steroids
- Compresses if weeping

Alternative
- Unna boot
- Surgery

Course and Complications

Stasis dermatitis is a chronic and slowly progressive disease unless treated. Dusky erythema in areas of stasis dermatitis is the harbinger of leg ulceration.

Allergy to topical preparations may occur in 60% of patients with stasis dermatitis. The compromised epidermal barrier from stasis allows sensitization to occur more easily than in normal skin. Contact dermatitis can easily be misdiagnosed as a flare-up of stasis dermatitis. Topical antibiotics are particularly prone to cause allergic contact dermatitis.

> Avoid the prolonged use of topical antibiotics since allergic contact dermatitis is frequent.

Pathogenesis

Venous incompetence results in increased venous pressure of the lower legs. This increased hydrostatic pressure results in swelling and edema. Capillary proliferation and leakage of red blood cells and vascular fluids result in inflammation. If the condition is unchecked, fibrin deposition will occur around the capillaries, resulting in tissue hypoxia, sclerosis, and necrosis with ulceration.

UNCOMMON ECZEMATOUS-APPEARING DISEASES

Darier Disease

Darier disease, also known as *keratosis follicularis*, is a rare, auto-somal dominantly inherited genodermatosis. It is characterized by a chronic waxing and waning course beginning in child-hood and lasting a lifetime. The eruption (Fig. 8.18) involves the scalp, face, neck, trunk, and extremities with accentuation in the seborrheic areas. It has tan, pink, brown, rough-feeling papules that coalesce into large plaques that can become sec-ondarily infected, resulting in crusting and weeping. The skin biopsy is diagnostic, demonstrating epidermal suprabasilar clefts with acantholytic keratinocytes. Mutations in the *ATP2A2* gene result in markedly reduced calcium-dependent epidermal adhesion molecules.

Glucagonoma Syndrome

Glucagonoma syndrome is a multisystem disorder character-ized by migrating erythematous, scaling, and crusted papules, patches, and plaques along with the occasional vesicle and pustule (Fig. 8.19). The skin biopsy demonstrates characteris-tic superficial epidermal necrosis. Hence, this condition is also known by the descriptive name, *necrolytic migratory erythema*. The eruption is periorificial, flexural, and acral, with associated glossitis. It is caused by a pancreatic tumor of the islet alpha cell, which secretes raised plasma glucagon levels. Besides the skin findings, patients with this syndrome also have weight loss, anemia, diarrhea, and diabetes.

Langerhans Cell Histiocytosis

Langerhans cell histiocytosis is a neoplasm of Langerhans cells that affects the skin and extracutaneous organs, particularly bone, bone marrow, spleen, liver, lungs, central nervous system, and lymph nodes. It can be acute and disseminated, chronic and multifocal, and localized. The acute, disseminated form (Fig. 8.20) typically presents in infancy and involves the scalp, trunk, and intertriginous areas (recalcitrant diaper dermati-tis). There are tan, pink, sometimes hemorrhagic, papules, and

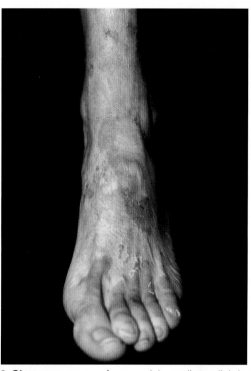

Fig. 8.19 Glucagonoma syndrome—pink, scaling, slightly crusted patches.

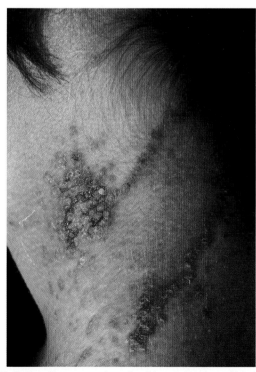

Fig. 8.18 Darier disease—red patch with annular crusted border.

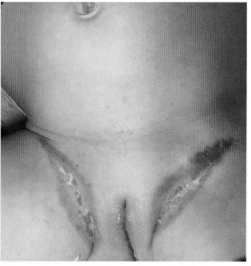

Fig. 8.20 Langerhans cell histiocytosis—red, slightly eroded patches.

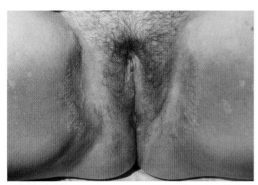

Fig. 8.21 **Lichen sclerosus**—red, slightly whitish, confluent macules and plaques.

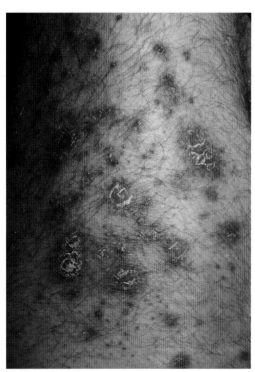

Fig. 8.22 **Pemphigus foliaceus**—red, slightly scaling papules and small plaques.

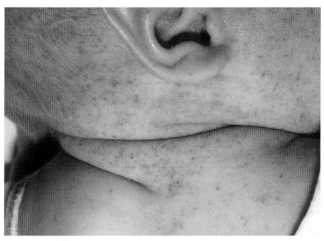

Fig. 8.23 **Wiskott–Aldrich syndrome**—diffuse pink and petechial papules and macules.

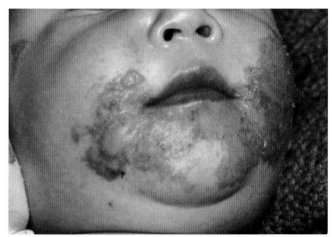

Fig. 8.24 **Zinc deficiency**—reddish perioral erosion.

scaling, slightly eroded, patches. The skin biopsy demonstrates a proliferation of Langerhans cells in the epidermis and dermis that stain with S-100 antibody and are seen on electron microscopy to contain Birbeck granules.

Lichen Sclerosus

Lichen sclerosus can initially be confused with a pruritic eczematous patch, especially in the anogenital region of females (Fig. 8.21). On close inspection, or with time, the typical ivory white papules and atrophic patches are seen (see Chapter 13).

Pemphigus Foliaceus

This rare, milder form of pemphigus affects the superficial epidermis, causing erythematous scaling with some crusting (Fig. 8.22), and a few flaccid bullae and erosions. Like pemphigus vulgaris (see Chapter 10), a skin biopsy with immunofluorescence is diagnostic. This reveals subcorneal/granular layer acantholysis with intercellular IgG staining.

Wiskott–Aldrich Syndrome

Wiskott–Aldrich syndrome is a rare X-linked recessive disorder that may appear like atopic dermatitis. Recurrent, severe infections suggest an immunodeficiency that is characterized by increased IgA and IgE levels, decreased IgM concentration, and impaired cell-mediated immunity. Petechiae (Fig. 8.23) and bleeding episodes are a manifestation of thrombocytopenia, as well as platelet dysfunction. Infection, bleeding, and lymphoreticular malignancy are causes of childhood death in these patients.

Zinc Deficiency

Zinc deficiency is an inherited (acrodermatitis enteropathica) or acquired (parenteral nutrition) condition characterized by perioral (Fig. 8.24), genital, and acral dermatitis plus diarrhea. It usually begins in infancy, with the diagnosis confirmed by low serum zinc levels. Essential fatty acid and biotin deficiencies have a similar dermatitis appearance.

SELF-ASSESSMENT

Case 1—Papulovesicular Rash (Fig. 8.25)
What Is Your Differential Diagnosis?

This acute eczematous eruption confined to the area beneath the dressing is typical of contact dermatitis. A less likely cause would be a fungal or bacterial infection since pustules are absent.

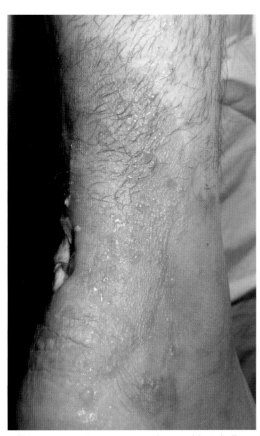

Fig. 8.25 This 40-year-old man was using povidone-iodine ointment dressings on a nonhealing wound. Two weeks after starting this therapy, he developed a markedly pruritic eruption under the dressing. The physical examination revealed a 3-cm necrotic ulcer with a surrounding erythematous, papulovesicular rash conforming to the rectangular area covered by the povidone-iodine dressing.

How Would You Treat This Patient?

The dermatitis cleared when the povidone-iodine dressings were replaced with saline compresses and a topical steroid cream.

How Would You Prove Your Diagnosis?

The patient had no history of iodine sensitivity. However, he had been applying the povidone-iodine dressing for 2 weeks, which is sufficient time to develop sensitivity to this compound. A patch test to 10% povidone-iodine solution was positive, confirming the diagnosis of allergic contact dermatitis.

IMPORTANT POINTS

1. Topical medicaments are an important cause of allergic contact dermatitis and should be suspected when an eczematous eruption occurs in areas that conform to application of the medication.
2. Avoidance of the allergen is the treatment of choice. Topical steroids hasten the resolution of allergic contact dermatitis.
3. Patch testing confirms the diagnosis of allergic contact dermatitis.

9

Scaling, Papules, Plaques, and Patches

CHAPTER CONTENTS

Algorithm of scaling rashes

Scaling Papules, Plaques, and Patches

INFECTIOUS

Fungal Infections
Pityriasis Rosea
Secondary Syphilis

NONINFECTIOUS

Discoid Lupus Erythematosus
Mycosis Fungoides
Psoriasis

Uncommon

Erythema Annulare Centrifugum

Ichthyosis

Parapsoriasis

Pityriasis Rubra Pilaris

ABSTRACT

Scale is the common characteristic of the diseases discussed in this chapter. Scaling disorders have also been called papulosquamous (squamous means scaly) diseases. As previously emphasized, *scale* represents thickened stratum corneum and is to be distinguished from *crust*, which represents the dried surface fluid, as found in the vesicular and pustular disorders. The elevation of scaling papules and plaques results from thickening of the epidermis (acanthosis) or underlying dermal inflammation. A *patch* is a scaling macule. It is flat because it has no epidermal thickening (the epidermis may even be atrophic) and little dermal inflammation.

KEY POINTS

1. Scaling disorders have multiple causes—immunologic, infectious, and neoplastic.
2. Borders are usually distinct, in contrast to eczema.
3. Scaling (stratum corneum) is not crusting (dried fluids and blood).

The papulosquamous disorders have diverse causes, as seen in Table 9.1. The lesions, in addition to being scaly, are sharply demarcated. The latter feature helps to distinguish them from scaling lesions of eczematous dermatitis, in which the borders are usually indistinct. Exceptions are *nummular (coin-shaped)*

TABLE 9.1 Scaling Papules, Plaques, and Patches[a]

	Frequency (%)[b]	Etiology	Physical Examination		Differential Diagnosis	Laboratory Tests
			Appearance of Lesions	Characteristic Distribution		
Lupus, discoid	0.2	Autoimmune	Red to *purplish* papules and plaques with adherent scale and *follicular plugging*; older lesions atrophic	Sun-exposed areas favored	Psoriasis Lichen planus Subacute cutaneous lupus erythematosus	Biopsy with immunofluorescence; antinuclear antibodies
Fungus	2.5	Infection (dermatophyte)	*Annular* patches with elevated borders surmounted by scale	Anywhere	See Table 9.2	Potassium hydroxide preparation; fungal culture
Mycosis fungoides	0.2	Neoplastic (lymphoma)	*Yellowish-red* or *violaceous*, irregularly shaped patches and plaques with only slight scale	*Asymmetric*; girdle area is often the first area involved	Psoriasis Parapsoriasis Eczema Erythroderma	Biopsy
Pityriasis rosea	1.1	Human herpesvirus 6 and 7	Tannish-pink *oval* papules and patches with delicate *collarette of scale*; rash preceded by *herald patch*	"Christmas tree" pattern on trunk; spares face and distal extremities	Secondary syphilis Tinea corporis Lichen planus Pityriasis lichenoides chronica Guttate psoriasis	
Psoriasis	5.2	Unknown	Erythematous plaques with *silvery scales*	Anywhere; scalp, elbows, knees, and *intergluteal cleft* are favored locations; nails are often involved	Seborrheic dermatitis Tinea cruris Candidiasis Intertrigo Pityriasis rosea Tinea corporis Dermatitis T-cell cutaneous lymphoma Onychomycosis	
Secondary syphilis	<0.1	Infection (spirochete)	*Red-brown* or *copper-colored* scaling papules and plaques, sometimes annular in shape	Generalized; *palms* and *soles* often included; mucous membranes sometimes involved	Pityriasis rosea Viral exanthem Drug eruption Sarcoidosis	Serologic test for syphilis

[a]See also discussions of seborrheic dermatitis (Chapter 8), lichen planus (Chapter 11), and tinea versicolor (Chapter 13).
[b]Percentage of new dermatology patients with this diagnosis seen in the Hershey Medical Center Dermatology Clinic, Hershey, Pennsylvania.

eczema, which can resemble tinea corporis, and *seborrheic dermatitis*, which in the scalp can be confused with psoriasis and on the chest can be confused with tinea corporis. *Lichen planus* is often also included in the papulosquamous disorders, but usually the scale is not readily evident, so we have designated this disease as a papular disorder (see Chapter 11). *Tinea versicolor* can appear as finely scaling patches, but patients more often present with lesions that appear as white spots; hence, this disease is discussed in Chapter 13.

The diagnostic approach to scaling diseases should include consideration of the distribution of the lesions and sometimes also the presence or absence of nail and mucous membrane involvement. Of the laboratory tests that are listed, the one that should be done most frequently is a potassium hydroxide (KOH) preparation of the scale to look for fungal elements. The general rule for scaling rashes of uncertain etiology is: "If it scales, scrape it!"

> In papulosquamous lesions, the borders are sharply demarcated; in eczematous lesions, they are usually not.

> For rashes of uncertain etiology, "If it scales, scrape it!"

DISCOID LUPUS ERYTHEMATOSUS

KEY POINTS

1. Atrophic, scaling, scarring plaques with hyperpigmented borders in sun-exposed areas.
2. A small proportion have systemic lupus erythematosus (SLE).
3. Skin biopsy is diagnostic.

Definition

Discoid lupus erythematosus (DLE) is one of several rashes that can occur in lupus. DLE is a rash that scales and scars. Immunoglobulins are found in the skin in this autoimmune disease. Clinically, the lesions appear as disk-shaped plaques surmounted by a white adherent scale that also involves the hair follicles. DLE may be limited to the skin, or it may be one of the manifestations of SLE.

> DLE may be limited to the skin or may be a manifestation of SLE.

Incidence

The disease affects primarily young and middle-aged adults and is two to three times more common in females than males. It is uncommon, but the exact incidence in the general population is not known. Of all the new patients seen in the authors' dermatology clinic, 2 per 1000 were seen for DLE.

History

The eruption may be slightly pruritic but is more often asymptomatic. Patients may give a history of exacerbations after exposure to sunlight. In patients with DLE, a history should be taken for symptoms of possible SLE, including photosensitivity, hair loss, nasal and oral ulcerations, Raynaud phenomenon, arthritis, and other extracutaneous organs.

Physical Examination

The earliest lesion is a purplish-red plaque, which accumulates scale as it matures. The scale is white and usually cohesive, so it can often be removed in one piece. When this is done, the underside of the scale may show small, spiny projections. These have been called "carpet tacks," and they represent the keratinous plugs that had been present in dilated hair follicles. The oldest lesions appear as *depressed*, atrophic plaques, often with pigmentary change, usually hypopigmentation in the center with a hyperpigmented rim (Fig. 9.1).

The distribution of the DLE lesion favors sun-exposed areas (i.e., the face, neck, upper trunk, and dorsal arms). An occasional patient has widespread cutaneous involvement. Erosions in the oral cavity, particularly of the palate, are occasionally found in patients with DLE. The scalp is frequently involved with scarring alopecia (see Chapter 20).

Differential Diagnosis

Psoriasis may be the most common misdiagnosis. The finding of atrophy helps to differentiate the two. *Lichen planus* lesions are

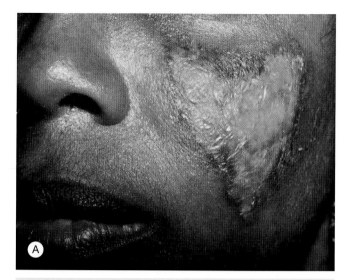

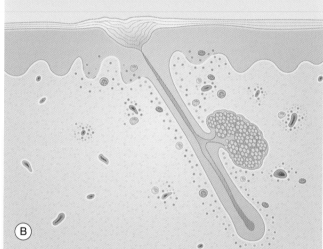

Fig. 9.1 Discoid lupus erythematosus. (A) Red and whitish, scaling, atrophic plaque with hyperpigmented (darker brown) border. (B) Epidermis—hyperkeratosis with follicular plugging; vacuolar degeneration of the basal cell layer. Dermis—perivascular and periappendageal inflammatory cell infiltration.

also purplish, but they are usually small (papular), have scant scale, and do not result in depressed scars. The scaling patches and plaques that occur in *subacute cutaneous lupus erythematosus* (SCLE) also do not scar; frequently they are annular and are often accompanied by circulating anticytoplasmic antibodies—anti-Ro (SSA) and anti-La (SSB). Superficial fungal infection, sarcoidosis, and granuloma faciale may be considered in the differential diagnosis and will be confirmed with a KOH or biopsy.

DIFFERENTIAL DIAGNOSIS OF DLE

- Psoriasis
- Lichen planus
- SCLE
- Fungal infection
- Sarcoidosis
- Granuloma faciale

Laboratory and Biopsy

Skin biopsy establishes the diagnosis (Fig. 9.1B). In addition to the history and physical examination, a laboratory screen for SLE should be done on all patients with DLE. This includes a complete blood cell count, a renal function panel, a urinalysis, and an antinuclear antibody (ANA) test. If the latter is positive, an anti-DNA antibody test should be ordered. Patients with DLE who have positive ANA tests or persistent complete blood cell count abnormalities are more likely to develop SLE subsequently.

> Patients with DLE should be screened for SLE with:
> 1. Complete blood cell count
> 2. Renal function panel
> 3. Urinalysis
> 4. Antinuclear antibody test

Therapy

Topical therapy is usually adequate. Steroids, applied topically or injected intralesionally, are used most often. Sun protection is important, and sunscreens that protect against both short ultraviolet B (UVB) and long ultraviolet A (UVA) light should be strongly recommended to all patients. Patients with extensive or recalcitrant disease sometimes require systemic therapy; antimalarials, such as chloroquine (Aralen) 250 mg daily or hydroxychloroquine (Plaquenil) 200–400 mg daily, are used most often. Patients receiving these antimalarial drugs should undergo ophthalmologic examination at baseline and then annually after 5 years of use, or yearly from the start if major risk factors are present. This is to monitor for the retinal toxicity that is rarely encountered with the dosages used in DLE. For patients with DLE not responding to the above measures, alternative systemic therapies, including retinoids (isotretinoin or acitretin), dapsone, thalidomide, azathioprine, mycophenolate mofetil, methotrexate, and oral gold, may be used.

THERAPY FOR CUTANEOUS LUPUS

Initial
- Topical steroids (e.g., clobetasol cream 0.05% b.i.d.)
- Sunscreens (Anthelios) and sun-protective clothing

Alternative
- Antimalarials (e.g., hydroxychloroquine 200 mg b.i.d., chloroquine 250 mg daily)
- Retinoids (e.g., isotretinoin, acitretin)
- Thalidomide
- Azathioprine
- Mycophenolate mofetil
- Methotrexate
- Dapsone
- Gold

Course and Complications

The course of the disease is chronic but, with therapy, usually controllable. New lesions may continue to appear over the course of years as old ones become inactive. Eventual remission occurs spontaneously in approximately 50% of patients. Scarring and postinflammatory hypopigmentation and hyperpigmentation are common and may result in disfigurement, particularly in Black patients. In the scalp, the scarring leads to permanent alopecia; if extensive, this can be a cosmetic problem. In patients presenting with only DLE lesions, the risk of subsequently developing SLE is 5%–10%.

> About 5%–10% of patients presenting with DLE subsequently develop SLE.

Pathogenesis

Lupus erythematosus has been classified as an autoimmune disease because of the autoantibodies found in the disease. In DLE, these are in the form of IgG and IgM deposited at the dermal–epidermal junction. The cause of this deposition and the role that these immunoglobulins play in the pathogenesis of the skin lesions are not clear. UV light has been implicated as a pathogenic factor. Circumstantial evidence for this includes the localization of lesions mainly in sun-exposed areas, the finding that many patients note that sun exposure exacerbates their skin disease and the experimental induction of skin lesions with UV light. A sequence of pathogenic events has been proposed as follows. UV light damages epidermal cells, releasing their nuclear antigens. These diffuse to the dermal–epidermal junction, where they combine with antibodies from the circulation, initiating an inflammatory reaction resulting ultimately in the clinical lesion.

T-cell dysregulation has also been implicated in the pathogenesis of cutaneous lupus. For example, increased activity of the Th2 subset of helper T cells has been found in lesional skin. The main function of these cells is to augment humoral immunity. Genetic predisposition to DLE is possible, but familial disease and association with specific HLA phenotypes have been reported more frequently with SLE than with DLE. Current evidence suggests that most patients with DLE have a genetically different disease from that in patients with SLE, a concept that accounts for the observation that most patients with DLE never develop SLE.

FUNGAL INFECTIONS

KEY POINTS
1. If it scales, consider scraping it for a KOH preparation.
2. Superficial fungi, dermatophytes, cause tinea infections.

Definition

These disorders result from infection of the skin by fungal organisms collectively called dermatophytes (*phyte* is the Greek word for plant). Various clinical lesions can result, but the most common are scaling, erythematous papules, plaques, and patches, which often have a serpiginous or worm-like border. The word *tinea* (Latin for worm) is used for these superficial fungal infections. It is followed by a qualifying term that

TABLE 9.2	**Fungal Infections**			
	Prevalence in General Population (Rate per 1000)[a]	**Location**	**Clinical Appearance**	**Differential Diagnosis**
Tinea capitis[b]		Scalp	Round, scaling area of alopecia Diffuse scaling Red, boggy, swollen area with pustules (kerion)	Alopecia areata Seborrheic dermatitis Bacterial infection
Tinea corporis		Body	Annular, "ringworm"	Nummular eczema Pityriasis rosea (herald patch) Psoriasis Impetigo Erythema annulare centrifugum Granuloma annulare
Tinea cruris	7	Groin	Sharply demarcated area with elevated, scaling, serpiginous borders	Psoriasis Seborrheic dermatitis Intertrigo Candidiasis Erythrasma
Tinea faciale		Face	Slightly scaling, erythematous patches and plaques; border may not be well demarcated in all areas	Photodermatitis Lupus erythematosus Seborrheic dermatitis Contact dermatitis
Tinea manuum		Hand	Diffuse dry scaling, usually on only one palm	Contact dermatitis Xerosis Psoriasis
Tinea pedis	39	Feet	Interdigital maceration Diffuse scaling on soles and sides of feet (moccasin) Vesicles and pustules on instep	Maceration Xerosis (dry skin) Contact dermatitis Dyshidrotic eczema Pustular psoriasis
Tinea unguium (onychomycosis)[c]	22	Nails	Subungual debris with separation from the nail bed	Psoriasis Trauma
Tinea versicolor[d]	8	Trunk	White, tan, or pink patches with fine desquamating scale	Vitiligo (white) Seborrheic dermatitis (tan or pink)

[a]Data from the US National Health Survey, 1978.
[b]See Chapter 20.
[c]See Chapter 21.
[d]See Chapter 13.

denotes the location of the infection on the body. For example, *tinea capitis* is a fungal infection of the scalp, and *tinea pedis* is a dermatophyte infection of the feet. *Tinea versicolor* is the only exception; its name derives from the several shades of color that lesions may have in this disease.

Synonyms for fungal infection of the skin:
1. Dermatophytosis
2. Tinea
3. Ringworm

Incidence

Dermatophytic infections are common, in aggregate representing 2.5% of the authors' new patients. The incidence is higher in

warmer, more humid climates. Table 9.2 gives the prevalence of four of the more common skin infections in the general US population.

History

In most dermatophytic infections, the patient presents with a scaling rash. Pruritus is common and often the chief complaint. A history of exposure to infected persons or other mammals (e.g., dogs, cats, cattle) may be elicited.

Physical Examination

The physical findings and differential diagnosis vary with the different tineas. The findings in *tinea capitis* are discussed in Chapter 20, and those in *tinea unguium* are discussed in Chapter 21. Because *tinea versicolor* most often presents as white spots, it is discussed in Chapter 13. The physical findings and differential diagnosis of the remaining dermatophyte infections are considered below.

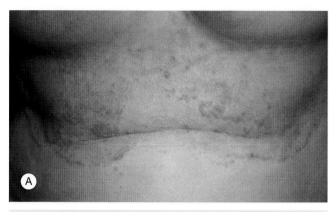

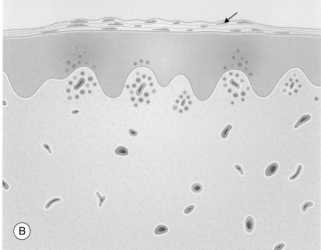

Fig. 9.2 (A) Tinea corporis—red, scaling patches with serpiginous borders. (B) Tinea. Epidermis—thickened stratum corneum infiltrated with fungal hyphae (*arrow*). Dermis—inflammation.

Tinea Corporis

> **KEY POINTS**
> 1. Annular patch with clear center and scaling, serpiginous border
> 2. Scrape the border scales for the KOH preparation

Tinea corporis is the classic "ringworm." Often, patients have a history of exposure to an infected animal such as a pet dog or cat.

Physical Examination

The typical lesion is annular, with an elevated, scaling border and a tendency for central clearing. One or several lesions may be present. In patients predisposed to chronic infection, the eruption may be widespread, and not all the lesions may be annular. In these instances, the finding of elevated serpiginous borders in some of the lesions is a helpful clue (Fig. 9.2).

Differential Diagnosis

The coin-shaped lesions of *nummular eczema* are usually multiple and located on the extremities. They are often mistaken by the patient, and sometimes by the physician, as ringworm. In nummular eczema, one usually sees no central clearing, and the KOH preparation is negative.

Pityriasis rosea starts with a single herald patch, which is frequently mistaken for tinea. The correct diagnosis usually

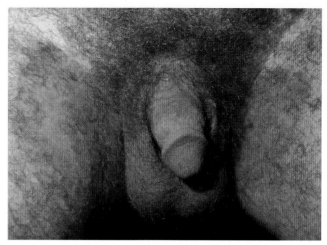

Fig. 9.3 **Tinea cruris**—sharply marginated oval red groin patches. Note typical sparing of the penis and scrotum.

becomes evident when the generalized eruption develops within a few weeks. Although occasionally annular, lesions of *psoriasis* are usually thicker and more scaly than those of fungal infections. More typical lesions of psoriasis are also usually found, and, of course, the KOH examination is negative.

Uncommonly, *impetigo* presents in an annular configuration (see Fig. 3.8). The finding of vesicles, pustules, and crusts in annular lesions should lead one to suspect a bacterial, rather than fungal, cause.

Erythema annulare centrifugum and *granuloma annulare* (see Chapter 18) are two uncommon diseases that may be confused with ringworm. Clinically, the differences are that in erythema annulare centrifugum, the scale is inside the elevated border and the KOH preparation is negative. In granuloma annulare, the border is more indurated and is *not* scaling. A skin biopsy is helpful in confirming the diagnosis of these two disorders. Both conditions are idiopathic and are usually localized but occasionally generalized. The generalized form of erythema annulare centrifugum is called *erythema gyratum repens*, a rare condition that is almost always associated with an internal malignant disease. Generalized granuloma annulare is sometimes associated with diabetes mellitus.

> **DIFFERENTIAL DIAGNOSIS OF TINEA CORPORIS**
> - Nummular eczema
> - Pityriasis rosea
> - Psoriasis
> - Impetigo
> - Erythema annulare centrifugum
> - Granuloma annulare

Tinea Cruris

> **KEY POINTS**
> 1. Erythematous patch with a serpiginous scaling border.
> 2. Scrotum and penis are not involved.

A groin rash has several common causes (Fig. 9.3); dermatophytic infection is one. Patients with tinea cruris (jock itch) frequently also have tinea pedis (athlete's foot). The perspiration that occurs with exercise is probably the most common predisposing denominator in these "athletic" rashes.

Physical Examination

Dermatophytic infection in the groin may not appear as an annular lesion, but the border is elevated, serpiginous, and scaling. Often, lesions have a tendency for central clearing. The scrotum and penis are seldom involved.

Differential Diagnosis

In addition to dermatophytic infection, there are two other common causes of a groin rash. *Candidiasis* appears as a bright, intensely erythematous (beefy red) eruption with poorly defined borders and satellite papules and pustules. The scrotum is often affected. *Intertrigo* represents simple irritant dermatitis, most often found in obese patients in whom moisture accumulates between skin folds in the inguinal area or other body folds and, along with friction, causes skin irritation. The eruption is not as red as that of candidiasis and not as sharply demarcated as tinea cruris. The KOH preparation is positive in tinea cruris and candidiasis but negative in intertrigo. On occasion intertrigo can be complicated by a candidal infection.

> Three major causes of a groin rash:
> 1. Tinea cruris
> 2. Candidiasis
> 3. Intertrigo

Less often, *psoriasis* and *seborrheic dermatitis* selectively affect the groin. *Erythrasma* is an uncommon disease of intertriginous skin caused by *Corynebacterium minutissimum*. Clinically, it appears as a velvety patch with fine scale that, under Wood's light examination, fluoresces a diagnostic coral pink.

DIFFERENTIAL DIAGNOSIS OF TINEA CRURIS

- Candidiasis
- Intertrigo
- Psoriasis
- Seborrheic dermatitis
- Erythrasma

Tinea Faciale

KEY POINTS
1. Look for a sharp serpiginous border
2. When in doubt, do a KOH preparation

This is an uncommon but often missed fungal infection of the skin (Fig. 9.4).

Physical Examination

Tinea faciale appears as an erythematous, usually asymmetric, eruption on the face. An annular pattern is frequently not evident, but usually at least some of the borders are well demarcated and are often serpiginous, providing a clue to the fungal origin. Pustules may be present and may further obscure the clinical diagnosis (Fig. 9.5).

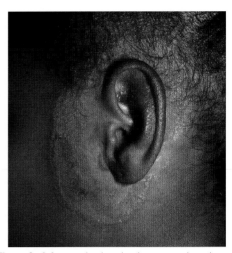

Fig. 9.4 Tinea faciale—oval, sharply demarcated, red, and hypopigmented (whitish) patch with slightly scaling inflammatory border and cleared center.

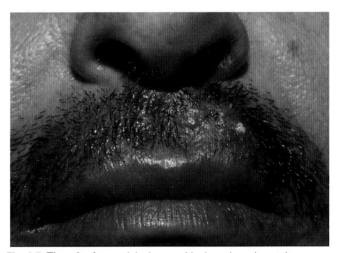

Fig. 9.5 Tinea barbae—pink plaque with alopecia and pustule.

Differential Diagnosis

The lesions in *seborrheic dermatitis* are usually symmetric and are not well demarcated.

Rashes resulting from sunlight (*photodermatitis*) are distinguished by their distribution, which is usually symmetric, sparing areas that are relatively protected from the sun, such as the eyelids and under the chin. *Contact dermatitis* may also be confused with tinea faciale.

Occasionally, tinea faciale can appear as a butterfly rash, resembling that of *lupus erythematosus*. The finding of sharp serpiginous borders should heighten the suspicion of a fungal origin. However, for any of these conditions, if there is scale and any doubt, scrape it!

DIFFERENTIAL DIAGNOSIS OF TINEA FACIALE

- Seborrheic dermatitis
- Photodermatitis
- Contact dermatitis
- Lupus erythematosus

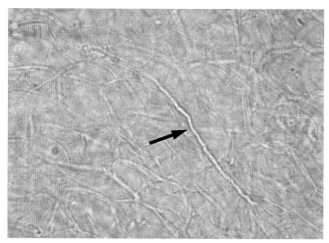

Fig. 9.6 **Tinea**—positive potassium hydroxide examination showing hyphae (*arrow*).

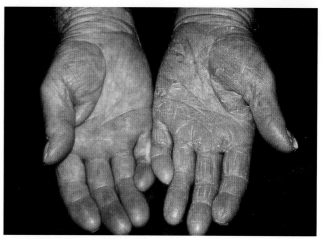

Fig. 9.7 **Tinea manuum**—diffuse scaling faint pink patch of only one (left) hand in a patient with tinea pedis—the "one hand, two feet" syndrome.

Laboratory Tests

The single most important laboratory test for all of these fungal infections is the KOH preparation (Fig. 9.6). The details of this procedure are outlined in Chapter 3. The finding of hyphae on a KOH preparation is diagnostic of a dermatophytic infection, whereas a candidal infection will have hyphae and oval yeast on microscopic examination. Usually, the clinical presentation distinguishes between the two, with *Candida* having satellite pustules around a beefy red patch and tinea having an annulare scaling patch with a clear center.

If desired, one can also obtain scales for fungal culture. Cultures distinguish between candidal and dermatophytic infections and are sometimes helpful in patients in whom dermatophytic infections are suspected, but the KOH examination is negative.

A skin biopsy is not indicated. If a biopsy is done to rule out other disorders, the dermatopathologist may miss the fungal elements in the stratum corneum (Fig. 9.2B). Contrary to some misconceptions, a Wood's light (black light) is of no help in diagnosing dermatophytic infection of the skin. A Wood's light fluoresces infected scalp hairs in one type of tinea capitis, but infected skin does not show fluorescence.

Tinea Manuum

KEY POINTS

1. One hand, two feet are typically involved.
2. For the hand with the "dry" scaling unilateral palm, do a KOH preparation.

Dermatophytic infection of the palm is uncommon but not rare. It virtually always occurs in a patient who has coexisting tinea pedis.

Physical Examination

Typically, tinea manuum involves only one hand, resulting in the "one hand, two feet" syndrome (Fig. 9.7). It appears as diffuse scaling of the palmar surface, much like the plantar scaling type of tinea pedis. The border on the wrist side is often sharply demarcated.

Differential Diagnosis

Chronic contact dermatitis and dry skin or *xerosis* can also appear as chronic scaling of the palms. However, these conditions usually involve both palms, and the border is generally not well demarcated.

Psoriasis can affect the palms with sharply demarcated scaling plaques. Usually, these plaques are bilateral and are more elevated and inflamed than in tinea manuum; often, lesions of psoriasis elsewhere on the body support the diagnosis. KOH preparation is necessary in cases of doubt.

DIFFERENTIAL DIAGNOSIS OF TINEA MANUUM

- Contact dermatitis
- Xerosis
- Psoriasis

Tinea Pedis

KEY POINTS

1. Interdigital, diffuse, plantar scaling, and vesiculopustular forms
2. Onychomycosis (nail tinea) occurs frequently with tinea pedis

As noted in Table 9.2, the feet are most often involved with dermatophytic infection. Tinea pedis affects approximately 4% of the general population and occurs in three forms, each of which has a different appearance.

Physical Examination

Interdigital tinea pedis appears as a macerated scaling process between the toes. It is most common in patients with sweaty feet.

Diffuse plantar scaling is extremely common in older patients. It is usually asymptomatic. The skin of the feet appears dry, with diffuse scaling on the soles extending onto the sides of the feet (Fig. 9.8A). The border may or may not be sharply demarcated. The distribution of this process on the feet has been likened to a "moccasin." Often, patients have accompanying nail involvement.

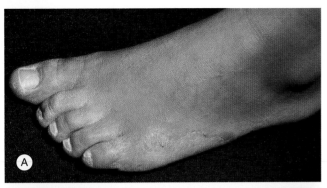

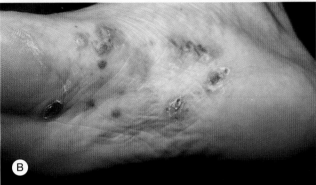

Fig. 9.8 Tinea pedis. (A) Diffuse plantar scaling faint pink and hypopigmented patch, which extends onto the side of the foot and is usually associated with onychomycosis. (B) Acute vesiculopustular form.

The *vesiculopustular* form (Fig. 9.8B) is the least common type of tinea pedis and the one that is most often misdiagnosed. Vesicles and pustules on the instep of the feet should lead to suspicion of this type of tinea pedis. A KOH preparation of the roof of the vesicle or pustule reveals fungal hyphae.

Differential Diagnosis

Patients with sweaty feet (hyperhidrosis) may develop *maceration* between the toes, simply as a result of retained moisture in these occluded areas. This then provides a good culture medium for the fungus to become secondarily involved. Clinically, simple maceration may be indistinguishable from interdigital tinea pedis. A KOH preparation enables one to diagnose fungal infection, but in both situations, measures to decrease sweating are also important.

Diffuse plantar scaling is most often passed off as *dry skin*. *Contact dermatitis* and *dyshidrotic eczema* are the two diseases most often confused with the vesiculopustular type of tinea pedis. In contact dermatitis and dyshidrotic eczema, however, the vesicles are usually smaller and rarely progress to pustules. *Pustular psoriasis* of the palms and soles is an uncommon disease that can also be confused with vesiculopustular tinea pedis. If doubt exists, a KOH preparation should be performed.

DIFFERENTIAL DIAGNOSIS OF TINEA PEDIS

- Maceration
- Xerosis
- Contact dermatitis
- Dyshidrotic eczema
- Pustular psoriasis

Therapy

For dermatophyte infections involving limited areas, the authors recommend one of the over-the-counter creams, which include clotrimazole (Lotrimin), miconazole (Micatin), and terbinafine (Lamisil). The patient is instructed to apply the topical antifungal to the infected area until the skin is clinically clear and then to apply it for 1–2 weeks longer in the hope of preventing recurrence.

Dermatophytes are unresponsive to nystatin.

Chronic *tinea pedis* is notoriously refractory to curative therapy, particularly when the patient has nail involvement. For suppressive therapy, an antifungal powder, such as miconazole powder (Zeasorb), should be used daily on an indefinite basis after the skin has been clinically cleared.

For patients with a disease that is either widespread or resistant to topical measures, systemic therapy is indicated. Systemic treatment is also most effective for treating scalp and nail infections. Oral systemic agents include griseofulvin, itraconazole (Sporanox), fluconazole (Diflucan), and terbinafine (Lamisil). For dermatophytic infection, griseofulvin was the standard treatment. Adult patients are treated with either microsized griseofulvin (e.g., Fulvicin U/F), 500 mg twice daily, or ultramicrosized griseofulvin (e.g., Gris-PEG), 250 mg twice daily for 4–6 weeks. The newer systemic antifungals, however, can achieve better results with shorter courses of treatment (and fewer side-effects). For example, most dermatophyte infections of the skin can be treated with a 1–2 week course of terbinafine (250 mg daily). Doses for children are adjusted downward according to body weight.

Initial therapy:
1. Limited skin involvement—topical antifungals
2. Hair, nails, and extensive skin involvement—systemic therapy

---

Treatment of *tinea capitis* requires 4–8 weeks of systemic therapy. Adjunctive twice-weekly use of a dandruff shampoo containing selenium sulfide (Selsun) can shorten the time course of this infection.

THERAPY FOR DERMATOPHYTE INFECTIONS

Initial (for Limited Skin Disease)
- Azoles—miconazole 2% or clotrimazole 1% cream, gel, spray, or powder b.i.d.
- Allylamines—terbinafine 1% cream or gel daily

Alternative (for Scalp, Nails, or Extensive Skin Involvement)
- Griseofulvin—microsize: 20 mg/kg daily, 250 mg twice a day
- Terbinafine:
  - <20 kg: 62.5 mg daily
  - 20–40 kg: 125 mg daily
  - >40 kg: 250 mg daily

Course and Complications

Some acute dermatophytic infections resolve spontaneously. Even in these patients, however, the time course can be shortened by the use of the therapy mentioned above.

Complications are rare. Secondary bacterial infections are uncommon. Recognizing that fungal infections can produce pustules (particularly when hair follicles are affected), one must be cautious about misdiagnosing such pustules as being bacterial in origin. KOH examinations and cultures clarify the matter if one is in doubt. Intertriginous tinea pedis can allow bacteria to gain access to deeper tissues. This is a common portal of entry in patients with recurrent cellulitis of the lower extremities, so treatment of the dermatophyte infection can prevent subsequent episodes of cellulitis.

Pathogenesis

The three genera of dermatophytes are *Trichophyton*, *Microsporum*, and *Epidermophyton*. Some of these organisms grow only on human hosts (anthropophilic), whereas others can also exist in soil (geophilic) or on animals (zoophilic). All the dermatophytes are keratinophilic (i.e., they feed on keratin). They all produce keratinases, a necessary requirement for their keratinophilia. Stratum corneum, hair, and nails are attractive substrates for these fungi, not only because of their keratin composition but perhaps also because of their low density of bacterial inhibitors and competitors. Dermatophytes form hyphae through which nourishment is obtained from the keratin-rich host environment.

The clinical appearance and behavior of a fungal infection of the skin depend partly on the host response. Slow-growing dermatophytes infecting only the outermost layers of the stratum corneum may not elicit an inflammatory response. The diffuse plantar scaling type of tinea pedis is an example. The clinical reaction may also be influenced by the type of dermatophyte; some are more likely than others to elicit an inflammatory reaction. In general, zoophilic dermatophytes provoke more inflammation than anthropophilic ones. Tinea corporis from *Microsporum canis* (*canis*, Latin for canine, or relating to the dog) is an example of an infection from a zoophilic dermatophyte that produces an inflammatory red, scaling annular lesion.

Human dermatophytic infections may resolve spontaneously, probably as a result of cellular immune responses provoked by antigenic material from the organisms. Persistent infections occur in patients who do not mount this immune reaction, either because the fungus has failed to provoke it (e.g., in chronic tinea pedis, in which the fungus growth remains superficial in the thick stratum corneum and does not gain access to the circulation) or because of dermatophyte-specific host immune deficiency. Dermatophytic infections do not invade beyond the epidermis because of their dependence on keratin for nutrition and the fungistatic properties of transferrin and β-globulin in human serum.

MYCOSIS FUNGOIDES

KEY POINTS

1. Cutaneous T-cell lymphoma
2. Survival decreases with the progression of skin involvement from patches to plaques to tumors
3. Treatment is usually palliative, not curative.
4. Prognosis for patients with early-stage disease is excellent. The most common cause of death in patients with advanced disease is infection.

Definition

Mycosis fungoides is not a fungal infection; rather, it is a cutaneous T-cell lymphoma with a misleading label. The skin lesions result from the proliferation in the dermis of malignant T lymphocytes, which have a propensity to migrate into the epidermis. The clinical appearance of the lesion depends on the stage of the disease, which may evolve from patch through plaque to noduloulcerative lesions, reflecting the progressive increase of the cellular infiltrate in the skin.

Mycosis fungoides is a cutaneous T-cell lymphoma, not a fungal infection.

Incidence

Mycosis fungoides is uncommon. In the United States, mycosis fungoides accounts for less than 1% of all lymphomas and fewer than 200 deaths per year. The disease primarily affects adults, most often those in the older age groups.

History

In the usual case, the eruption slowly evolves over a period of years. It often starts as a nonspecific rash, which may be diagnosed as "atypical" psoriasis or eczema. *Parapsoriasis*, an uncommon idiopathic disorder characterized by salmon-colored, slightly scaling patches, may be a precursor. With evolution, the lesions become more elevated and indurated. Most patients with mycosis fungoides have pruritus, ranging from mild to severe. Severe pruritus should raise suspicion of extracutaneous (particularly hematogenous) involvement.

Physical Examination

The key to the diagnosis rests with the following features: the lesions are irregular in shape, peculiar in color (often reddish brown, violaceous, or orange), and asymmetric in distribution (Fig. 9.9). The degree of elevation of the lesions depends on the stage of the disease. In the patch stage, the lesions are flat, surmounted by a slight scale, and sometimes accompanied by epidermal atrophy, which clinically appears as "cigarette paper" wrinkling of the surface. Other lesions may show *poikiloderma*, a term used to describe a reticulate pattern of hyperpigmentation, hypopigmentation, and erythema with telangiectasia. In poikiloderma, the epidermis also shows atrophy. As the disease progresses, increased cellular infiltration of the skin occurs, expressed clinically as elevated, indurated plaques. These plaques are generally more widespread (Fig. 9.10). In advanced disease, nodules appear and frequently ulcerate (see Fig. 19.3). Lymphadenopathy is also often found in more advanced diseases and can be reactive, or more rarely, indicative of malignant infiltration of the lymph node.

Mycosis fungoides should be suspected in rashes with lesions that are:
1. Irregular in shape
2. Peculiar in color and polymorphic (i.e., presence of both atrophic patches and thicker plaques in a single patient)
3. Resistant to therapy for eczema or psoriasis

Sézary syndrome represents a leukemic variant of cutaneous T-cell lymphoma with some features similar to mycosis fungoides; this syndrome is characterized by total body erythema (erythroderma), lymphadenopathy, and a high number of

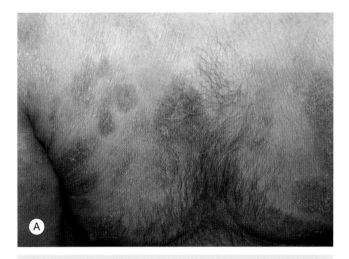

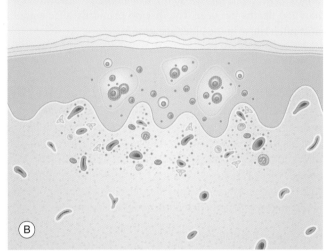

Fig. 9.9 Mycosis fungoides. (A) Red to violaceous and brownish, slightly scaling and wrinkled, irregularly shaped patches. (B) Epidermis—hyperkeratosis; epidermal atrophy (especially in patch stage); exocytosis of malignant lymphocytes, sometimes in focal collections (Pautrier microabscesses). Dermis—mild to marked infiltrate of mixed inflammation cells, including cerebriform lymphocytes.

atypical lymphocytes (or Sézary cells) in the peripheral circulation (see Fig. 14.20).

Differential Diagnosis

Mycosis fungoides may appear as *parapsoriasis* (see Fig. 9.23), *atypical eczema*, or *psoriasis*. In patients with nodular disease, other malignant tumors may be considered. In patients with Sézary syndrome, the differential diagnosis includes other causes of generalized erythema (see Chapter 14).

> Mycosis fungoides should be considered in patients with "atypical" eczema or psoriasis.

DIFFERENTIAL DIAGNOSIS OF MYCOSIS FUNGOIDES

- Parapsoriasis
- Eczema
- Psoriasis
- Other forms of cutaneous lymphoma
- Erythroderma

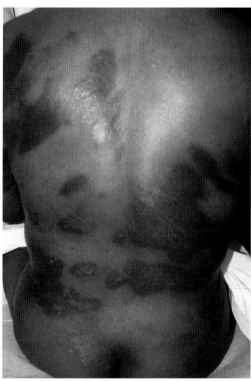

Fig. 9.10 Mycosis fungoides—irregularly shaped, asymmetric, deep red/purple hyperpigmented indurated plaques.

Laboratory and Biopsy

The most important laboratory test is the skin biopsy. Frequently, multiple biopsies must be performed before a histologic diagnosis can be secured, particularly in patients with early, patch-stage disease.

> Multiple skin biopsies, often over time, may be needed to establish the diagnosis.

The most important histologic feature is the presence of *Pautrier microabscesses* within the epidermis (Fig. 9.9B). These represent collections of lymphocytes, many of which are atypical. Atypical lymphocytes are also found in varying numbers in the dermal infiltrate. With high-power examination, the nuclei of these lymphocytes are characteristically highly convoluted or cerebriform. In the early stages of the disease, they may be present only in small numbers; in the nodular stage, a dense infiltrate of malignant cells is seen.

The malignant cells in mycosis fungoides are derived from a monoclonal proliferation of helper T cells and, less commonly, suppressor T cells. The *T-cell receptor gene rearrangement test* may be used to determine monoclonality in T-cell infiltrates in skin and other tissues. Differentiated helper T cells have specific cell surface receptors that possess specificity that is determined by the rearrangement of the receptor gene. A T-cell receptor gene rearrangement test detects a population of cells with the same rearrangement, thereby determining monoclonality, a finding that is supportive of malignancy. This test has been used as an aid in diagnosing mycosis fungoides in skin, blood, and lymph nodes. False-positive results occasionally occur. A newer assay, termed *high-throughput T-cell receptor gene rearrangement*, has improved sensitivity and specificity for the detection of malignant clones compared to traditional, polymerase chain reaction–based assays and may be useful in certain cases.

A complete blood cell count, with careful examination of the peripheral smear, should also be performed when looking for circulating mycosis fungoides cells. If lymph nodes are enlarged, an excisional lymph node biopsy should be performed.

Therapy

For disease localized to the skin, external therapy is preferred: (1) topical steroid, (2) UV light, either UVB or UVA in combination with psoralens (PUVA), (3) nitrogen mustard gel, (4) bexarotene (rexinoid) and retinoids, (5) imiquimod, and (6) electron beam therapy. Orally administered low-dose methotrexate, retinoid or rexinoid, vorinostat or romidepsin (a histone deacetylase inhibitor), and intramuscular interferon-α have been used in patients with recalcitrant skin disease.

In patients with advanced systemic disease, combination immunotherapy (e.g., a retinoid or rexinoid plus interferon-α), histone deacetylase inhibitors (oral vorinostat or intravenous romidepsin), targeted monoclonal antibody therapy (e.g., brentuximab vedotin, mogamulizumab), or single-agent chemotherapy is usually used, sometimes in combination with one of the topical modalities. Some patients with Sézary syndrome have also been successfully treated with extracorporeal photochemotherapy. In this treatment, white blood cells are removed from the patient several hours after psoralen ingestion, externally exposed to UVA, and reinfused into the circulation. Treatments are given on 2 back-to-back days, either monthly or twice monthly. Response rate can be increased by combining this extracorporeal photochemotherapy with bexarotene and/ or interferon-α.

THERAPY FOR MYCOSIS FUNGOIDES

Initial
- Steroids (e.g., clobetasol cream 0.05% b.i.d.)
- UVB
- Nitrogen mustard gel
- Compounded topical carmustine
- Radiotherapy (electron beam)
- Bexarotene and retinoids
- Imiquimod

Alternative
- PUVA
- Radiotherapy (total skin electron beam therapy)
- Methotrexate
- Retinoids (e.g., isotretinoin) or rexinoid (e.g., bexarotene)
- Pegylated interferon α-2a
- Extracorporeal photochemotherapy
- Histone deacetylase inhibitors (vorinostat, romidepsin)
- Targeted monoclonal antibodies (brentuximab vedotin, mogamulizumab, alemtuzumab, pembrolizumab)
- Single-agent chemotherapy (pralatrexate, liposomal doxorubicin, gemcitabine, etoposide, etc.)

Course and Complications

In most patients, mycosis fungoides is a chronic, smoldering disease with slow progression over many years. Treatment in the early stages can result in complete clearance of the skin lesions, although relapses are common after therapy is discontinued. Systemic involvement develops in advanced disease, usually affecting the lymph nodes first and the internal organs later. Mean survival for patients with systemic involvement is approximately 2 years.

Pathogenesis

Mycosis fungoides is a neoplastic disease of helper (CD4+) T cells and, less commonly, suppressor (CD8+) T cells. Its first manifestation usually appears in the skin. The ongoing debate is whether the process is malignant from the start, or whether it begins as a chronic inflammatory condition in which activated T cells eventually undergo malignant transformation. Either way, the end result is a monoclonal proliferation of helper or suppressor T cells in the skin.

> In mycosis fungoides, there is a monoclonal proliferation of helper (CD4+) or suppressor (CD8+) T cells in the skin.

The initiating events in this disease are not well established. Langerhans cells in the epidermis have been implicated as participating in the initial phases, perhaps themselves stimulated by external factors and, in turn, interacting with T cells, which are subsequently activated. Environmental chemicals have been implicated as a causative factor in some patients, but this has not been well proven. However, for most patients with mycosis fungoides, the underlying origin remains unknown, and the pathogenetic pathway is a matter of debate.

PITYRIASIS ROSEA

KEY POINTS
1. Herald patch is the harbinger of a more generalized eruption.
2. Oval, slightly scaling patches on the neck, trunk, and proximal extremities.
3. Reconsider the diagnosis if the condition lasts for more than 2–3 months.

Definition

Pityriasis rosea (*pityriasis* means "bran-like scale" and *rosea* means "rose colored") is an acute, self-limiting, inflammatory dermatosis that may be caused by human herpesviruses 6 and 7. It is characterized clinically by oval, minimally elevated, scaling patches, papules, and plaques that are located mainly on the trunk (Fig. 9.11).

Incidence

The exact incidence is not known, but the disease is relatively common. It is the third most common papulosquamous disease, affecting 1% of the new patients seen in the authors' dermatology clinic. The disease affects mainly older children and young adults and occurs with some seasonal variations, being least common during the summer months.

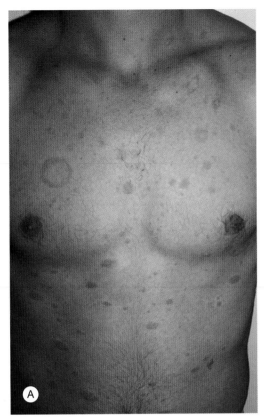

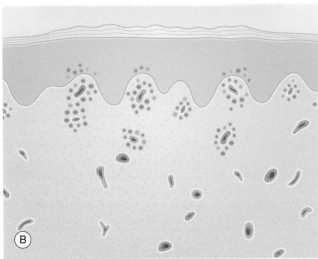

Fig. 9.11 **Pityriasis rosea**. (A) Oval pink patches with delicate scaling near border. (B) Epidermis—slight hyperkeratosis and acanthosis with focal spongiosis and scattered lymphocytes. Dermis—moderate perivascular lymphocytic infiltrate.

History

Characteristically, the generalized eruption is preceded by a single lesion, called the "herald patch." This is frequently misdiagnosed as ringworm. The herald patch is followed after several days to weeks by the generalized rash. The patient usually feels well. Itching is often present and ranges in severity from mild to moderate.

A "herald patch" precedes the generalized eruption.

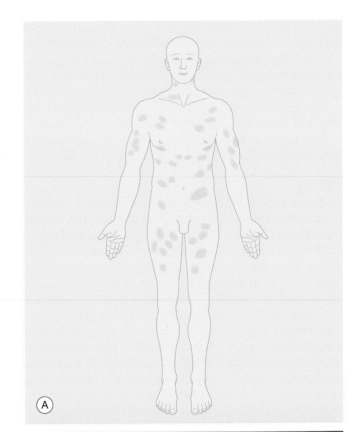

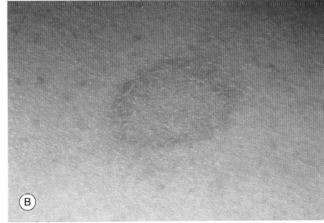

Fig. 9.12 **Pityriasis rosea**. (A) Distribution has been likened to that of a Christmas tree. (B) Herald patch.

Physical Examination

The herald patch, the largest of the lesions, ranges from 2 to 5 cm (Fig. 9.12B). The multiple lesions that follow resemble the herald patch but are smaller. They are typically tannish pink or salmon colored, round to oval, and surmounted by a delicate scale, which in the mature lesion is located near the border. Typically, oval lesions on the neck and trunk follow the skin cleavage lines in a pattern that, with imagination, has been likened to that of a "Christmas tree." The rash is distributed mainly on the trunk and neck and sometimes on the proximal extremities. In children, the face may also be affected. In addition, in children, papular or vesicular variants of the disease can occur. Oral lesions, although not prominent, have been described and range from pink macules to hemorrhagic puncta to small ulcerations.

Differential Diagnosis

Although the diagnosis of pityriasis rosea is usually straightforward, sometimes other disorders must be considered in the differential diagnosis. In *tinea corporis*, patients usually have only a few lesions. If doubt exists, however, a KOH preparation should be done. The explosive onset of the small lesions of *guttate psoriasis*, distributed mainly on the trunk, can be confused with pityriasis rosea. However, the scale in psoriasis is thicker and more silvery, and the course is more prolonged. Uncommonly, generalized *lichen planus* can resemble pityriasis rosea. *Pityriasis lichenoides chronica* is an uncommon disorder in which the lesions may resemble those of pityriasis rosea but (as the name implies) are chronic rather than transient. *Drug eruptions* should be considered in any patient with acute generalized dermatosis. Usually, however, a drug eruption is more brightly red, more confluent, less scaling, and itchier than pityriasis rosea.

The most important diagnosis to consider in the differential is *secondary syphilis*, particularly if the eruption is atypical; for example, if the patient has no herald patch, if the distal extremities (particularly the palms and soles) are involved, or if the patient is systemically ill. In all cases of "atypical" pityriasis rosea, a serologic test for syphilis should be ordered.

DIFFERENTIAL DIAGNOSIS OF PITYRIASIS ROSEA

- Tinea corporis
- Guttate psoriasis
- Lichen planus
- Pityriasis lichenoides chronica
- Drug eruption
- Secondary syphilis

For patients with "atypical" pityriasis rosea, a serologic test for syphilis must be performed to rule out secondary syphilis.

Laboratory and Biopsy

The diagnosis is made based on the characteristic history and physical findings. Skin biopsy is nonspecific and rarely indicated. If it is performed, the findings will include mild hyperkeratosis with focal parakeratosis, minimal acanthosis with focal spongiosis, and a moderate dermal inflammatory infiltrate, with a few of the cells migrating into the epidermis (Fig. 9.11B).

Therapy

Treatment is usually not necessary for this self-limiting disease. Occasionally, antihistamines are needed for pruritus and moisturizing creams for the dry scaling that occurs as the lesions evolve. UV light therapy (UVB), acyclovir, or erythromycin appears to accelerate resolution, but these are usually not needed.

THERAPY FOR PITYRIASIS ROSEA

Initial
- None unless symptomatic

Alternative
- UV light
- Acyclovir 400–800 mg five times a day for 1 week
- Erythromycin 500 mg b.i.d. for 2 weeks

Course and Complications

The disease involutes spontaneously in a time course ranging from 2 weeks to 2 months, with an average time of approximately 6 weeks. It recurs in only approximately 2% of patients. No complications occur, except for occasional postinflammatory hypopigmentation or hyperpigmentation, which resolves slowly over time, often months.

Pityriasis rosea clears spontaneously within 2 months.

Pathogenesis

The rash appears to be mediated by a cellular (type IV) immune reaction. A possible viral trigger, human herpesviruses 6 and 7, has been implicated. However, the disease does not occur endemically, and its occurrence in household contacts is uncommon.

PSORIASIS

KEY POINTS
1. Well-demarcated red, silvery, scaling plaques.
2. Elbows, knees, and scalp are typically involved, as well as other sites.
3. Inflammation and epidermal proliferation provide opportunities for therapeutic intervention.

Definition

Psoriasis is an inflammatory rash with increased epidermal proliferation (acanthosis) resulting in an accumulation of stratum corneum (scale). The etiology is unknown but appears to be multifactorial, resulting in inflammation and epidermal proliferation. The clinical appearance is that of sharply demarcated red papules, patches, and plaques, surmounted by silvery scales (Fig. 9.13).

Incidence

Some 2%–5% of patients of European descent and 0.1%–0.3% of the Asian populations are affected by psoriasis. Onset may occur at any age but is most common in adults, with an average age of 35 years.

History

The disease usually starts gradually, although occasionally it is explosive in onset or exacerbation. The sudden appearance of multiple small (guttate) lesions of psoriasis in a generalized

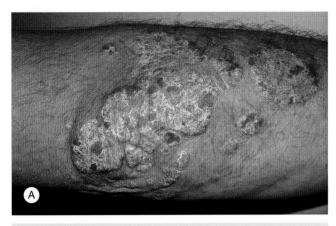

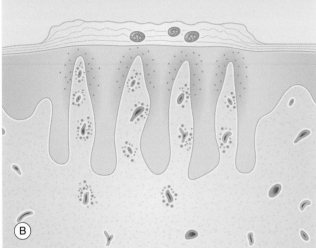

Fig. 9.13 Psoriasis. (A) Well-demarcated pink/red plaques with white scales involving the elbow. (B) Epidermis—hyperkeratosis, acanthosis with elongated rete pegs, and infiltration by neutrophils, forming micro-abscesses in the stratum corneum. Dermis—capillary proliferation with perivascular inflammation.

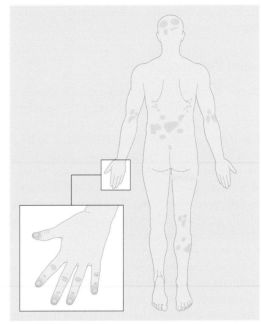

Fig. 9.14 Typical distribution of psoriasis—elbows, knees, scalp, intergluteal cleft, and nails.

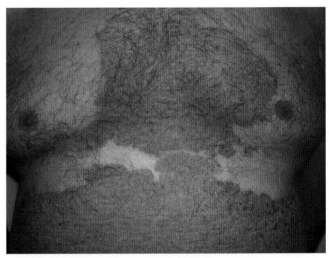

Fig. 9.15 Psoriasis—widespread red plaques.

distribution is often preceded by a streptococcal throat infection. In patients with severe sudden onset or rapidly worsening large-plaque psoriasis, a predisposing human immunodeficiency virus (HIV) infection should be considered: 1% of patients with acquired immune deficiency syndrome (AIDS) develop severe psoriasis, and sometimes the psoriasis is the presenting manifestation of AIDS. Other aggravating factors that have been implicated in psoriasis include trauma to the skin that precipitates a psoriatic lesion (Koebner phenomenon) and emotional stress, which, although difficult to document scientifically, is believed by many patients to be a contributing factor. A few drugs have been found to aggravate psoriasis. Lithium is the best-proven culprit, but beta-blockers and nonsteroidal antiinflammatory drugs have also been implicated. Itching (*psoriasis* is derived from the Greek word for "itching") ranges from mild to severe. A family history of psoriasis can be elicited from approximately one-third of patients.

> Think of infection with sudden onset or worsening of psoriasis.

Physical Examination

The lesions are sharply demarcated, and depending on skin tone, red, pink, or dark brown papules, patches, and plaques are surmounted by scale, which is characteristically silvery. In intertriginous areas, maceration prevents scales from accumulating, but the lesions remain red or dark brown and sharply defined. Psoriasis is classically distributed on the scalp, elbows, and knees (Fig. 9.14). The intergluteal cleft is also a common site and is frequently overlooked. Although these are typical sites, psoriatic lesions can occur anywhere and may cover the entire skin surface (Fig. 9.15).

Nail involvement (see Chapter 21, Fig. 21.4) is present in as many as 50% of patients with psoriasis and can be associated with involvement of the hands (Fig. 9.16). The nails may be pitted with small, ice pick–like depressions in the nail plate.

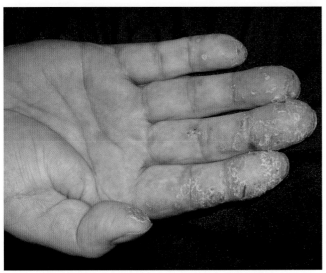

Fig. 9.16 Psoriasis—pink, scaling, fissured patches on the hand, often associated with nail involvement.

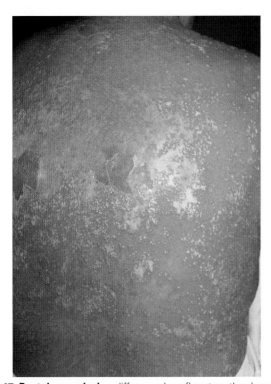

Fig. 9.17 Pustular psoriasis—diffuse and confluent erythroderma (red) studded with pustules.

Onycholysis (separation of nail plate from nail bed) can also occur. This condition is caused by a plaque of psoriasis in the distal nail bed with an accumulation of scale, which lifts the plate from the nail bed. The nails may be thick, irregular, and discolored (yellowish).

Pustular psoriasis is an uncommon variant. In this form of the disease, superficial pustules occur in one of three presentations: (1) pustules studding more typical plaques, (2) pustules confined to the palms and soles, and (3) a rare generalized eruption in which the pustules erupt abruptly on large areas of red skin and are accompanied by fever and leukocytosis (Fig. 9.17).

Deficiency of the interleukin 1 (IL-1) receptor antagonist and of the IL-36 receptor antagonist causes severe neonatal-onset and variable age-onset pustular psoriasis with systemic inflammation, respectively.

Differential Diagnosis

The diagnosis is usually not difficult, especially when the lesions have the characteristic silvery scale and involve typical locations. It may be more difficult when the scale is not present, as in extremely early lesions or in intertriginous areas.

Intertriginous lesions may be confused with *tinea cruris*, *candidiasis*, and *intertrigo* (see Tinea Cruris, above). Psoriasis of the scalp is most often confused with *seborrheic dermatitis*, in which the scaling is usually finer, yellower, and more diffuse with indistinct borders. Guttate psoriasis on the trunk is sometimes confused with *pityriasis rosea* or *tinea corporis*. *Chronic dermatitis* and *T-cell cutaneous lymphoma* can mimic psoriasis occasionally. Nail involvement may be clinically indistinguishable from a *fungal infection*; a positive KOH preparation, periodic acid–Schiff stain of a nail clipping, or fungal culture enables diagnosis of the latter.

DIFFERENTIAL DIAGNOSIS OF PSORIASIS
• Tinea cruris
• Candidiasis
• Intertrigo
• Seborrheic dermatitis
• Pityriasis rosea
• Tinea corporis
• Chronic dermatitis
• Cutaneous T-cell lymphoma
• Onychomycosis

Laboratory and Biopsy

A biopsy is usually not necessary; in fact, the clinical picture is often more characteristic than the histologic findings. If a biopsy is performed, the pathologic examination shows hyperkeratosis, parakeratosis, decreased granular layer with an acanthotic epidermis, and an inflammatory infiltrate in the dermis that includes neutrophils, and some of which may migrate into and through the epidermis, forming small collections within the stratum corneum (Munro abscesses) (Fig. 9.13B).

Therapy

The goal of therapy is to decrease epidermal proliferation and the underlying dermal inflammation. Five types of topical agents are used: steroids, tar and anthralin preparations, calcipotriene (a vitamin D derivative), tazarotene (a vitamin A derivative), and UV light.

Topical steroids are both antimitotic and antiinflammatory. Over-the-counter hydrocortisone preparations are usually ineffective, requiring stronger prescription steroids (see Chapter 4). These agents are expensive but useful for patients with limited areas of involvement. A good response is usually noted within several weeks, but tachyphylaxis (loss of effect with continued use of a drug) may develop. Therefore for long-term use of topical steroids, we instruct patients to use an intermittent regimen (e.g., use the agent for only 2 of every 3 weeks or skip days when doing well). This practice may also reduce the potential for developing steroid atrophy of the skin. Psoriasis also responds to systemic steroids, but these should be avoided because of their well-known long-term side-effects and because psoriasis may rebound badly after the drug is discontinued.

Topical tars and *anthralin* are older, less commonly used medications that are hydrocarbons with antimitotic activity; tars can also be antiinflammatory. These products can stain skin (temporarily) and fabrics (permanently) and are slow to produce a response, although the responses that are achieved tend to last longer and tachyphylaxis is less likely to develop than with topical steroids. Tar oil added to a bath is a convenient way to apply tar to the total skin surface. The patient should be advised, however, that these tar oils stain plastic (but not porcelain) bathtubs. Tar preparations applied directly to the skin may be more effective than tar baths but are messier to use. Hence, we instruct patients to apply tar at bedtime. Commercial tar preparations are available, but we more often prescribe a compounded preparation containing a tar liquid—5% liquor carbonis detergens—contained in Aquaphor. To this, 3% salicylic acid may be added as a keratolytic to help remove thick scales if they are present. Anthralin is commercially available in a cream preparation, ranging in concentration from 0.1% to 1.0%. Because of potential irritancy, this therapy is initiated with low concentrations and advanced as tolerated. A 30-minute short-contact regimen can be used, but we usually suggest an overnight application. Skin irritation and staining are the main disadvantages of anthralin therapy.

Calcipotriene ointment, cream, and lotion are vitamin D derivatives with antimitotic activity. It is applied twice daily and requires several months of use for full effect. Some patients respond well but many do not. It is expensive and may cause irritation but is otherwise safe for long-term use in limited plaque disease. We sometimes do alternate weekly treatments with topical steroids and calcipotriene to reduce the side-effects of steroids and maintain disease control.

Tazarotene (0.05% and 0.1%) is a retinoid (vitamin A derivative). In general, retinoids promote differentiation and inhibit proliferation—desirable effects for an antipsoriatic drug. Topical tazarotene is applied at bedtime, often in conjunction with a topical steroid applied in the morning. It is effective for many patients, but it is expensive and may cause irritation (which is ameliorated by the morning steroid). Tazarotene is also rated as category X for pregnancy, so it should not be used in women with childbearing potential.

UV light therapy can be used alone or in combination with other therapies. The least expensive source of UV light is the sun. However, this is often impractical. Tanning salons are another source of UV light, which the patient can use three or four times weekly. Intensive UV light therapy (narrowband UVB) can be provided in the offices of many dermatologists. Some patients find it convenient to purchase an expensive commercial UV light unit for their use at home, although home UV light should be used only with a clinician's guidance.

> Systemic agents for psoriasis are reserved for patients with moderate-to-severe disease.

PUVA has mostly been replaced by narrow-band UVB. The psoralen drug intercalates between the DNA strands and binds to them during irradiation with UVA. Therefore when the drug is taken by mouth, it reaches all the tissues of the body, and only those tissues that receive the UVA radiation (i.e., the skin and the eyes, unless shielded) are affected. This treatment could result in cataracts, so the eyes must be protected with special glasses. The major long-term concerns involve premature aging of the skin and the development of skin cancer, including melanoma. Narrow-band UVB that does not require taking psoralen and appears to be safer—less carcinogenesis—is now the preferred UV light therapy.

Methotrexate, a folate antagonist, inhibits cellular proliferation and is effective in many patients with psoriasis. It is administered on a weekly schedule. Complete blood cell counts and liver and renal function need to be monitored at frequent intervals. The major long-term concern is liver toxicity, so regular liver function blood tests and intermittent screening for cirrhosis are required. Familiarity with methotrexate and careful follow-up with patients are necessary to avoid serious side-effects of this drug. Some side-effects can be minimized with the addition of folic acid, taken every day of the week except the day the methotrexate is given.

Acitretin (Soriatane) is a retinoid with profound effects on keratinization. It is administered orally on a daily basis and is particularly effective for pustular psoriasis. Acitretin often improves but seldom clears the more common plaque-type psoriasis. It can be used in conjunction with UV light for an additive effect. Acitretin is a *teratogen* and is not safe for use in women with childbearing potential. Additional common side-effects include drying of skin and mucous membranes, hair loss, peeling of palms and soles, and numerous other less common problems, including effects on bones, eyes, liver, and blood lipids.

Systemic *cyclosporine* (Neoral) is also approved for treating psoriasis and is very effective in this role. It is, however, potentially nephrotoxic and requires careful monitoring.

Biologic agents that suppress the inflammatory response by inhibiting tumor necrosis factor (TNF), and interleukins (IL-12/23, IL-36, and IL-17) are quite effective in treating psoriasis without some of the serious side-effects of other systemic treatments. The main concerns with them are an increased potential for infections and a very small risk of lymphoma. These agents include the following: TNF inhibitors—etanercept (Enbrel), adalimumab (Humira), infliximab (Remicade); IL-12/23 inhibitors—ustekinumab (Stelara), guselkumab (Tremfya), risankizumab (Skyrizi), tildrakizumab (Ilumya); IL-17 inhibitors—secukinumab (Cosentyx), and ixekizumab (Taltz); and IL-36 inhibitor—spesolimab-sbzo (Spevigo). They are administered subcutaneously, intramuscularly, or intravenously.

Apremilast (Otezla) and roflumilast are oral agents that block the enzyme phosphodiesterase-4 (PDE-4) and are effective for mild-to-moderate psoriasis. They do not require laboratory testing. However, they have frequent gastrointestinal side-effects, and apremilast may be associated with depression.

Janus kinase (JAK) inhibitors (tyk2—deucravacitinib) are the newest therapeutic agents for the treatment of moderate-to-severe psoriasis.

Apremilast or biologics are the authors' preferred alternative treatment when topical steroids and/or UV light fail to control psoriasis.

THERAPY FOR PSORIASIS

Initial
- Steroids—mid-potency to strong potency (e.g., triamcinolone 0.1% or clobetasol 0.05% b.i.d.)
- Tars and anthralin
- Calcipotriene ointment, cream, or solution b.i.d.
- Tazarotene gel 0.05% or 0.1% daily
- UV light—sunlight, tanning salon

Alternative
- UV light—narrow-band UVB, PUVA
- Methotrexate
- Acitretin
- Cyclosporine
- Biologics (TNF, IL-17, IL-12/23, IL-36 inhibitors)
- PDE-4 inhibitors
- JAK inhibitors

Course and Complications

Psoriasis is a chronic condition that waxes and wanes, frequently without obvious cause. Perhaps because of the favorable influence of sunlight, many patients note that their psoriasis is better in summer and worse in winter. With the use of the above therapies, the disease can usually be controlled, although not cured. This skin disease, like many others, can be socially stigmatizing and, in some individuals, physically disabling. The impact on quality of life can be enormous, with disruption of activities of daily life, impaired interpersonal relationships, and diminished self-esteem.

Psoriatic skin may be colonized with *Staphylococcus aureus*. With scratching, secondary infections occasionally occur. Uncommonly, psoriasis affects the total body surface, resulting in erythroderma with its associated complications, which include loss of heat, fluid, and protein; hospitalization may be required.

Arthritis accompanies psoriasis in approximately 5% of patients, and psoriatic arthritis is often diagnosed years after the skin findings are present, so patients must be asked about joint pain at each visit. It classically affects the distal interphalangeal joints but more often occurs as asymmetric arthritis involving small- and medium-sized joints. Ankylosing spondylitis can also occur in psoriatic arthritis. Psoriatic arthritis is usually treated with nonsteroidal antiinflammatory drugs, although these sometimes aggravate the skin lesions. Methotrexate and biologics are useful for psoriatic arthritis and are indicated particularly in the rapidly destructive type—arthritis mutilans (Fig. 9.18). Moderate-to-severe cutaneous psoriasis appears to be a risk factor for cardiac disease.

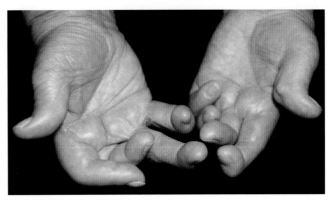
Fig. 9.18 Psoriatic arthritis mutilans.

Arthritis accompanies psoriasis in approximately 5% of patients. Five clinical types are recognized:
1. Asymmetric small- and medium-sized joint involvement
2. Distal interphalangeal joint disease
3. Rheumatoid arthritis–like
4. Ankylosing spondylitis
5. Mutilating

Pathogenesis

Many patients with psoriasis are genetically predisposed. Some 35% have a family history of psoriasis; in identical twins, the disease occurs concurrently in 80%. The precipitating factors responsible for unmasking this genetic predisposition include streptococcal infection, stress, smoking, drugs, and physical trauma.

Others have implicated the dermal inflammatory process as being primary in the evolution of a psoriatic lesion and epidermal hyperplasia. Clinical observations, laboratory studies, and targeted therapies support the immunologic basis of psoriasis. Many experimental data now suggest that psoriasis may be a T-cell-mediated autoimmune disease driven by T helper cell (Th1) and 17 cytokines. The therapeutic effectiveness of cyclosporine and biologic agents, which are T-cell-targeted drugs, supports this theory. The understanding of the immunopathogenesis of psoriasis has translated into the development of therapeutic biologic agents that reduce the number of pathogenic T cells, inhibit T-cell activation and migration, or block the activity of inflammatory cytokines. Investigators have noted that neutrophils extravasated from the superficial dermal capillaries invade the epidermis. Raised levels of leukotrienes (one of the products of arachidonic acid metabolism) have been found in psoriatic skin, where, as mediators of inflammation (TNF-α, IL-12 and IL-23), they may attract neutrophils and may provoke epidermal proliferation.

Psoriasis is an inflammatory disease that provides opportunities for therapeutic intervention.

Whatever the provocation, the end result for the epidermis is an accelerated cell cycle or an increased number of cycling cells recruited from the normal resting cell population. This leads to an increased number of dividing cells, culminating in an orgy of epidermal proliferation. Cellular turnover is increased seven-fold, and the transit time from the basal layer to the top of the stratum corneum is decreased from the normal 28 days to 3 or 4 days. This process is too fast for the cells to be shed, so they accumulate, resulting in the characteristic scale.

> In a psoriatic plaque, epidermal cell production is increased sevenfold.

SECONDARY SYPHILIS

KEY POINTS

1. *Treponema pallidum* is causative.
2. Involvement of the palms and soles is typical.
3. Serologic tests for syphilis are nontreponemal (rapid plasma reagin [RPR] or Venereal Disease Research Laboratory [VDRL]) and treponemal specific (fluorescent treponemal antibody-absorption [FTA-ABS] or *T. pallidum* enzyme immunoassay [TP-EIA]).

Definition

The rash of secondary syphilis represents an inflammatory response in the skin and mucous membranes to the hematog-enously disseminated *T. pallidum* spirochete. Clinically, the rash may appear in various ways, but the most common is scaling papules and plaques.

Incidence

Despite the availability of penicillin, secondary syphilis is still present in our society, and its incidence has been increasing in recent years, certainly in the general population, but dispropor-tionately more so in men who have sex with men and people with HIV.

History

The secondary phase of syphilis starts 6–12 weeks after the appearance of the primary chancre. The chancre has usually (but not always) healed by the time the secondary phase develops, but it may be remembered by the patient. Systemic symptoms are usually present, and they include fever, headache, myalgia, arthralgia, sore throat, and malaise. Pruritus, once thought not to occur in secondary syphilis, is noted occasionally.

Physical Examination

The rash of secondary syphilis is a great imitator. It may appear as macules, nonscaling papules and annular plaques, scaling papules, patches, and plaques, and, occasionally, pustules or nodules. Vesicles or bullae are not present, however, except in newborns with congenital disease and occasionally in patients with HIV. The most common lesions are scaling papules and small plaques, in which the color is a clue. Lesions are most frequently not just red but rather reddish brown (ham colored) or yellowish (copper colored). The eruption is often general-ized, but palmar and plantar involvement with lesions of these colors is particularly noteworthy (Fig. 9.19). Other possible mucocutaneous features include (1) white mucous patches in

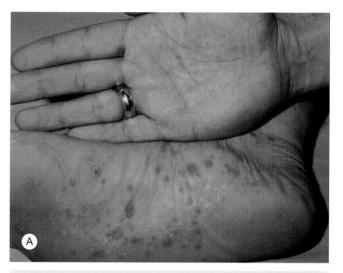

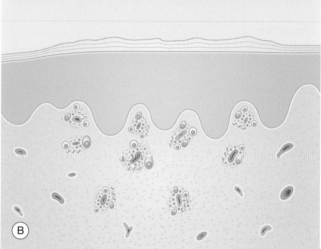

Fig. 9.19 Secondary syphilis. (A) Characteristic plantar and pal-mar, "ham"-colored (reddish), slight scaling patches and macules. (B) Epidermis—slight hyperkeratosis. Dermis—perivascular infiltrate with lymphocytes, plasma cells, and spirochetes (with silver stain).

the mouth; (2) condylomata lata, which are flat-topped, moist, warty-appearing lesions in the genital areas; and (3) spotty alo-pecia of the scalp, which has been described as "moth-eaten" in appearance. The general physical examination usually reveals the presence of lymphadenopathy.

> The rash of secondary syphilis is a great imitator. Involvement of the palms and soles suggests this diagnosis.

Differential Diagnosis

As mentioned, the rash of secondary syphilis can mimic many other skin disorders, the most common of which is *pityriasis rosea*, as has been discussed; *drug eruption, viral exanthem,* and *sarcoidosis* (for the annular lesions seen especially in Black patients). A general guideline to remember is that, for patients with a generalized rash of unknown origin and systemic complaints, secondary syphilis should be considered and the patient should be tested for it.

> In patients with fever and rash of unknown origin, a serologic test for syphilis should be done.

DIFFERENTIAL DIAGNOSIS OF SECONDARY SYPHILIS

- Pityriasis rosea
- Drug eruption
- Viral exanthem
- Sarcoidosis

Laboratory and Biopsy

In secondary syphilis, the nontreponemal serologic tests for syphilis (STS), RPR, or VDRL are always positive in immunocompetent hosts and usually present in high titers. The treponemal-specific tests, FTA-ABS test and TP-EIA, are more specific tests for syphilis. Screening can be done with a treponemal-specific test (TP-EIA) and then confirmed with a nontreponemal test. The positivity of these two blood tests secures the diagnosis. False-positive tests, usually in low titers, occur in some patients with SLE.

The STS may be negative in a patient with coexisting HIV infection and secondary syphilis. If syphilis is suspected in this setting, a darkfield examination or biopsy of a skin lesion can confirm the diagnosis. These procedures visualize the spirochetes in serous fluid obtained from the lesion or in special stains of biopsy material. The histologic findings are otherwise frequently nonspecific, showing simply an inflammatory infiltrate and, in lesions with scale, hyperkeratosis and mild acanthosis. Plasma cells are often present in the inflammatory infiltrate and may suggest the diagnosis (Fig. 9.19B). Patients diagnosed with syphilis should also be tested for HIV infection because the presence of the former indicates a risk factor for acquiring the latter.

Therapy

Penicillin remains the treatment of choice for syphilis. For primary and secondary syphilis in immunocompetent hosts, a single intramuscular injection of 2.4 million units of benzathine penicillin G is adequate therapy. HIV-positive patients require more intensive therapy, either with benzathine penicillin injections weekly for 3 weeks or with a course of intravenous aqueous penicillin or intramuscular ceftriaxone. Immunocompetent patients who are allergic to penicillin may be treated with a 14-day course of either tetracycline 500 mg q.i.d. or doxycycline 100 mg b.i.d. With therapy, many patients experience a febrile reaction (Jarisch–Herxheimer reaction) beginning within 12 hours and resolving within 1 day.

> In patients with HIV, syphilis progresses rapidly and requires more intensive therapy.

THERAPY FOR SECONDARY SYPHILIS

Initial
- Benzathine penicillin G 2.4 million units IM

Alternative
- Doxycycline 100 mg b.i.d. or tetracycline 500 mg q.i.d. for 2 weeks

Course and Complications

Without therapy, the lesions of secondary syphilis resolve spontaneously in 1–3 months in immunocompetent patients. With therapy, the lesions resolve promptly, and the titer of the nontreponemal STS is reduced markedly by 12 months. The treponemal-specific test often remains positive indefinitely.

In the secondary phase, the treponemal organism spreads not only to the skin but also to other organs. Hepatitis occurs in approximately 10% of the patients, bone and joint disease in approximately 4%, and nephritis even less often. Central nervous system involvement, as reflected by abnormal cerebrospinal fluid findings, occurs in approximately 10% of immunocompetent patients but is much more frequent in patients living with HIV, in whom rapid progression to symptomatic neurosyphilis may occur.

Approximately one-third of untreated immunocompetent patients develop late (years later) complications of syphilis (tertiary), of which the most important are the cardiovascular and central nervous system manifestations. In people with HIV, progression to tertiary syphilis is more frequent and can occur within months after the primary infection.

Pathogenesis

The disease is caused by the spirochete *T. pallidum*. The organism is traumatically inoculated into mucous membranes or skin, most often during sexual intercourse. After a 10- to 90-day incubation period, the *primary* lesion appears as an ulcer (chancre). After another brief latent period, during which the organism continues to multiply, hematogenous dissemination occurs (*secondary* syphilis). Organisms infecting the skin provoke an immunologic response, which is clinically manifested by a variety of inflammatory lesions.

UNCOMMON SCALING DISORDERS

ERYTHEMA ANNULARE CENTRIFUGUM

This annular or polycyclic eruption is characterized by waxing and waning patches with a "trailing" scale that is chronic and recurrent over months and years (Fig. 9.20). For most, it is idiopathic. However, occasionally it has been associated with dermatophyte infections, foods, medications, and, rarely, malignancy. Treatment is symptomatic with topical steroids.

ICHTHYOSIS

The ichthyoses are a heterogeneous group of distinct genodermatoses characterized by generalized scaling seen at birth or shortly thereafter. Genetic mutations resulting in abnormal

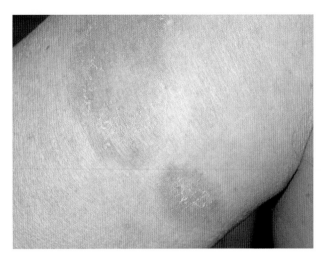

Fig. 9.20 Erythema annulare centrifugum—polycyclic pink patches with a "trailing" scale.

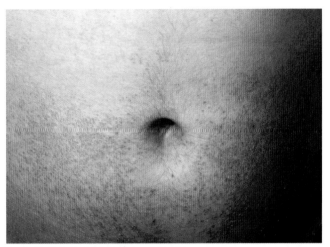

Fig. 9.21 X-linked ichthyosis—"dirty" brown scaling, more prominent on lower abdomen.

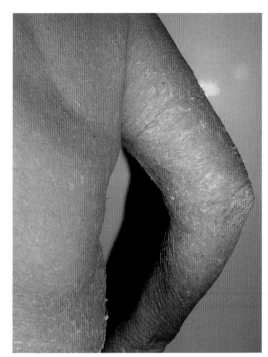

Fig. 9.22 Acquired ichthyosis—diffuse, fine, whitish scaling in a generalized distribution. Look for a systemic association with lymphoma, metabolic disorder, or medications.

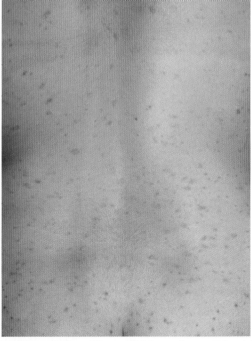

Fig. 9.23 Parapsoriasis—diffuse, slightly scaling, mildly pink, small patches and thin plaques.

epidermal cornification cause the dry scaling of the skin. Severity ranges from mild "dry" skin involvement (*ichthyosis vulgaris—filaggrin mutation*) to severe, thick, plate-like scaling (*lamellar ichthyosis—transglutaminase 1 decreased/absent activity*) to blistering at birth followed by thick, horny, spine-like scaling prominent in flexures (*epidermolytic ichthyosis—keratin 1 and 10 mutations*). *X-linked* ichthyosis is characterized by "dirty"-appearing, large brown scales, most prominent on the extensor extremities and trunk of males (Fig. 9.21). It is caused by the deletion of the *steroid sulfatase* gene on the X-chromosome and is inherited as a recessive trait. Mothers carrying the gene often have a history of failure of labor to begin or progress. Corneal opacities and cryptorchidism are frequent findings. *Acquired ichthyosis* (Fig. 9.22) begins in adults and is associated with malignancy (e.g., lymphomas), metabolic disease (e.g., hypothyroidism), and drugs (e.g., retinoids).

Parapsoriasis

Parapsoriasis is a group of confusing scaling disorders that is most easily divided into small and large-plaque parapsoriasis.

Both groups have fairly well-demarcated, slightly scaling, erythematous to tan patches, and thin plaques, which are asymptomatic and chronic. Small plaque parapsoriasis (Fig. 9.23) appears very similar to pityriasis rosea but lasts longer than 2–3 months and has a benign course. Large-plaque parapsoriasis has an irregularly shaped, well-demarcated, and sometimes

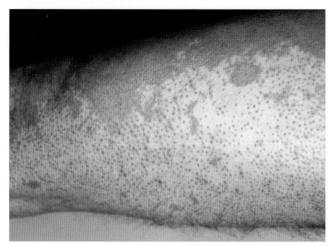

Fig. 9.24 **Pityriasis rubra pilaris**—red, slightly scaling, follicular papules and plaques.

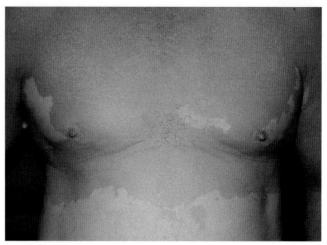

Fig. 9.25 **Pityriasis rubra pilaris**—red, slightly scaling, confluent plaques with islands of normal skin.

wrinkled appearance, which in about 10% of cases evolves into mycosis fungoides. Skin biopsies are nondiagnostic and treatment with UV light is usually successful.

Pityriasis Rubra Pilaris

Pityriasis rubra pilaris is a chronic idiopathic disorder characterized by scaling follicular papules (Fig. 9.24), diffuse and confluent, yellowish-pink, well-demarcated plaques with islands of normal-appearing skin (Fig. 9.25), and thick scaling palms and soles (Fig. 9.26). It affects all ages and is generally mildly pruritic. Painful fissuring of the palms and soles can cause significant disability. A skin biopsy demonstrates characteristic findings. First-line therapies for adults and children include the IL-17 and IL-23 inhibitor classes of biologics. Alternative therapies include methotrexate and oral retinoids but are not as effective as the biologics.

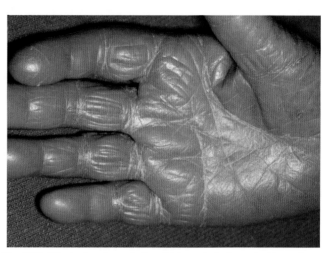

Fig. 9.26 **Pityriasis rubra pilaris**—thickened, dusky red, shiny palms.

SELF-ASSESSMENT

Case 1—Scaling Rash (Fig. 9.27)

What Is Your Differential Diagnosis?

The differential diagnosis would include any of the papulosquamous disorders, although pityriasis rosea, secondary syphilis, and DLE are not likely. Mycosis fungoides must still be considered for these irregularly shaped, asymmetric plaques, especially in light of the patient's history. Partially treated psoriasis is also possible. For a scaling rash of uncertain origin (especially one in which the lesions have sharp, serpiginous borders), fungal infection is the first diagnosis to exclude.

What Test Would You Do Next?

A KOH preparation should be the first test. A positive result in this case is diagnostic for a superficial fungal infection.

IMPORTANT POINTS

1. This case illustrates the general rule: if the diagnosis is uncertain and if the rash scales, scrape it.
2. Because the eruption was widespread, a systemic antifungal agent was prescribed, and the rash cleared.

Case 2—Scaling Rash on Head, Neck, Trunk, and Arms (Fig. 9.28)

What Is Your Differential Diagnosis?

A widespread scaling eruption suggests a differential diagnosis of psoriasis, tinea, pityriasis rosea, secondary syphilis, lupus, T-cell cutaneous lymphoma, and dermatitis. The chronic course eliminates pityriasis rosea and syphilis.

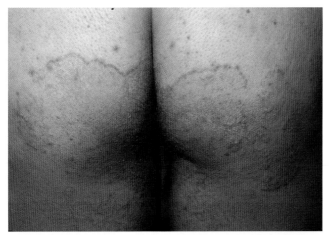

Fig. 9.27 This 50-year-old man was initially seen in dermatology consultation for generalized dry, red, itchy skin of many years' duration. Three skin biopsies were performed, which showed an inflammatory infiltrate with some atypical lymphocytes, but not in sufficient numbers to diagnose mycosis fungoides (Sézary syndrome). The patient was treated with a topical steroid cream applied to the entire skin surface. At follow-up 2 weeks later, much of the rash had improved, but a sharply demarcated, scaling eruption persisted on the buttocks and feet.

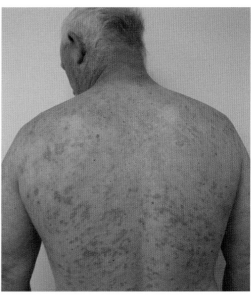

Fig. 9.28 This 48-year-old man developed pruritic, pink, slightly scaling papules and plaques 3 years ago on the head, neck, trunk, and arms. His review of systems and previous medical history were unremarkable. It was uncertain whether the eruption was exacerbated by sunlight.

What Would You Do Now?

A KOH preparation was negative for fungal elements. A skin biopsy helped make diagnosis, and it revealed pathologic changes in lupus erythematosus. Further laboratory testing resulted in normal antinuclear antibody, double-stranded DNA, complete blood cell count with platelet count, urinalysis, and complete metabolic profile. Testing for SSA was positive and SSB was negative. All these tests confirm the diagnosis of cutaneous lupus erythematosus.

How Would You Treat This Patient?

Sun protection is the first and foremost, even with the patient's questionable history of sun sensitivity. Topical steroids such as triamcinolone cream 0.1% in large volumes may suppress the lupus. The next step would be an antimalarial such as hydroxychloroquine 200 mg twice daily. If these interventions fail, then systemic immunosuppressants are warranted.

IMPORTANT POINTS

1. Scaling eruptions in a sun-exposed distribution suggest the possibility of lupus erythematosus.
2. A skin biopsy is diagnostic of lupus.
3. The medical history, general physical and laboratory examinations will separate cutaneous versus systemic involvement.

Vesicles and Bullae

CHAPTER OUTLINE

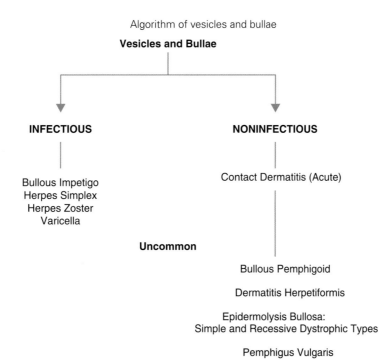

Algorithm of vesicles and bullae

Vesicles and Bullae

INFECTIOUS

Bullous Impetigo
Herpes Simplex
Herpes Zoster
Varicella

Uncommon

NONINFECTIOUS

Contact Dermatitis (Acute)

Bullous Pemphigoid

Dermatitis Herpetiformis

Epidermolysis Bullosa:
Simple and Recessive Dystrophic Types

Pemphigus Vulgaris

Porphyria Cutanea Tarda

ABSTRACT

Vesicles and bullae, when intact, are easily recognized primary lesions (Table 10.1). Crusts (dried serum and blood) are secondary lesions that should lead one to suspect a preceding vesicle/bulla or pustule. The etiology of vesicular and bullous diseases includes viral and bacterial infections; allergic and irritant contact dermatitis; and autoimmune, genetic, and metabolic diseases. Pathogenesis of blister formation is helpful in understanding the location of the lesion within the skin. The blister may occur within the epidermis (intraepidermal) or beneath it (subepidermal).

KEY POINTS

1. Blistering is an easily recognized primary lesion.
2. Weeping and crusting suggest a blistering process.
3. There are multiple causes of blistering.

Where blisters occur in the skin helps in making the diagnosis
1. Intraepidermally
2. Subepidermally

TABLE 10.1   Common Blistering Diseases

Disease	Frequency[a]	Etiology	History	Physical Examination	Differential Diagnosis	Laboratory Test
Bullous impetigo	0.1	*Staphylococcus aureus*	Pruritus	Circular yellow crusts, purulent bullae Head, neck, extremities	Contact dermatitis Herpes simplex Superficial fungus Pemphigus vulgaris Staphylococcal scalded skin syndrome	Gram stain Culture
Contact dermatitis	2.8	Allergen Irritant	Irritant: exposure occurs hours to days before rash Allergic: exposure occurs 1–4 days before rash	Papulovesicles Conforms to the area of contact with sharp margins Often has a geometric or linear configuration	Atopic dermatitis Bullous impetigo Herpes simplex Superficial fungal infection	Patch test
Herpes simplex	1.5	Herpes simplex virus	Itching or pain prodrome	Grouped vesicles Perioral and perineal location most frequent	Impetigo Superficial fungal infection Contact dermatitis	Tzanck smear Culture Immunofluorescent staining
Herpes zoster	0.4	Varicella-zoster virus	Itching or pain prodrome	Grouped vesicles Dermatomal distribution	Herpes simplex in a dermatomal configuration	Tzanck smear Culture Immunofluorescent staining
Varicella	<0.1	Varicella-zoster virus	Marked pruritus	Macules, papules, vesicles, pustules Generalized	Rickettsialpox Smallpox Disseminated herpes simplex and herpes zoster Coxsackievirus, echovirus Monkeypox	Tzanck smear Culture Immunofluorescent staining

[a]Percentage of new dermatology patients with this diagnosis seen in the Hershey Medical Center Dermatology Clinic, Hershey, Pennsylvania.

The following diseases illustrate the pathogenetic mechanisms involved in blister formation at the different levels of the skin. Detachment of the horny layer by an epidermolytic toxin produced by *Staphylococcus aureus* causes a subcorneal blister. Invasion of epidermal cells by the herpesvirus causes degenerative changes and intraepidermal vesicles. Intercellular edema caused by contact dermatitis results in stretching of the intercellular bridges (spongiosis) until they burst, forming intraepidermal vesicles. Dissolution of the intercellular adhesion molecules secondary to autoantibodies in pemphigus vulgaris causes loss of epidermal cohesion (acantholysis) and blisters within the epidermis.

Damage to the structures within the basement membrane zone causes a loss of coherence between basal cells and the dermis. These subepidermal bullae are characteristic of bullous pemphigoid, dermatitis herpetiformis, and porphyria cutanea tarda.

Blisters usually rupture, producing crusting and weeping. If they become filled with purulent material, they are called *pustules*.

BULLOUS IMPETIGO

KEY POINTS

1. Fragile, clear, or cloudy bullae
2. *S. aureus* toxin causes the blister
3. Treat with a penicillinase-resistant antibiotic

Definition and Etiology

Bullous impetigo is an intraepidermal (subcorneal) bacterial infection of the skin caused by certain strains of *S. aureus* (Fig. 10.1). Impetigo is also discussed in Chapter 12.

Incidence

Bullous impetigo occurs most frequently in preschool-aged children.

History

Crowding, poor hygiene, chronic dermatitis, and neglected injury to the skin are predisposing factors in the development of impetigo. An initial site of involvement is followed by multiple sites that may be pruritic.

Physical Examination

Fragile, clear, or cloudy bullae (Fig. 10.1A) are characteristic of bullous impetigo. A thin, varnish-like crust occurs after the rupture of the bulla. A delicate, collarette-like remnant of the blister roof is often present at the rim of the crust. Gyrate 0.05- to 2-cm crusted patches may be formed with clear centers and active margins. Autoinoculation results in satellite lesions. The face, neck, and extremities are most often affected. Regional

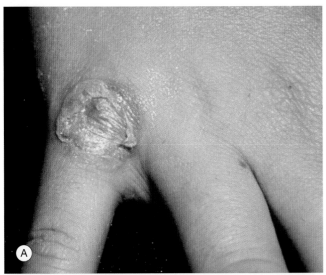

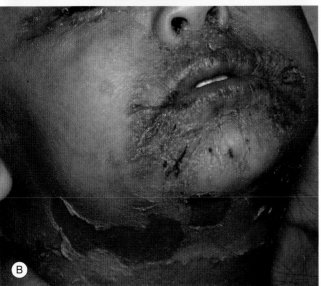

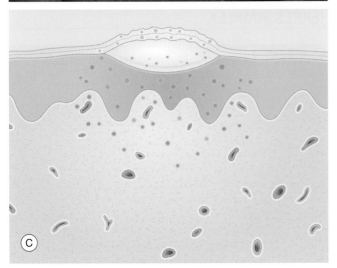

Fig. 10.1 **Bullous impetigo**. (A) Red fragile bullae. (B) Staphylococcal scalded skin syndrome—denuded and crusted, red, scalded-appearing patches involving the typical distribution: periorbital, perioral, and neck. (C) Subcorneal bulla, inflammation.

adenopathy may be present, but patients have no systemic symptoms.

Differential Diagnosis

Contact dermatitis, herpes simplex virus (HSV) infection, and occasionally *superficial fungal infections* (see Fig. 9.8B) may produce vesiculobullous or crusted lesions similar to those of impetigo. The history, patch tests, Tzanck and potassium hydroxide (KOH) preparations, and appropriate cultures differentiate these entities. *Pemphigus vulgaris* may also produce crusted lesions and should be suspected in patients with chronic, apparently impetiginized, patches that have not responded to appropriate antibiotics.

Staphylococcal scalded skin syndrome (Fig. 10.1B) is an uncommon disorder affecting primarily infants and young children. It is characterized by the sudden onset of fever, skin tenderness, and erythema, followed by the formation of large, flaccid bullae and shedding of large sheets of skin, leaving a denuded, scalded-appearing surface. In contrast to bullous impetigo, in which *S. aureus* may be recovered, the bullae of staphylococcal scalded skin syndrome are sterile. The usual source of infection is in the conjunctiva, nose, ear canals, or pharynx. In the newborn, an infected umbilical stump may be the source.

DIFFERENTIAL OF BULLOUS IMPETIGO

- Contact dermatitis
- Herpes simplex
- Superficial fungal infection
- Pemphigus vulgaris
- Staphylococcal scalded skin syndrome

Laboratory and Biopsy

Gram staining of the clear or cloudy fluid from a bulla reveals gram-positive cocci. *S. aureus* grows out in more than 95% of the cultures. Biopsy of impetigo, which is usually not done because the diagnosis is obvious, reveals a subcorneal pustule or blister (Fig. 10.1C).

Therapy

Most *S. aureus* cultured from impetigo lesions is penicillin resistant. Therefore a cephalosporin, such as cefalexin, or penicillinase-resistant semisynthetic penicillin, such as dicloxacillin, should be chosen. A triple antibiotic, retapamulin, or mupirocin ointment applied three times daily is as effective as oral antibiotics in treating impetigo that is limited to a small area. For community-acquired methicillin-resistant *S. aureus* (MRSA), trimethoprim–sulfamethoxazole or doxycycline can be used as alternative treatments.

General hygiene should also be implemented to prevent its spread. Cleansing with an antibacterial cleanser and gentle removal of crust hasten healing. Daily changing of items that contact the area of impetigo, such as towels, washcloths, and shavers, is recommended. For widespread or recurrent impetigo, bleach baths can be helpful.

THERAPY FOR BULLOUS IMPETIGO

Initial
Antibiotics
- Cefalexin: 25–50 mg/kg daily in oral suspension, 500 mg b.i.d.
- Dicloxacillin: 500 mg b.i.d.
- Triple antibiotic, mupirocin, or retapamulin ointment applied b.i.d. or t.i.d.

General Hygiene
- Antibacterial soap: chlorhexidine gluconate
- Changing of towel, washcloth, shaver, and so on, daily
- Bleach baths: ¼–½ cup of bleach in ½ tub of water daily

Alternative — for MRSA
- Trimethoprim–sulfamethoxazole one double-strength table b.i.d. or 4–6 mg/kg b.i.d.
- Doxycycline 100 mg b.i.d.

Course and Complications

Even without treatment, impetigo heals spontaneously in 3–6 weeks. Antibiotics hasten healing (within 1 week of starting therapy) and reduce contagiousness.

Pathogenesis

An epidermolytic toxin targeting desmoglein 1, a desmosomal adhesion molecule, causes the subcorneal cleavage characteristic of bullous impetigo and staphylococcal scalded skin syndrome. This toxin is from pathogenic phage group II *S. aureus*. In bullous impetigo, the toxin is produced at the site of the lesion. In staphylococcal scalded skin syndrome, it is produced remotely and then carried hematogenously to the skin.

Epidermolytic toxin causes bullae.

CONTACT DERMATITIS (ACUTE)

Because acute contact dermatitis is characterized by a vesicular eruption (Fig. 10.2A), it is mentioned briefly here. In Chapter 8, it is discussed in more detail, along with other eczematous eruptions.

Contact dermatitis is an inflammatory reaction of the skin caused by an irritant or allergenic chemical. It may be an acute or chronic process. Intraepidermal vesicles are the hallmark of acute contact dermatitis. Additional characteristics are weeping, crusting, edema, and erythema. The areas involved frequently have sharp margins with geometric and linear configurations. Poison ivy and other plants characteristically cause linear streaks of papulovesicles. Treatment is with steroids (topical or systemic), antihistamines, and wet dressings or soaks. The biopsy of acute contact dermatitis reveals spongiosis and intraepidermal vesicle formation with inflammation (Fig. 10.2B).

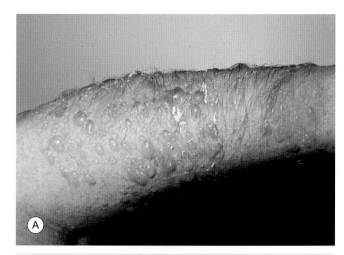

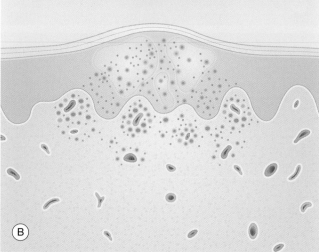

Fig. 10.2 Acute contact dermatitis. (A) Multiple bullae in the area of contactant—poison ivy. Note the sparing area covered by the watch band. (B) Epidermis—bulla, spongiosis. Dermis—perivascular infiltrate.

HERPES SIMPLEX

KEY POINTS

1. Recurrent grouped vesicles in the same location.
2. Tzanck smear is diagnostic.
3. Treatment is suppressive, not curative.

Definition

Herpes simplex is an acute, self-limiting, intraepidermal vesicular eruption caused by infection with HSV (Fig. 10.3). HSV is a DNA virus that replicates within the nucleus. Based on culture and immunologic characteristics, it is divided into two types: HSV-1 and HSV-2. Usually, HSV-1 causes oral infection and HSV-2 causes genital infection. Primary infections with these viruses are characteristically followed by recurrent attacks.

Incidence

Infection with HSV is common worldwide. It is estimated that in the United States more than 50% of adults are seropositive for HSV-1 and more than 20% for HSV-2.

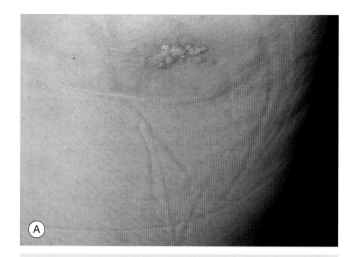

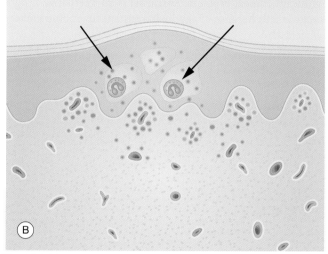

Fig. 10.3 **Herpes simplex**. (A) Grouped vesicles on an erythematous base. (B) Epidermis—bullae, multinucleated giant cells (*arrows*). Dermis—perivascular inflammation.

History

Primary infection with HSV-1 usually occurs in children, in whom it is subclinical in 90% of cases. The remaining 10% of infected children have acute gingivostomatitis. In contrast, HSV-2 primary infection usually occurs after sexual contact in postpubertal individuals, and it produces acute vulvovaginitis or progenitalis. Primary infections are frequently accompanied by systemic symptoms that include fever, malaise, myalgia, headache, and regional adenopathy. Localized pain and burning may be so severe that drinking and eating, or urinating, may be compromised.

Infection of the lips (herpes labialis) is usually caused by HSV-1, whereas the genitals and buttocks are more often infected with HSV-2. The risk of a woman developing genital herpes on exposure to an infected man is estimated to be 80%–90%. The risk of recurrence after primary genital infections is less with HSV-1 (14%) than with HSV-2 (60%). Recurrent attacks are preceded by localized itching or burning and are characterized by their occurrence in the same location. This prodrome usually begins within 24 hours before the appearance of the eruption and occurs in approximately two-thirds of patients.

Herpes should be suspected if a vesicular eruption is:
1. Recurrent in the same location
2. Preceded by a prodrome

HSV infections are not limited to the lips and genital area; either type can infect any area of the skin. Therefore a history of a vesicular eruption recurring in the *same* location should lead to a suspicion of HSV infection.

Physical Examination

Indurated erythema followed by grouped vesicles on a red, inflamed base is typical of herpes infections. The vesicles quickly become pustules, which rupture, weep, and crust. Affected skin sometimes becomes necrotic, resulting in punched-out ulceration.

Grouped vesicles on a red base are characteristic of HSV infection.

Primary infections—gingivostomatitis or vulvovaginitis—are characterized by extensive vesiculation of the mucous membranes. This results in erosions, necrosis, and a marked purulent discharge. Herpes infection can develop in any area where inoculation has occurred. *Recurrent herpes* infections are characterized by localized grouped vesicles in the same location. *Herpetic whitlow* is an infection of the fingers. This is an occupational hazard for medical and dental personnel that can be prevented by wearing gloves. Traumatic herpes simplex has been reported in epidemics among wrestlers (herpes gladiatorum). *Eczema herpeticum* is a generalized cutaneous infection with HSV in individuals with predisposing skin diseases such as atopic dermatitis. It is accompanied by severe toxic symptoms and may be fatal.

Differential Diagnosis

Impetigo, *contact dermatitis*, and, less often, *superficial fungal infections* may be confused with herpes simplex and can be ruled out by the history, Gram staining and culture of the blister fluid, patch testing with suspected allergens, and KOH preparation test of the blister roof.

DIFFERENTIAL DIAGNOSIS OF HERPES SIMPLEX

- Impetigo
- Contact dermatitis
- Superficial fungal infection

Laboratory and Biopsy

The occurrence of grouped vesicles on an erythematous base is characteristic of HSV infection. Polymerase chain reaction (PCR) assay is the preferred method to diagnose herpes infections, being rapid, specific, and sensitive.

A Tzanck smear, which reveals multinucleated giant cells (Fig. 10.4), is a simple yet reliable method of confirming a herpetic infection. Smears from the base of the lesion stained with Giemsa, Wright, or toluidine blue demonstrate multinucleated giant cells, which are diagnostic of HSV infection. A detailed description of preparing a Tzanck preparation is presented in Chapter 3. The positivity of the Tzanck preparation varies with the lesion sampled: vesicle, 67%; pustule, 55%; and crust–ulcer, 16.7%. A high correlation exists between Tzanck preparation and viral culture. However, when performed properly, the culture has greater positivity: vesicle, 100%; pustule, 73%; and crust–ulcer, 33%. Direct immunofluorescent staining of vesicle smears compares favorably with viral cultures. Although usually not necessary, the biopsy (Fig. 10.3B) reveals an intraepidermal blister with multinucleated epidermal giant cells and an acute inflammatory process. Patients with genital herpes should be screened for other sexually transmitted diseases.

> Tzanck smear revealing multinucleated giant cells confirms a herpetic infection.

> PCR of vesicle base/fluid is an effective and efficient diagnostic test for herpes viral infections.

Therapy

Acyclovir (Zovirax), valacyclovir (Valtrex), famciclovir (Famvir), penciclovir (Denavir), and docosanol (Abreva) are the drugs of choice for HSV infections. Their low toxicity and specificity for HSV have resulted in widespread acceptance. Their unique mechanism of action accounts for their selectivity against HSV. Acyclovir is a synthetic acyclic purine nucleoside analog. Phosphorylation of acyclovir depends on HSV-specific thymidine kinase. This enzyme converts acyclovir to acyclovir monophosphate, which is further converted into acyclovir triphosphate by cellular enzymes. Acyclovir triphosphate inhibits viral DNA polymerase and replication of viral DNA. It is effective against replicating viruses but does not eliminate latent viruses. Valacyclovir is a prodrug that is better absorbed than its metabolite acyclovir. Famciclovir, also a prodrug, is metabolized to penciclovir, a synthetic acyclic guanosine derivative. Penciclovir shares similar activation pathways with acyclovir that depend on viral thymidine kinase to form penciclovir triphosphate, which halts DNA synthesis. In active infections, these antiviral drugs

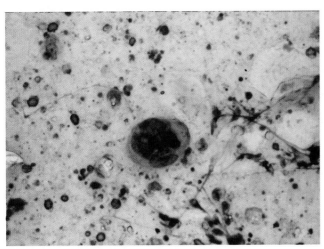

Fig. 10.4 Tzanck smear—multinucleated giant cell.

decrease the duration of viral shedding, accelerate healing of the lesions, and may reduce local and systemic symptoms. For genital herpes infection, condom use can prevent the transmission of HSV-2 by 50% and should be encouraged for individuals with active and asymptomatic shedding of the virus.

> Condom use decreases the transmission of HSV-2.

Intravenous acyclovir is indicated in the treatment of severe primary HSV, including eczema herpeticum, and in initial and recurrent infections in severely immunocompromised patients. The most important adverse reactions are the deposition of drug crystals in the renal tubules of patients with inadequate hydration or impaired renal function. Resistant strains of HSV have emerged in immunocompromised patients and have posed a significant clinical problem. Foscarnet is an alternative drug if acyclovir fails because of acyclovir-resistant thymidine kinase–deficient HSV.

THERAPY FOR HERPES SIMPLEX

Initial
First Episode—Primary
- Acyclovir: 400 mg t.i.d. for 7 days, 5–10 mg/kg IV every 8 hours for 5–7 days
- Valacyclovir: 1000 mg b.i.d. for 7 days
- Famciclovir: 250 mg t.i.d. for 7 days

Recurrent
- Acyclovir: 800 mg t.i.d. for 2 days, 5% ointment every 2 hours for 7 days
- Valacyclovir: 2000 mg b.i.d. for 1 day
- Famciclovir: 1 g b.i.d. for 1 day
- Acyclovir 5% ointment: six times daily for 7 days
- Penciclovir 1% cream: every 2 hours while awake for 4 days
- Docosanol 10% cream: five times daily until healed

Chronic Suppressive
- Acyclovir: 400 mg b.i.d.
- Valacyclovir: 1000 mg daily
- Famciclovir: 250 mg b.i.d.

Alternative
- Foscarnet 40 mg/kg every 8–12 hours for 1–2 weeks

Course and Complications

The incubation period after contact with HSV is approximately 1 week. The clinical course of the primary herpes infection lasts approximately 3 weeks. A prodrome of 1–2 days is followed by a vesiculopustular eruption that continues for about 10 days. This phase is followed by crusting, ulceration, and healing after a further 10 days. For most patients, HSV is an asymptomatic chronic infection of the sensory ganglia. Overt eruptions recur in a minority of infected persons after varying periods of latency, during which the virus remains dormant within the dorsal nerve root ganglion corresponding to the site of infection. Recurrences have a shorter course of 1–2 weeks. Several factors, including fever, ultraviolet light, physical trauma, menstruation, and emotional stress, are attributed to initiating recurrence. Asymptomatic, subclinical shedding of the HSV is common and is instrumental in transmitting HSV to others.

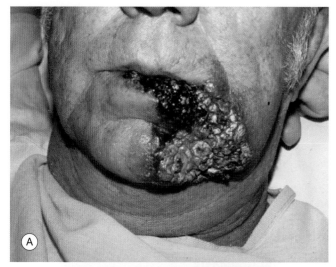

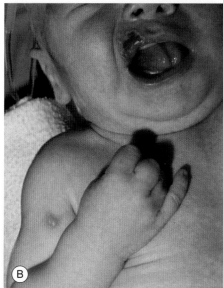

Fig. 10.5 (A) Chronic cutaneous herpes simplex—red crusted plaque. (B) Neonatal herpes simplex—grouped vesicles on an red base on the lip and arm.

The immunocompromised host is most at risk of developing complications from HSV infections. These complications include chronic ulcerative herpes simplex (Fig. 10.5A), which lasts for weeks to months; generalized acute mucocutaneous herpes simplex; and systemic infection involving the liver, lung, adrenal glands, and central nervous system.

> Untreated neonatal herpes is frequently fatal and has severe morbidity.

HSV infection of the neonate, *neonatal herpes* (Fig. 10.5B), is a devastating but fortunately uncommon disease. The fatality rate without treatment is more than 50%, and at least 50% of the survivors have significant neurologic sequelae. A significant reduction in mortality and morbidity occurs with acyclovir treatment. For women who have evidence of an active HSV infection at delivery, a cesarean section is recommended. Complicating neonatal HSV infection, however, are the findings that (1) cultures to screen women immediately before delivery

do not predict infection for the fetus; (2) more than 70% of mothers of babies with neonatal HSV have no history of genital HSV infection; and (3) symptomatic disease may not occur for as long as 1 month after delivery. Two-thirds of affected infants have mucocutaneous manifestations of HSV infection.

> In most cases of neonatal herpes, the mother has no history of genital disease, and it may take up to 1 month after delivery for symptoms to develop.

A relatively uncommon complication of HSV infection is *erythema multiforme*. Immune complexes composed of antibodies and HSV antigens have been found in the serum of patients with erythema multiforme after HSV infection. These immune complexes may be the pathogenesis of the vascular changes seen in erythema multiforme. In addition, HSV DNA has been found in the lesions of erythema multiforme associated with HSV infection.

> Erythema multiforme may occur after HSV infection.

Pathogenesis

HSV is a highly contagious virion spread by direct contact with infected individuals who are often asymptomatically shedding the virus. Studies of shedding and survival of HSV from patients with herpes labialis have detected herpesvirus in their saliva (78%) and on their hands (67%), with virus viability on skin, cloth, and plastic for 2–4 hours.

The virus penetrates the epidermal cell, in which a complex series of steps occurs. The virus undergoes a replicative cycle and induces protein and DNA synthesis with the assembling of intact virions and eventual lysis of the host cell membrane. New copies of viral DNA are packaged into capsids, which are then covered with an amorphous tegument. The viral envelope, which contains virus-specific glycoproteins, is formed by budding through the host nuclear membrane. This process requires an intact host cellular metabolism for substrate synthesis and replication. The destructive effect on epidermal cells results clinically in intraepidermal vesicles.

Latent HSV, undetectable by tissue culture, electron microscopy, and immunofluorescence, presumably resides in the dorsal nerve root sensory or autonomic ganglia in a nonreplicative state. Outbreaks recur with reactivation of the replicative cycle, production of a new virus, and spreading back down the nerve. Latency within the ganglion cells is possible, apparently because the HSV genomes within these cells are relatively well protected from immunologic attacks.

HERPES ZOSTER

KEY POINTS

1. Grouped vesicles in a dermatome
2. Vaccinate
3. Treat early in the middle-aged and elderly people to prevent severe postherpetic neuralgia

Definition

Herpes zoster (shingles) is an intraepidermal vesicular eruption occurring in a dermatomal distribution (Fig. 10.6). It is caused by the reactivation of latent varicella-zoster virus in people who have had varicella.

Vesicular dermatomal eruption is distinctive for herpes zoster.

Incidence

Some 30% of individuals develop herpes zoster during their lifetime. Two-thirds of these individuals are older than 50 years. The attack rate is age-dependent, with a rate of 1 case per 1000 among healthy people less than 20 years old; 3 cases per 1000 in patients between 20 and 49 years old; and a peak of 11 cases per 1000 at age 80–89 years. Patients with cancer and AIDS have a higher incidence than the general population (e.g., 8%–25% of patients with Hodgkin disease develop herpes zoster). The frequency of second attacks may be 5%. However, what is thought to be recurrent zoster may be HSV in a dermatomal distribution.

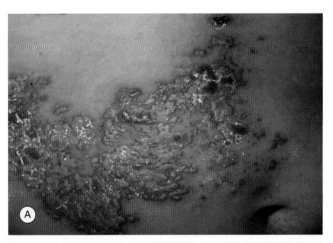

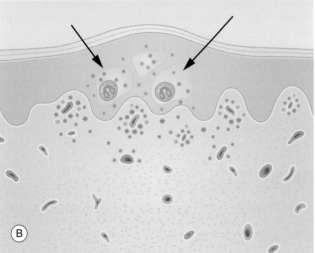

Fig. 10.6 Herpes zoster. (A) Grouped, cloudy, and hemorrhagic vesicles on a red base in a dermatomal distribution. (B) Epidermis—bullae, multinucleated giant cells (*arrows*). Dermis—perivascular inflammation.

History

A prodrome of radicular pain and itching precedes the eruption. It can simulate migraine, pleurisy, myocardial infarction, or appendicitis.

The prodrome may mimic migraine, pleurisy, myocardial infarction, or appendicitis.

Physical Examination

The eruption is characterized by groups of vesicles on a red base situated unilaterally along the distribution of a cranial or spinal nerve. Bilateral involvement is rare. Frequently, the eruption involves the immediately adjacent dermatomes.

Differential Diagnosis

The dermatomal distribution of herpes zoster is diagnostic. However, *herpes simplex* may occur in a dermatomal fashion.

DIFFERENTIAL DIAGNOSIS OF HERPES ZOSTER

* Herpes simplex in a dermatomal configuration

Laboratory and Biopsy

Usually, no laboratory tests are necessary. The Tzanck preparation, direct immunofluorescent staining of vesicle smears, PCR (most sensitive test), biopsy (Fig. 10.6B), and culture are confirmatory in unusual cases. Although herpes zoster has a higher incidence in patients with established malignant disease, patients presenting with herpes zoster who are otherwise healthy do not have a higher incidence of occult cancer and therefore do not need a screening laboratory examination for malignancy. In patients at risk for HIV infection, herpes zoster may be the presenting sign, and serologic testing for HIV is indicated.

Herpes zoster is not a marker for an occult malignant disease. It may be the presenting sign of an HIV infection.

Therapy

Prevention with Zoster Vaccine Recombinant, Adjuvanted (Shingrix) is very effective and indicated in individuals older than 50 years of age. When the vesiculopustules of herpes zoster rupture, crusting and weeping are reduced with astringent (Domeboro) compresses. Analgesics commensurate with the amount of pain experienced by the patient are indicated. Acyclovir (Zovirax), at a dosage of 10 mg/kg every 8 hours intravenously or 800 mg five times daily orally for 7–10 days, halts the progression of herpes zoster in *immunocompromised* patients and is most effective when started within 3 days of the beginning of the eruption. The effects include less cutaneous and visceral dissemination, cessation of new vesicle formation, and reduced pain. The modest benefit of acyclovir, valacyclovir (Valtrex), and famciclovir (Famvir) for *otherwise healthy* patients may not justify the expense, except in severe infections and in patients older than 50 years of age, to reduce postherpetic neuralgia. The use of corticosteroids in otherwise healthy patients to prevent postherpetic neuralgia has been advocated but has not been convincingly proven to be worthwhile. Amitriptyline (Elavil) at a dosage of 50–100 mg daily, or gabapentin (Neurontin) 100–300 mg three times daily, may be helpful in managing postherpetic neuralgia once it occurs. Capsaicin analgesic cream 0.075% (ZostrixHP), used topically three or four times daily on affected skin, can also provide pain relief. Caution must be maintained to avoid inadvertent contact with the eyes or unaffected skin, because capsaicin normally produces transient burning. Foscarnet is indicated for resistant herpes zoster.

THERAPY FOR HERPES ZOSTER

Prevention
- Zoster vaccine

Initial
Antivirals*
- Acyclovir: 800 mg five times daily for 7 days, 10 mg/kg IV every 8 hours for 5–7 daysValacyclovir: 1 g t.i.d. for 7 days
- Famciclovir: 500 mg t.i.d. for 7 days

Compresses
- Aluminum acetate

Pain Medication
- Analgesics
- Amitriptyline: 25–100 mg at bedtime
- Gabapentin: 100–300 mg t.i.d.

Alternative
- Foscarnet 40 mg/kg every 8 hours for 10 days

*Treatment is optional in individuals (1) with mild rash and pain, (2) with eruption >72 hours, and (3) younger than 50 years of age.

Course and Complications

The succession of lesions begins with macules, which develop into vesicles. Over the next several days, pustules develop and are followed by crusting and eventual healing in 2–3 weeks. Hemorrhagic bullae and gangrenous changes may occur and may result in scarring.

Cutaneous dissemination of herpes zoster from the original dermatome develops in some patients, particularly immunocompromised patients, in whom the condition is more likely to be severe and prolonged. It occurs within 5–7 days of the initial eruption and may be accompanied by fever, malaise, and prostration. The immunocompromised patient is susceptible to visceral involvement of the liver, lung, and central nervous system.

Postherpetic neuralgia is uncommon in patients younger than 40 years of age, but 27%, 47%, and 73% of untreated adults older than 55, 60, and 70 years of age, respectively, develop this complication, which is frequently difficult to control and very troubling to the patient. Besides older age, the risk of developing postherpetic neuralgia increases if you are female, have a prodrome, and have more severe acute pain and eruptions.

However, 80% of patients with postherpetic neuralgia become asymptomatic within 12 months.

The nasociliary branch of the ophthalmic division of the trigeminal nerve innervates the eye and the tip of the nose. Therefore herpes ophthalmicus should be suspected when herpes zoster involves the tip of the nose. Scarring of the cornea and conjunctiva may occur; thus this finding requires urgent treatment. Other occasional complications of herpes zoster are full-thickness skin necrosis and Bell palsy.

> When herpes zoster involves the tip of the nose, suspect eye involvement.

Pathogenesis

After primary varicella infection (which the patient often does not recall), the virus becomes latent within the sensory nerve ganglia. With reactivation, replication again occurs with the migration of the virus along the nerve to the skin. Viremia frequently occurs, sometimes resulting in disseminated lesions.

VARICELLA

KEY POINTS
1. Generalized pruritic vesicles.
2. Lesions in all stages.
3. Treatment is usually symptomatic.

Definition

Varicella (chickenpox) is an acute, highly contagious, intraepidermal vesicular eruption caused by varicella-zoster virus. Clinically, it appears as a generalized vesicular eruption (Fig. 10.7A).

Incidence

Varicella is predominantly a childhood disease, with 90% of cases occurring before the age of 10 years. Investigators estimated that 3.5–4.0 million cases occurred annually in the United States prior to the advent of vaccination. Chickenpox occurs throughout the year, but the incidence peaks sharply in March, April, and May. Varicella vaccine has reduced the incidence of hospitalization greatly since its introduction.

History

After a 2- to 3-week incubation period, a 2- to 3-day prodrome of chills, fever, malaise, headache, sore throat, anorexia, and dry cough precedes the onset of the markedly pruritic vesicular eruption. The patient is infectious for approximately 1 week (1–2 days before the rash and a further 4–5 days until the vesicles have become crusted).

Physical Examination

Varicella is a generalized pruritic eruption that is most prominent on the trunk but also involves the head; the extremities, including palms and soles; and the mucous membranes of the mouth and conjunctiva. It is characterized by successive crops of rapidly progressive lesions over an 8- to 12-hour period. The lesions begin as macules, which quickly develop into papules, vesicles, and pustules. Crusting and, sometimes, necrosis precede healing. Characteristically, all types of lesions are present at the same time. The vesicles are 2–3 mm in diameter, occur on an erythematous base, and have a "dewdrop on a rose petal" appearance (Fig. 10.7B). They are often umbilicated and hemorrhagic.

> Chickenpox has all types of lesions: macules, papules, vesicles, pustules, and crusts.

Differential Diagnosis

Before its eradication, smallpox, which is characterized by a febrile prodrome, lesions in the same stage of development, and centrifugal distribution, was the most important disease to exclude. The presence of lesions in all stages of varicella helped to differentiate it from *smallpox*, in which all lesions are in the *same stage* of development. *Disseminated herpes simplex* and *herpes zoster, coxsackievirus, echovirus, rickettsialpox*, and *Mpox* can produce vesicular eruptions similar to those of varicella. Diagnosing varicella is usually not difficult, but if there is any doubt, PCR and cultures can rule out these other infections.

DIFFERENTIAL DIAGNOSIS OF VARICELLA (CHICKENPOX)

- Smallpox
- Disseminated herpes simplex and herpes zoster
- Coxsackievirus, echovirus
- Rickettsialpox
- Mpox

Laboratory and Biopsy

The diagnosis of varicella is usually obvious. A Tzanck preparation reveals multinucleated giant cells typical of herpesvirus infection. Viral cultures, direct fluorescent antibody staining of vesicle smears, biopsy (Fig. 10.7C), and serologic studies may also be done to confirm the diagnosis, although usually these are not necessary. Culture of the varicella-zoster virus is difficult; therefore direct identification of the virus in vesicle smears by immunofluorescent staining is the preferred test. The biopsy, which is rarely done, reveals an intraepidermal blister with multinucleated giant cells (Fig. 10.7C).

Therapy

Treatment for chickenpox is largely symptomatic. Antihistamines and topical agents such as calamine lotion are used to reduce itching. Bathing with colloidal oatmeal (Aveeno) can be used for its soothing, cleansing, and antiinflammatory benefits. Aspirin should be avoided in children because of its association with Reye syndrome. Acyclovir or valacyclovir reduces complications in adults and immunosuppressed children. The use of antivirals in immunologically normal children generally is not indicated unless rare visceral involvement is present, such as varicella pneumonia.

Varicella vaccination (Varivax) is safe and effective in healthy children and adults, especially in preventing moderately severe and severe cases. Passive immunization with varicella-zoster

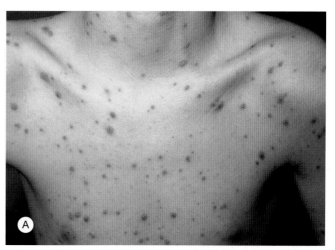

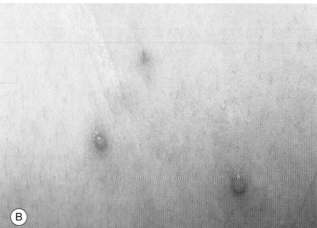

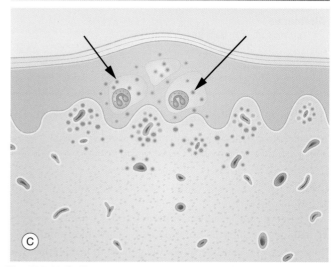

Fig. 10.7 Varicella. (A) Individual red and crusted vesicles in a generalized distribution. (B) "Dewdrop" vesicle on a "rose petal" erythematous base. (C) Epidermis—bullae, multinucleated cells (*arrows*). Dermis—perivascular inflammation.

immune globulin (VZIG; VariZIG) is used in high-risk patients. VZIG is prepared from plasma containing high titers of varicella-zoster antibody. It is effective in preventing or modifying varicella infection in immunodeficient patients if it is administered shortly after exposure. VZIG is not given to patients with active disease. Patients with leukemia or lymphoma, those with congenital or acquired immune deficiency, those receiving immunosuppressive medication, and newborns of mothers who have varicella are candidates for treatment.

THERAPY FOR VARICELLA

Prevention
- Varicella virus vaccine
- VZIG

Initially for Symptomatic Infection
Antihistamines
- Diphenhydramine: 25–50 mg q.i.d.; elixir—12.5 mg/5 mL, 5 mg/kg daily in four divided doses
- Hydroxyzine: 10–25 mg q.i.d.; syrup—10 mg/5 mL, 2 mg/kg daily in four divided doses
- Oatmeal bath
- Calamine lotion

Alternative for Adults, Severe Infection, Immunosuppression
- Acyclovir or valacyclovir

Course and Complications

Approximately 100 deaths occurred each year in the United States as the result of varicella before the vaccination was instituted in 1995. The major complications (pneumonia, encephalitis, and hepatitis) are disproportionately high in adults, very young children, and immunocompromised individuals. Nowadays, with vaccination, the complications, hospitalizations, and death rates from varicella have dropped significantly.

Morbidity and mortality rates are greatly increased in immunocompromised patients.

Varicella during pregnancy poses an approximately 10% risk of intrauterine infection of the fetus, resulting in congenital varicella syndrome or neonatal varicella, with devastating effects on the child.

Pathogenesis

Varicella primary infection begins in the nasopharynx. After local replication, viremia seeds in the reticuloendothelial tissue. Secondary viremias cause dissemination to the skin and viscera. Varicella-zoster virus then enters a latent phase in the sensory ganglia.

UNCOMMON BLISTERING DISEASES

Bullous pemphigoid, dermatitis herpetiformis, epidermolysis bullosa, pemphigus vulgaris, and porphyria cutanea tarda are rare, blistering disorders that are important because of their significant mortality or morbidity (Table 10.2). They should be considered when the more common causes of blistering disease

---

TABLE 10.2   Uncommon Blistering Diseases

Disease	Pathogenesis	Physical Examination	Blister Location	Laboratory Test	Therapy
Bullous pemphigoid	Autoimmune	Tense bullae on inflamed or noninflamed skin Flexor surfaces	Subepidermal	DIF (+) IgG and C3 basement membrane zone IIF (+)	Prednisone Doxycycline Azathioprine Methotrexate Mycophenolate mofetil Rituximab
Dermatitis herpetiformis	Immune complex	Excoriated, crusted papules, vesicles, and urticarial plaques Elbows, knees, back, buttocks	Subepidermal	DIF (+) IgA dermal papillae IIF (+)	Dapsone Sulfapyridine Gluten-free diet
Epidermolysis bullosa simplex	Gene mutation	Tense bullae on hands and feet	Intraepidermal	Biopsy	Prevent trauma, wound care
Pemphigus vulgaris	Autoimmune	Flaccid bullae, erosions, and crusts Generalized	Intraepidermal	DIF (+) IgG and C3 intercellular in epidermis IIF (+)	Prednisone Rituximab Azathioprine Methotrexate Mycophenolate mofetil Gold
Porphyria cutanea tarda	Metabolic	Tense bullae, crusted erosions, milia Dorsum of hands	Subepidermal	Raised urinary uroporphyrin DIF (+)—usually not done IIF (−)	Phlebotomy Antimalarials

C3, Complement; *DIF*, direct immunofluorescence; *IgA*, immunoglobulin A; *IgG*, immunoglobulin G; *IIF*, indirect immunofluorescence; +, positive; −, negative.

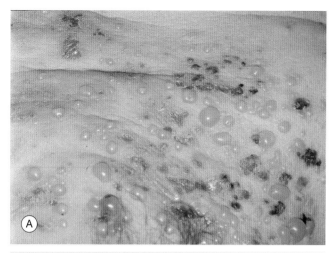

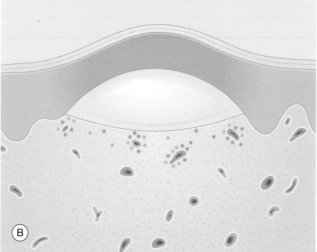

Fig. 10.8 **Bullous pemphigoid**. (A) Tense bullae on noninflammatory skin and crusted residual bullae. (B) Dermis—subepidermal bulla.

have been ruled out and appropriate laboratory data have been collected. Three of the five diseases—pemphigus vulgaris, bullous pemphigoid, and dermatitis herpetiformis—are examples of immunologically mediated disorders. Porphyria cutanea tarda is a metabolic disorder characterized by defective heme synthesis and excessive porphyrin production. Epidermolysis bullosa is a group of genetic disorders with mutations that produce structural defects in the epidermis or dermis.

BULLOUS PEMPHIGOID

Bullous pemphigoid is an autoimmune disorder characterized by large and tense blisters that occur on normal or erythematous/urticarial-appearing skin (Fig. 10.8A). Subepidermal bullae (Fig. 10.8B) are characteristic pathologic findings. The condition occurs in elderly patients (sixth, seventh, and eighth decades). The preferred sites of involvement are the groin, axillae, and flexural areas. Approximately one-third of patients have oral involvement. The bullae do not extend laterally (negative Nikolsky sign) like those of pemphigus vulgaris. Healing usually occurs without scarring.

> The bullae of bullous pemphigoid are tense, occurring on the normal or inflamed skin.

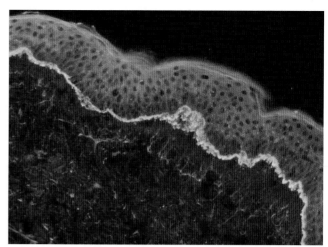

Fig. 10.9 **Bullous pemphigoid**—direct and indirect immunofluorescent staining shows a linear deposit of immunoglobulin G or complement at the dermal–epidermal junction.

Direct and indirect immunofluorescence studies reveal a linear band of immunoglobulin G (IgG) and complement C3 deposited along the basement membrane zone, where blister formation occurs (Fig. 10.9). The IgG autoantibodies are directed against two hemidesmosome-associated proteins (the bullous pemphigoid antigens BP230 and BP180) in the basement membrane zone. These antigens are found intracellularly in association with the hemidesmosome and extracellularly in the lamina lucida, which is the uppermost portion of the basement membrane zone between the epidermis and dermis.

The prognosis is excellent, and the disease usually subsides after months or years. The tendency for the blistered skin to heal results in a low mortality rate. However, the morbidity caused by widespread blistering requires treatment with systemic steroids, doxycycline, and immunosuppressive agents.

DERMATITIS HERPETIFORMIS

Dermatitis herpetiformis is a chronic, intensely pruritic, vesicular disease characterized by grouped (herpetiform) papules, vesicles, and urticarial plaques, which are distributed symmetrically on the elbows, knees, buttocks, low back, and shoulders (Fig. 10.10A). The vesicles are often not intact, secondary to scratching as a result of intense pruritus. The disease usually begins in early adulthood, and the general health of the patient is otherwise excellent.

> Because of scratching, excoriations, rather than vesicles, may be all that is seen in dermatitis herpetiformis.

The typical histologic change of dermatitis herpetiformis is a subepidermal blister (Fig. 10.10B) with neutrophilic abscesses in the dermal papillae. Direct immunofluorescence testing demonstrates granular deposits of IgA at the tips of the dermal papillae (Fig. 10.11). Indirect immunofluorescence testing for IgA antiendomysial antibodies is also sensitive and specific.

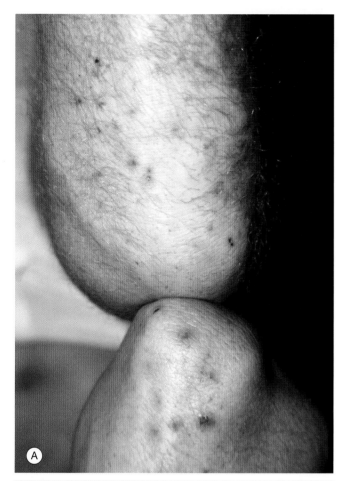

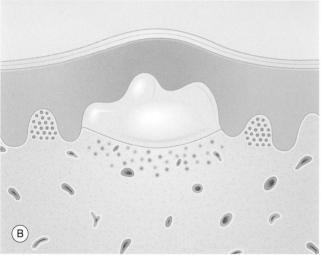

Fig. 10.10 Dermatitis herpetiformis. (A) Crusted vesicles on the elbow and knee—typical distribution. (B) Dermis—subepidermal bulla, neutrophils in dermal papillae.

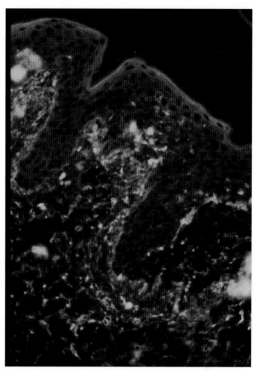

Fig. 10.11 Dermatitis herpetiformis—direct and indirect immunofluorescent staining shows granular deposits of immunoglobulin A in the tips of dermal papillae.

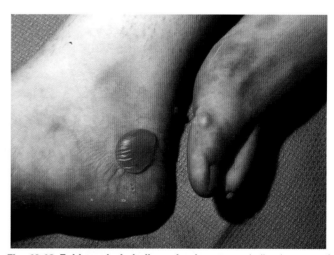

Fig. 10.12 Epidermolysis bullosa simplex—tense bullae in areas of friction on the feet.

Dermatitis herpetiformis characteristically clears rapidly after treatment with dapsone or sulfapyridine, although the disease recurs promptly when therapy is stopped. Approximately 75% of patients have an associated (but usually asymptomatic) gluten-sensitive enteropathy. In these patients, a strict gluten-free diet causes remission or allows a significant reduction of the medication dose.

EPIDERMOLYSIS BULLOSA: SIMPLEX AND RECESSIVE DYSTROPHIC TYPES

Epidermolysis bullosa is a group of disorders characterized by mutations in genes that encode for the structural proteins of the epidermis and dermis. This results in epidermal, junctional, and subepidermal blisters produced by minor friction or trauma. These genodermatoses range in severity from being relatively minor to being severely disabling and fatal. Epidermolysis bullosa simplex (Fig. 10.12) has blistering limited to the hands and feet and is caused by dominant keratin 5 and 14 gene mutations. This defect produces keratinocyte fragility and intraepidermal

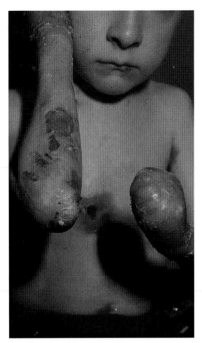

Fig. 10.13 Recessive dystrophic epidermolysis bullosa—erosions and "mitten" deformity of the hand.

TABLE 10.3   Pemphigus Vulgaris versus Pemphigus Foliaceus

	Pemphigus Vulgaris	Pemphigus Foliaceus
Autoantigen	Desmoglein 3	Desmoglein 1
Clinical features	Flaccid bullae, erosions, *oral lesions*	Scaling, few flaccid bullae, erosions
Histopathology	Suprabasal acantholysis, "tombstone" basal keratinocyte pattern	Subcorneal/granular layer acantholysis
Immunofluorescence	Intercellular IgG, C3	Intercellular IgG, C3

C3, Complement; *IgG*, immunoglobulin G.

cleavage. Recessive dystrophic epidermolysis bullosa (Fig. 10.13) results from mutations in the gene encoding type VII collagen, *COL7A1*. The severe form is characterized by "mitten-like" deformity of the hands and feet, contractures, blistering and scarring of the mouth and eyes, esophageal strictures, growth retardation, anemia, and nutritional deficiency. Treatment of epidermolysis bullosa is symptomatic and supportive, including protection from trauma, good wound care, treatment of infections, and nutritional supplements.

> Epidermis bullosa can be mild to severe, depending on which structural protein is defective.

PEMPHIGUS VULGARIS

Pemphigus vulgaris (Table 10.3) is an autoimmune disease characterized by blistering of the skin and mucous membranes. It occurs predominantly in middle and old age, with an estimated incidence of 1 per 100,000. The bullae are flaccid and superficial and range from 1 to 10 cm in size. They rupture easily, leaving large denuded, bleeding, weeping, and crusted erosions (Fig. 10.14). Pressure applied laterally to the bulla results in extension (Nikolsky sign). The oral mucosa (erosions of the mouth) is almost always involved and is frequently the presenting site.

> The flaccid bullae of pemphigus vulgaris break easily, leaving erosions and crusts.

The bulla of pemphigus vulgaris occurs intraepidermally, just above the basal layer (Fig. 10.14B). It is formed by the loss of cohesion between epidermal cells (acantholysis). Direct

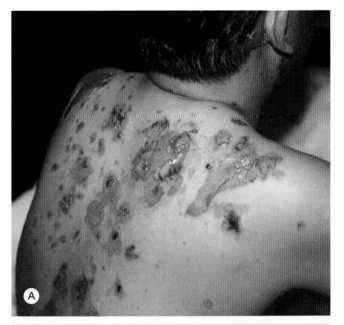

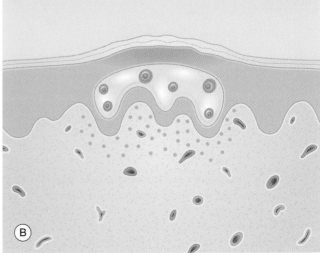

Fig. 10.14 Pemphigus vulgaris. (A) Flaccid bullae and erosions. (B) Epidermis—suprabasal bulla, acantholytic epidermal cells.

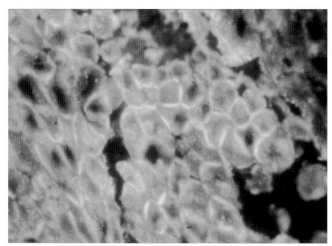

Fig. 10.15 **Pemphigus vulgaris**—direct and indirect immunofluorescent staining shows intercellular staining with immunoglobulin G and complement.

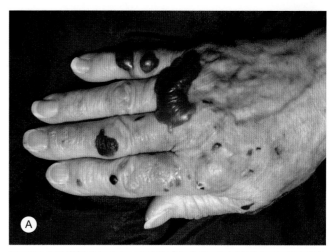

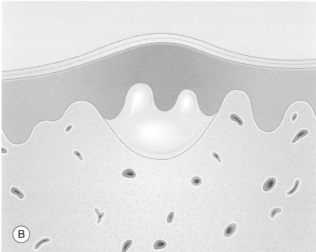

Fig. 10.16 **Porphyria cutanea tarda**. (A) Tense hemorrhagic bullae on the dorsal hand, the classic location. (B) Dermis—subepidermal bulla.

(with patient skin) and indirect (with patient serum) immunofluorescence studies are positive, showing deposits of immunoglobulins (predominantly IgG) or complement C3 between epidermal cells (intercellular space) (Fig. 10.15). Experimental evidence suggests that the interaction between the circulating IgG autoantibodies and epidermal cell surface antigens (adhesion molecule desmoglein 3) contained in intercellular adhering junctions (desmosomes) leads to blister formation. In addition, the production of proteolytic enzymes that hydrolyze the cell surface proteins causes a loss of adhesion between keratinocytes.

Before the introduction of systemic steroids, pemphigus vulgaris was associated with an extremely high mortality rate. Systemic steroids, rituximab, and immunosuppressive agents such as methotrexate, cyclophosphamide, azathioprine, mycophenolate mofetil, and gold are used. The overall mortality rate is 8%–10%, and death now occurs more frequently as a result of steroid-induced complications than from the disease. Two other major types of pemphigus are pemphigus foliaceus and paraneoplastic pemphigus. *Pemphigus foliaceus* (Chapter 8) often has an eczematous appearance with a few scattered small flaccid bullae and erosions and is caused by antibodies to desmoglein 1. *Paraneoplastic pemphigus* can clinically and histologically mimic a mixture of pemphigus vulgaris and erythema multiforme. It is associated with a variety of tumors, most frequently non-Hodgkin lymphoma and chronic lymphocytic leukemia.

> Untreated pemphigus vulgaris has a high mortality rate.

PORPHYRIA CUTANEA TARDA

The porphyrias are a group of disorders characterized by abnormalities in the heme biosynthetic pathway resulting in abnormal porphyrin metabolism and excessive accumulation of various porphyrins. Porphyria cutanea tarda is the most common form of porphyria. It is characterized by subepidermal blisters on the hands and excessive uroporphyrin excretion in the urine. Bullae, vesicles, erosions, crusts, milia, and mild scarring occur on sun-exposed skin, especially the dorsum of the hands (Fig. 10.16A). Facial hair, predominantly on the temples and cheeks, and mottled facial pigmentation resembling melasma also occur.

The bullae of porphyria cutanea tarda occur subepidermally (Fig. 10.16B). Direct immunofluorescence reveals immunoglobulin and complement around the dermal blood vessels and at the dermal–epidermal junction. The metabolic changes in porphyria cutanea tarda are diagnostic, so immunofluorescence testing is not warranted. Characteristically, urinary levels of uroporphyrins and coproporphyrins are markedly raised, with a ratio of uroporphyrin to coproporphyrin of at least 3:1. Liver function test results and serum iron levels are usually increased. The urine is dark brown and fluoresces orange-red under Wood's light. *Variegate porphyria* and *hereditary coproporphyria* have neurologic and abdominal symptoms as well as the same cutaneous findings as porphyria cutanea tarda. The ratio of urinary uroporphyrin to coproporphyrin is 1:1 in variegate porphyria, and further serum or fecal porphyrin measurements are necessary to diagnose hereditary coproporphyria.

> Variegate porphyria, hereditary coproporphyria, and porphyria cutanea tarda have identical skin findings.

Porphyria cutanea tarda is familial or sporadic. It is often precipitated by alcohol, hepatitis C, or hormones (contraceptive pills). It is also strongly associated with hereditary hemochromatosis. The biosynthetic pathway for heme requires the conversion of uroporphyrinogen to coproporphyrinogen by the enzyme uroporphyrinogen decarboxylase. When this enzyme is absent, uroporphyrins accumulate and produce porphyria cutanea tarda. The treatment of choice is phlebotomy or very low-dose antimalarials, such as hydroxychloroquine, given in single doses a few times per week.

SELF-ASSESSMENT

Case 1—Recurrent Vesicles (Fig. 10.17)

What Is Your Diagnosis?

These grouped vesiculopustules on an erythematous base are typical of HSV infection. In addition, the history of a recurrent vesicular eruption in the same place is classic for this viral infection. No other diagnosis should be seriously considered.

What Laboratory Tests Would You Do?

A Tzanck preparation is all that is necessary to confirm the clinical diagnosis. If you are still in doubt, a viral culture can be obtained.

What Are Your Recommendations to This Patient?

Acyclovir, valacyclovir, or famciclovir may be used in patients with frequent recurrences. These medications reduce the duration of viral shedding and time to healing of lesions when administered early in the course of a recurrent episode.

Case 2—Crusted Erosions on the Dorsum of the Hands and Forearms (Figs. 10.18 and 10.19)

What Is Your Differential Diagnosis?

Erosions suggest a blistering disease. The configuration, distribution, and history make an infectious cause such as herpes and impetigo unlikely. Acute contact dermatitis causes vesicles and bullae. However, there is no evidence of dermatitis surrounding the crusts. Uncommon blistering diseases such as pemphigus, bullous pemphigoid, epidermolysis bullosa, and porphyria should be considered. Hypertrichosis of his temples suggests the diagnosis of porphyria cutanea tarda.

What Would You Do Now?

A simple test is to fluoresce the patient's urine with a Wood's light (Fig. 10.19). This is a quick screen for

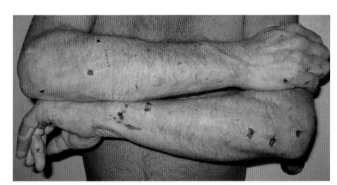

Fig. 10.18 This 51-year-old man had a 10-year history of occasional blisters on his hands. In the last year, the blistering had become worse, with involvement of his arms, legs, and head. A trip to the beach flared the eruption.

IMPORTANT POINTS

1. A Tzanck preparation is an easy laboratory test that confirms the diagnosis of HSV infection.
2. Acyclovir, valacyclovir, and famciclovir are the current treatments of choice for HSV infection, but they are not curative.

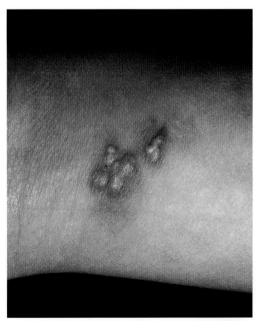

Fig. 10.17 This 32-year-old woman had a history of a recurrent vesicular eruption. It started 5 years before, and it recurs five or six times yearly. A tingling sensation precedes the onset of the rash.

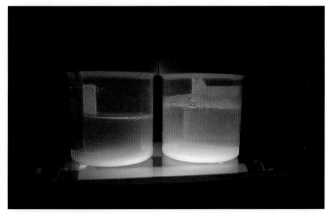

Fig. 10.19 Wood's light revealed coral red fluorescence of the patient's urine (*left*) compared with the normal lime green urine (*right*).

detecting elevated urine uroporphyrins. His laboratory tests revealed elevated liver enzymes, iron levels, and urine uroporphyrins. He had negative tests for hepatitis C, hemochromatosis, and HIV. His diagnosis is porphyria cutanea tarda.

How Would You Treat This Patient?

Treatment begins with preventing further liver and cutaneous damage by cessation of alcohol and precipitating medications, as well as starting sun protection. Phlebotomy is the first-line therapy. Low-dose antimalarials such as hydroxychloroquine can be used as an alternative treatment.

IMPORTANT POINTS

1. When there is crusting, look for blisters.
2. Consider a systemic disease in your differential diagnosis of skin symptoms.

Inflammatory Papules

CHAPTER CONTENTS

Algorithm of inflammatory papules

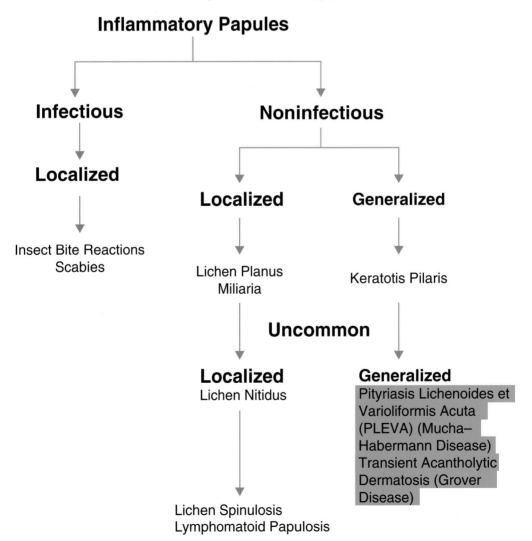

Inflammatory Papules

Infectious

Noninfectious

Localized

Insect Bite Reactions
Scabies

Localized

Lichen Planus
Miliaria

Generalized

Keratotis Pilaris

Uncommon

Localized
Lichen Nitidus

Generalized
Pityriasis Lichenoides et
Varioliformis Acuta
(PLEVA) (Mucha–
Habermann Disease)
Transient Acantholytic
Dermatosis (Grover
Disease)

Lichen Spinulosis
Lymphomatoid Papulosis

ABSTRACT

The common diseases discussed in this chapter are characterized by discrete, small, erythematous papules that do *not* become confluent. Most of these disorders are pruritic, and some are markedly so. As a result, the papules are often crusted secondary to excoriation. Papules are common primary lesions found in numerous skin diseases, including acne, eczematous diseases (e.g., atopic dermatitis), and scaling disorders (e.g., psoriasis). However, in these diseases, other features are present that allow for their characterization. For example, comedones and pustules accompany papules in acne, eczematous papules coalesce into plaques in atopic dermatitis, and plaques as well as papules located on extensor surfaces are present in psoriasis. The diseases in this chapter feature individual papules as the predominant finding or primary lesion (Table 11.1). History and physical examination often establish the diagnosis, but a biopsy, when needed, confirms the clinical suspicion. The diseases are organized by the categories of infectious versus noninfectious. The categories are further divided into the important finding of the distribution of lesions on physician examination: localized versus generalized. Think of generalized distribution presenting symmetrically, in other words, with one side of the body mirroring the other side of the body. Finally, some diseases with a localized distribution may present, more uncommonly, with a generalized distribution.

KEY POINTS

1. Itching is usually prominent.
2. Primary lesion is usually a papule.
3. Skin biopsy, when needed, confirms clinical suspicion.

INSECT BITE REACTIONS

KEY POINTS

1. Immediate hives after an insult suggest the diagnosis.
2. Develop only in people who are allergic.
3. Often appear in a localized distribution of groups of three (breakfast, lunch, and dinner!).
4. Insect stings, not insect bites, are a common cause of anaphylaxis.

Definition

Insect bites, stings, and infestations produce local inflammatory reactions (Fig. 11.1) in response to injected foreign chemicals and proteins. Acute skin reactions appear as hives or papular urticaria, and more chronic reactions appear as inflammatory papules. Insects that sting (usually when threatened) include bees, wasps, and fire ants. Insects that bite (usually out of hunger) include mosquitoes, fleas, flies, bedbugs, and lice. Spiders, ticks, and chiggers are other arthropods that sometimes attack human skin.

Incidence

Most insect bites are recognized as such and are not brought to a physician's attention. Anaphylactic reactions occur in 0.3%–3% of stings. Winged hymenoptera, mainly honeybees, bumblebees, and yellow jackets, are the most common cause of allergic insect sting reactions, including anaphylaxis. In the southern United States, fire ants are the leading cause of these reactions.

Insect bites and stings are primarily a seasonal phenomenon.

TABLE 11.1 Papules

	Frequency (%)[a]	Etiology	History	Physical Examination	Differential Diagnosis	Laboratory Test
Insect bite reactions	0.7	Stinging and biting arthropods	Insect often not seen by patient	Papules with central puncta and often *grouped* *Asymmetric* distribution	Urticaria Impetigo Mucha–Habermann disease	–
Keratosis pilaris	Not known	Unknown	Bothersome rough bumps	Follicular, monomorphic papules Extensor arms and thighs and facial cheeks	Acne Lichen nitidus Lichen spinulosus	–
Lichen planus	0.6	Unknown	–	Purple, polygonal flat-topped papules with Wickham striae Can be generalized: wrists, ankles, and *mucous membranes* favored	Lupus erythematosus Lichen planus–like drug eruption Graft-vs-host disease	Biopsy
Miliaria	0.1	Sweat duct occlusion	Fever or occlusion of affected skin	Numerous small papules Trunk, especially back, usually affected	Contact dermatitis Folliculitis Candidiasis	Biopsy (not usually necessary)
Scabies	1.5	Mite	Other close contacts often affected	*Burrows* (when found) diagnostic Generalized distribution sparing head Genitalia often affected	Atopic dermatitis	Scraping

[a]Percentage of new dermatology patients with this diagnosis seen in the Hershey Medical Center Dermatology Clinic, Hershey, Pennsylvania.

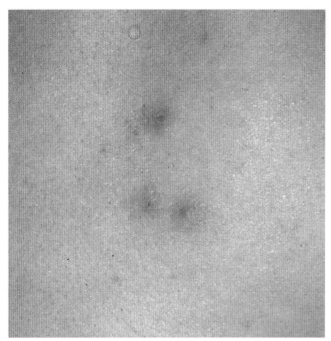

Fig. 11.1 Insect bites. Grouped red, crusted papules with red flare.

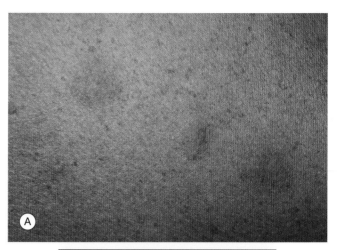

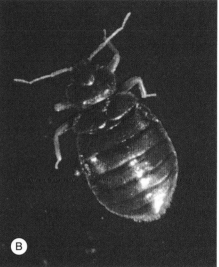

Fig. 11.2 (A) Bedbug insect bites—characteristic "breakfast, lunch, and dinner." (B) Recovered bedbug—*Cimex lenticularis*.

History

When someone is stung by an insect, the insult is usually remembered because the sting induces immediate pain. This is not always the case for biting insects; some delay may occur between the actual bite and the itching that follows. If the physical examination suggests insect bites (even when the patient is unaware of having been bitten), the history should be pursued carefully for possible exposures. For indoor exposure, fleas are common offenders. We inquire not only about pets currently living in the dwelling but also about whether pets recently occupied the premises. If a house had been previously occupied by flea-infested pets, the abandoned hungry fleas may form a welcoming party for the newly arrived human guests. We also ask about pets in homes visited by the patient. Spiders are sometimes responsible for indoor bites; their presence requires a careful search of the home. Bedbugs are becoming an increasingly recognized household insect that likes to bite in groups of three, commonly referred to as "breakfast, lunch, and dinner" (Fig. 11.2). Bedbugs often infest bats and birds and then hide in cracks and crevices, attacking the susceptible, sleeping victim in the early morning hours. Infestations with head lice often occur epidemically in school children, so a history of affected playmates should be sought and the school nurse consulted.

"Indoor" insects:
1. Fleas
2. Spiders
3. Bedbugs
4. Lice

Contrary to some misconceptions, it is not necessary for other persons dwelling in the same household, or even the same

bed, to be affected. For insect bite reactions, two factors are required: a biting insect and a host who is allergic to the bite. Not all people are sensitive, and not all people attract insects equally.

Papules and, in highly allergic individuals, bullae occur only in people who are allergic and who attract the insects (Fig. 11.3).

Physical Examination

The reaction to a sting is usually an immediate hive, often with a central punctum, that resolves within a few hours. The lesions are present in localized distribution. Large local reactions, manifesting as extensive erythema and swelling at the bite site, resolve after several days. Of the stinging insects, only the honeybee leaves behind its stinger, which on close inspection appears as a sharp barb projecting from the skin. If found, this stinger should be removed gently to prevent the release of additional venom from the attached venom sack. Fire ants produce multiple itching hives, which quickly

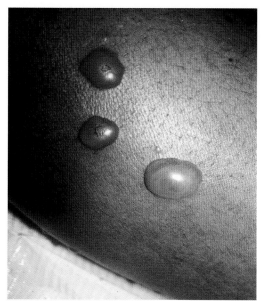

Fig. 11.3 **Insect bites**. Grouped bullae with central puncta from mosquito bites in susceptible host.

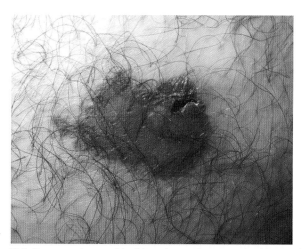

Fig. 11.4 **Brown recluse spider bite**—impending necrotic skin reaction.

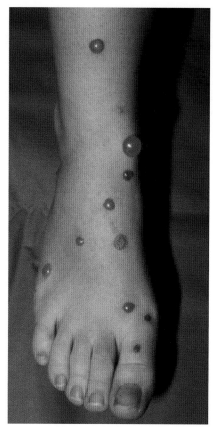

Fig. 11.5 **Insect bites**—multiple vesicles.

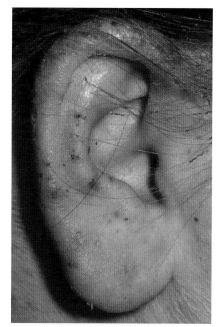

Fig. 11.6 **Lice**—multiple vesicles; excoriated papules and white nits in hair.

progress to painful papulovesicles and pustules. The bite of a recluse spider is unique in that it produces a severe local necrotic reaction with ulceration (Fig. 11.4). Although the bite may be "quiet," the reaction that ensues over the following days is not. Chiggers favor the legs and areas of tight-fitting clothing where they produce inflammatory papules and vesicles, and occasionally even bullae (Fig. 11.5). Ticks painlessly burrow their heads in the skin, and pubic lice (pediculosis pubis) attach to hair; both can be visualized macroscopically. Head lice (pediculosis capitis) may be difficult to find but should be suspected in the presence of itching of the scalp, particularly the occiput or peripheral scalp (Fig. 11.6). The eggs (nits) are most often found and appear as small, 2- to 3-mm, oval, translucent concretions affixed to hair shafts. Similar findings occur in body lice (pediculosis corporis) and pubic lice (crabs, pediculosis pubis).

Physicians are most often consulted for insect bites that produce itching papules. These are typically grouped and asymmetric. Flea bites frequently occur in streaks of three: "breakfast, lunch, and dinner." Sometimes, a central punctum can be

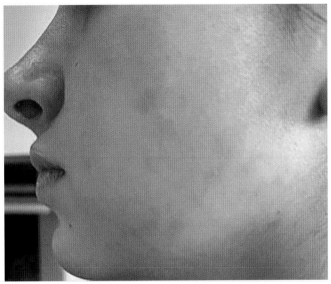

Fig. 11.7 Delusional parasitosis—multiple crusted papules and scars from chronic picking.

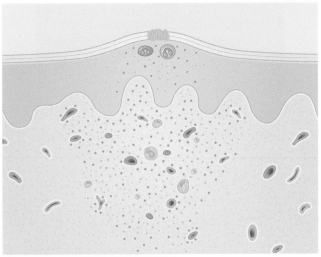

Fig. 11.8 Insect bite reaction. Epidermis—crust; spongiosis; inflammation cell infiltrate. Dermis—dense infiltrate of mixed inflammatory cells, often including eosinophils.

identified in the papule; this is diagnostic. If the offending insects remain in the environment, new lesions will continue to appear. Occasionally, only excoriations are found. Postinflammatory hyperpigmentation after insect bite reactions is commonly seen in patients with skin of color.

Differential Diagnosis

For patients with urticarial reactions, other causes of urticaria (see Chapter 16) may be considered. When the hive has a central punctum, its cause is an insect bite. *Other foreign bodies* can induce pruritic papules in the skin. Fiberglass is an example. This diagnosis can be suggested by the history and confirmed by the presence of a refractile material in the epidermis on biopsy or skin scraping. Delusional infestation (aka delusions of parasitosis) is a severe, chronic medical condition characterized by crusted papules and scars from "skin picking." Patients suffer from a false, fixed belief that "bugs are under my skin" and cannot be corrected by logic or reasoning. Diagnosis and treatment require building rapport and psychiatric evaluation and treatment (Fig. 11.7). *Dermatitis herpetiformis* (see Chapter 10) is in the differential diagnosis, particularly when only excoriations are found. Excoriation may also lead to secondary infection and a diagnosis of impetigo (see Chapter 12). An uncommon idiopathic disorder, pityriasis lichenoides, presents with scattered necrotic papules and vesicles that can resemble insect bites but are usually more generalized and symmetric. A skin biopsy helps to distinguish pityriasis lichenoides disease from an insect bite reaction.

DIFFERENTIAL DIAGNOSIS OF INSECT BITES
• Urticaria
• Delusional infestation
• Dermatitis herpetiformis
• Pityriasis lichenoides

Laboratory and Biopsy

The diagnosis is usually made clinically. Skin testing with commercial venom kits can be performed by an allergist. A biopsy, if performed, shows a wedge-shaped superficial and deep cellular infiltrate so dense that it may be mistaken for malignant lymphoma. An insect bite is suggested by virtue of a mixed inflammatory cell infiltrate, which includes numerous eosinophils (Fig. 11.8).

Therapy

The primary therapy is to remove the offending insect from the environment of the patient or vice versa. Insects that are attached to the skin can be gently removed with tweezers (e.g., ticks) or killed chemically (e.g., lice) with agents such as permethrin crème rinse (Nix). For lice, fomite transmission is proven, as adult lice can live away from a human host for 3 days and nits can live for 10 days. Most lice treatments are pediculicidal, but not ovicidal, and require a retreatment in 7–10 days. For fleas, not only must the pet be treated but also the house must be professionally fumigated. Insect repellent containing diethyltoluamide (DEET) remains a safe and effective deterrent to insect bites, especially ticks, with the lowest effective dose of approximately 30%. Permethrin application to clothing also repels ticks, agents responsible for Lyme disease (see Chapter 16) and Rocky Mountain spotted fever. Colognes, perfumes, and scented hair sprays can attract insects and should be avoided in sensitive individuals.

Successful treatment of flea bites includes fumigation of the home.

Treatment of the inflammatory reaction in the skin is symptomatic. Topical steroids, systemic antihistamines, and occasionally systemic steroids may be helpful in relieving the itching.

THERAPY FOR INSECT BITE REACTIONS

Initial

Separation of Host From Insect
- Lice: topical permethrin
- Fleas: house fumigation
- Bedbugs: house fumigation
- Ticks: DEET repellent and permethrin on clothing

Symptomatic Therapy for Itching
- Topical steroids (e.g., clobetasol 0.05% cream b.i.d. for 2 weeks)
- Antihistamines

Alternative
- Lice: topical benzyl alcohol and malathion
- Symptomatic therapy for itching: systemic steroids
- EpiPen for highly allergic individuals

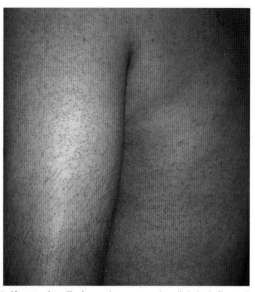

Fig. 11.9 Keratosis pilaris—minute, rough, slightly inflamed papules on the upper outer arm.

Course and Complications

In highly sensitive individuals, stings can produce serious anaphylactic reactions, mediated through immunoglobulin E, that occasionally result in death. Patients with anaphylactic reactions require prompt therapy with airway management, epinephrine, antihistamines, and systemic steroids, despite little evidence of systemic steroid benefit. Patients with severe reactions are likely to have severe reactions to future stings. Subsequent "desensitization" immunotherapy is frequently indicated for future prophylaxis. Immunotherapy is not necessary, however, in most children with urticarial reactions, even when these reactions are severe and generalized, as long as symptoms are confined to the skin. It is advisable, however, for such patients to have injectable epinephrine (Ana-Kit, EpiPen) readily available, especially when picnicking, hiking, or camping.

Most insect bite reactions resolve spontaneously and uneventfully. Secondary infection may occur, particularly when the patient has been scratching excessively. Scratching and infection can lead to scarring. A persistent local reaction to the bite of an infected deer tick is a characteristic finding in Lyme disease and is called *erythema migrans* (see Chapter 16).

Pathogenesis

Most insect bite reactions are the result of host allergies to injected secretions, including venoms (from stinging insects) and enzymes. Histamine, acetylcholine, and other vasoactive chemicals have also been isolated from the venom of stinging insects, and these, too, may play a role in the immediate reaction. However, the primary mechanism for insect bite reactions is allergy. The degree of host allergy determines the intensity of the reaction, which ranges from none to severe. As exemplified by *erythema migrans*, cutaneous reactions to insect bites may also be caused by microorganisms transmitted by the bite.

KERATOSIS PILARIS

KEY POINTS
1. Involves extensor arms and thighs and face
2. Follicular papules
3. Bothersome appearance

Definition

Keratosis pilaris is a disorder characterized by keratinized hair follicles. Monomorphic, follicle-based papules with a central horny spine are located predominantly on the extensor upper arms and thighs, with the cheeks of face less commonly affected (Fig. 11.9).

Incidence

Almost one-half of the population is affected by keratosis pilaris. It is most common in adolescents, especially those with a history of dry skin, as seen in patients with atopic dermatitis and ichthyosis vulgaris. A positive family history is often present.

History

Patients often report "rough bumps" that do not go away with washing, especially scrubbing. The condition is often mistaken for acne. Keratosis pilaris is not pruritic or painful. However, patients do not like their "bumpy" appearance. Signs and symptoms worsen in the winter and improve with age.

Physical Examination

Keratosis pilaris is characterized by individual, small, follicular papules with a central horny spine. The lesions can be noninflamed or inflamed. Keratosis pilaris is monomorphic. Common areas of involvement include the cheeks and extensor upper arms and thighs. With facial involvement, background erythema

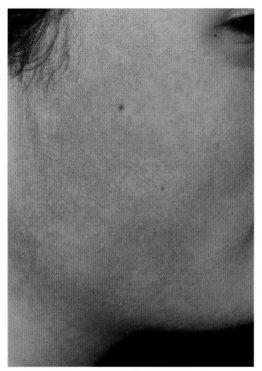

Fig. 11.10 Keratosis pilaris—minute rough papules, sometimes better felt than seen, with background erythema on a child's face.

is commonly seen (Fig. 11.10). The lesions are present in a symmetric distribution (e.g., both upper arms or cheeks are affected).

Differential Diagnosis

Clinical recognition makes the diagnosis straightforward. When keratosis pilaris occurs on the face, it is often diagnosed mistakenly as acne. To distinguish acne from keratosis pilaris involving the cheeks, look for pustules and comedones that are diagnostic of acne. Lichen spinulosus, which can appear clinically similar to keratosis pilaris, has a sudden onset, is located most commonly on the abdomen, extensor arms, knees, and neck, and may remit spontaneously after 1–2 years. The papules of lichen nitidus are flat-topped and not as rough as keratosis pilaris. In addition, koebnerization (linear streaks of papules) is seen in lichen nitidus, not keratosis pilaris.

DIFFERENTIAL DIAGNOSIS OF KERATOSIS PILARIS
• Acne
• Lichen spinulosus
• Lichen nitidus

Laboratory and Biopsy

Keratosis pilaris is a straightforward clinical diagnosis. Laboratory workup and biopsy are not necessary.

Therapy

Education and reassurance are the mainstays of treatment. It is important to recognize that keratosis pilaris can be cosmetically distressing. An emollient cream can soften the rough papules. Therapeutic emollients containing 20% urea (Carmol 20), salicylic acid 6% (Keralyt), and ammonium lactate 12% (LacHydrin, prescription only, or AmLactin, available over the counter) have keratolytic properties, thereby decreasing corneocyte adhesion. Tretinoin cream 0.05% (Retin-A) or over-the-counter adapalene gel 0.1% (Effaclar) can also be used successfully.

THERAPY FOR KERATOSIS PILARIS
Initial
• Reassurance and education
• Therapeutic emollients
• Urea 20%
• Salicylic acid 6%
• Ammonium lactate 12%
Alternative
• Tretinoin cream 0.05%
• Adapalene gel 0.1%

Course and Complications

Keratosis pilaris can improve with age but tends to be persistent, especially in individuals with a history of dry skin (e.g., ichthyosis vulgaris). It can be associated with postinflammatory hyperpigmentation in darker skin types. Complications are uncommon.

Pathogenesis

Although the etiology of keratosis pilaris is unknown, abnormal keratinocyte desquamation most likely leads to keratin plugging of the hair follicle.

LICHEN PLANUS

KEY POINTS
1. Purplish papules favor flexor wrists and distal lower extremities.
2. It can affect hair, skin, nails, and mucous membranes.
3. Biopsy confirms clinical suspicion.

Definition

Lichen planus is an idiopathic inflammatory disorder of the skin. Clinically, the papules are flat (planus) and are surmounted by subtle, fine, white dots and lines that, with imagination, resemble the appearance of lichen found in nature (Fig. 11.11).

Lichen planus is characterized by five Ps:
1. Purplish
2. Planar
3. Pruritus
4. Polygonal
5. Papule

Incidence

The disorder is uncommon but not rare. It is the presenting problem in 6 per 1000 of the authors' new dermatology patients.

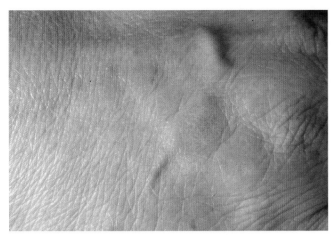

Fig. 11.11 Lichen planus—flat-topped (planar) purple papules with Wickham striae.

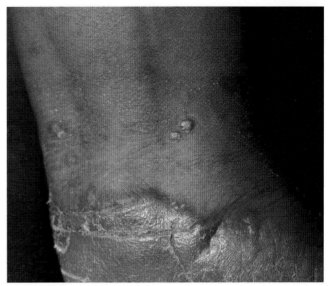

Fig. 11.13 Lichen planus—palmar plaque with characteristic papule involving flexor wrist.

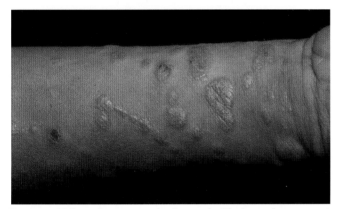

Fig. 11.12 Lichen planus—papules in streaks (Koebner phenomenon).

It is estimated that lichen planus affects less than 1% of the population. Lichen planus occurs in children and adults.

History

The major complaint is itching, which is often severe. Mucous membrane involvement sometimes results in painful erosions. Lichen planus–like eruptions can be induced by drugs, so a careful drug history should be elicited. Clinicians should have a high index of suspicion regarding lichen planus in patients with hepatitis C virus, although the cause and effect relationship remains uncertain.

Physical Examination

The primary lesion is a purple, polygonal, flat-topped papule. Its surface has a fine reticulate pattern of white dots and lines (Wickham striae) that can be visualized on *close* inspection. Wickham striae are more readily visible through a handheld lens after the application of a drop of oil on the surface of the papule. The papules are sometimes arranged in streaks, presumably resulting from the trauma of scratching (Koebner phenomenon; Fig. 11.12). The wrists and ankles are favored locations for lichen planus, but any area may be affected, including the palms, soles, and genitalia (Fig. 11.13). Patients may have only a few papules or innumerable ones in a generalized distribution. Uncommonly, individual lesions may attain plaque size. Residual hyperpigmented macules, more often appreciated

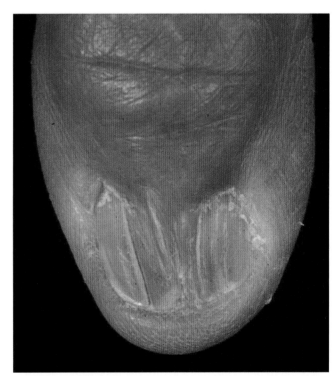

Fig. 11.14 Lichen planus—nail matrix involvement leads to dystrophic nail.

in dark-skinned individuals, typically result from the inflammatory process. The nails and hair follicles are occasionally involved with dystrophic changes and even scarring (Fig. 11.14).

Mucous membrane involvement is common and, in some patients, is the sole manifestation of the disease. Most often, this condition appears as white streaks in a reticulate pattern (see Chapter 22). Blisters and erosions also sometimes occur. The buccal mucosa is affected most often, but the tongue, lips, and gums may also be involved (Fig. 11.15). Remember that lichen planus can be present in both localized and generalized distribution.

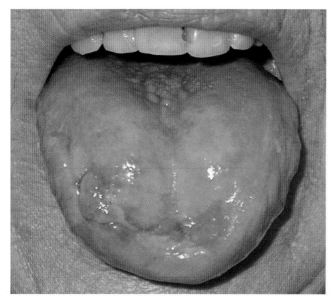

Fig. 11.15 Oral lichen planus—ulcers on the tongue require biopsy to exclude malignancy.

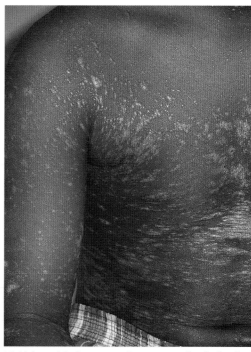

Fig. 11.16 Lichenoid drug eruption—generalized distribution with psoriasis-like (eczematous) papules and plaques.

Differential Diagnosis

The white lines on the surface of violet lichen planus papules are often subtle, so the disease usually does not appear as a scaling disorder. Occasionally, however, more scales can be present, in which case, the papulosquamous disorders (see Chapter 9) must be considered, including *psoriasis, pityriasis rosea*, and *discoid lupus erythematosus*. Of these, *discoid lupus* is the most commonly confused, and in some patients, the two diseases may overlap. Lichen planus presenting with only a few scattered papules can be confused with *insect bites*. *Lichenoid drug eruptions* can mimic lichen planus. Drugs that most often cause lichenoid eruptions are angiotensin-converting enzyme (ACE) inhibitors, beta-blockers, thiazide diuretics, antimalarials, quinidine, and gold salts. The lesions are generalized, often in a photodistribution, and more eczematous, leading to persistent signs of hyperpigmentation (Fig. 11.16). Lichen nitidus and lichen spinulosus, as previously discussed, do not have the purplish, flat-topped appearance of lichen planus. When the palms and soles are involved, a serologic test for syphilis should be performed to rule out *secondary syphilis*. Some patients with *graft-versus-host disease* also develop a skin eruption that closely resembles lichen planus both clinically and histopathologically. The differential diagnosis for mucous membrane involvement with lichen planus includes *"leukoplakia," candidiasis*, and *secondary syphilis* (see Chapter 22).

DIFFERENTIAL DIAGNOSIS OF LICHEN PLANUS

- Papulosquamous disorders (e.g., psoriasis, pityriasis rosea, discoid lupus erythematosus)
- Lichenoid drug eruption
- Lichen nitidus and lichen spinulosus
- Secondary syphilis
- Graft-versus-host disease

Drugs that can cause lichen planus–like eruptions:
1. Thiazide diuretics
2. ACE inhibitors
3. Beta-blockers
4. Gold salts
5. Antimalarial drugs (chloroquine, hydroxychloroquine)
6. Quinidine

Laboratory and Biopsy

If the clinical diagnosis is in doubt, a biopsy may be performed. In lichen planus, the histologic features are characteristic. The typical constellation of findings includes hyperkeratosis, thickened granular layer, degeneration of the basal cell layer, colloid bodies (necrotic basal cells), and a dense, "band-like" inflammatory infiltrate in the papillary dermis that obscures and disrupts the dermal–epidermal junction (Fig. 11.17).

Therapy

The treatment is nonspecific and often not totally successful. The inflammatory reaction is suppressed with steroids. Localized disease is treated with strong topical steroids such as fluocinonide 0.05% cream, especially in children. For severe widespread disease, a course of systemic steroids is sometimes required, but caution is advised when administering these agents on a long-term basis because of the well-known side-effects. Acitretin (Soriatane 25–50 mg daily) can clear cutaneous and oral lichen planus in more severe cases. Topical retinoids (e.g., tretinoin gel) and topical steroids (e.g., clobetasol gel) have been successful in some patients with mucous membrane lesions. Topical tacrolimus (Protopic) has also been used effectively for oral and cutaneous lichen planus. Phototherapy

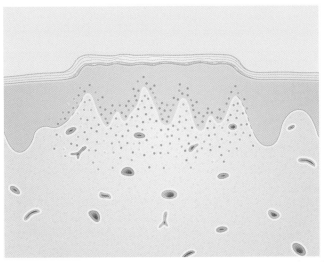

Fig. 11.17 Lichen planus. Epidermis—hyperkeratosis; degeneration of the basal cell layer; "saw-tooth" pattern of rete pegs. Dermis—dense, band-like, lymphocytic infiltrate in the upper dermis.

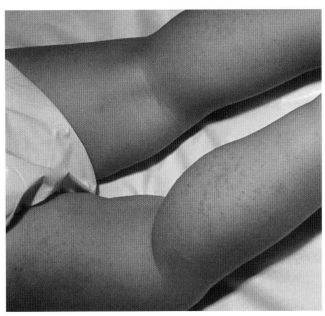

Fig. 11.18 Miliaria—multiple red papules in an infant.

(e.g., narrow-band ultraviolet B [UVB]) can be beneficial for generalized lichen planus and lichenoid drug eruptions. Off-label use of apremilast (Otezla) has shown promising results for lichen planus treatment in one small study. Cyclosporine has been used as a treatment of last resort in selected patients with severe disease.

THERAPY FOR LICHEN PLANUS
Initial
• Topical steroids (e.g., fluocinonide cream 0.1% b.i.d.)
Alternative
• Topical tacrolimus
• Systemic steroids
• Narrow-band UVB
• Retinoids (acitretin)
• Cyclosporine

Course and Complications

The course may be chronic, ranging from months to years. Almost two-thirds of patients experience spontaneous resolution within 1 year. Patients with mucous membrane involvement usually have a more prolonged course, often lasting years. Recurrences are uncommon, occurring in less than 20% of patients.

Serious complications are uncommon. Postinflammatory hyperpigmentation may be cosmetically unpleasing and can be treated with skin-lightening therapies but usually fades with time. Complications of mucous membrane lichen planus include candidiasis and squamous cell carcinoma, necessitating routine clinical follow-up and biopsy of changing oral lesions.

Pathogenesis

The cause of lichen planus remains unknown. Evidence that immune factors play a role includes (1) the finding of immunoglobulins at the dermal–epidermal junction in 95% of lichen planus lesions; (2) the observation that certain drug reactions can mimic lichen planus; and (3) the occurrence of lichen planus–like eruptions in patients who have undergone bone marrow transplantation and who are experiencing a graft-versus-host reaction.

MILIARIA

KEY POINTS
1. Miliaria rubra and miliaria crystallina seen commonly in infants
2. Caused by the occlusion of sweat ducts
3. Resolves with cooling and avoiding occlusion

Definition

Miliaria, or heat rash, represents an inflammatory reaction around a sweat duct. The reaction is caused by blockage of the duct along with extravasation of its contents into the surrounding tissue. Clinically, miliaria most often appears as multiple small papules (Fig. 11.18). The diagnosis of miliaria falls into three types, depending on the level of sweat duct occlusion in the skin layer: (1) crystallina—stratum corneum, (2) rubra—mid-epidermis, and (3) profunda—dermal–epidermal junction.

Incidence

Miliaria is an uncommon presenting complaint in the authors' outpatients. It is most commonly seen in neonates (miliaria crystallina) and in adults who live in warm, humid environments, particularly in skin that has been occluded (miliaria rubra). In infants, heat rash is recognized by the parents and seldom causes them to seek a dermatologic consultation. However, it is frequently seen on the backs of hospitalized patients who are in a constant, lying position.

History

In the ambulatory patient, miliaria is most commonly seen in neonates whose sweat ducts are not completely developed. Miliaria results from exposure to a hot, humid environment. In the bedridden patient, fever, sweating, and occlusion of the skin are predisposing factors. Strenuous physical activity can lead to miliaria. Pruritus is often the presenting complaint.

Physical Examination

Miliaria rubra, the most common form of miliaria, appears as multiple discrete, small, red papules. It is most often localized to the trunk, particularly the back. Although sweat ducts are not visible, miliaria is suspected when a patient has multiple small, discrete, uniform-sized papules not associated with hair follicles. Less common variants are *miliaria crystallina*, with superficial noninflamed vesicles containing crystal-clear fluid (dewdrops), commonly seen in infants with clear, fragile vesicles on the face and trunk (Fig. 11.19), and *miliaria pustulosa*, with erythematous pustules.

Differential Diagnosis

Miliaria rubra and pustulosa may be confused with *folliculitis*. In miliaria, the pustules are usually smaller and more numerous and do not have centrally placed hair. Sometimes, however, the two conditions coexist because they may share the same predisposing factor of occlusion. In infants, erythema toxicum neonatorum affects half of healthy newborns and is distinguished from miliaria by the red, broad flare around the papules on the face, trunk, and proximal extremities. The eruption resolves on its own within 10 days. Candidiasis also occurs in moist occluded skin, but the eruption is usually "beefy red," confluent, scaling, and surrounded by satellite papules and pustules. The word *milia* sounds similar to miliaria, but the condition it denotes is different. Milia are small, noninflamed, superficial, epidermal keratin cysts often found on the face of young infants and adults. Acne is distinguished from miliaria by the presence of comedones, characteristic age, and distribution of presentation.

> Miliaria is a heat rash—milia are small, keratin-filled cysts.

> **DIFFERENTIAL DIAGNOSIS OF MILIARIA**
> - Erythema toxicum neonatorum in infants
> - Folliculitis
> - Acne

Laboratory and Biopsy

The diagnosis is usually made clinically. For pustules, Gram staining and culture rule out bacterial folliculitis. A potassium hydroxide preparation enables the identification of *Candida*. If a biopsy is performed, serial sections must be done to reveal the intraepidermal portion of the sweat duct, which is surrounded by spongiosis and a chronic inflammatory cell infiltrate in the epidermis and superficial dermis (Fig. 11.20).

Therapy

Therapy is directed at removing the predisposing conditions. Most important are cooling measures and air exposure for occluded skin. For ambulatory patients, this is easily accomplished. For bedridden patients, this means ensuring that the bed is dry and the patient turns frequently. In infants, miliaria resolves on its own without intervention. A mild-to-mid-potency topical steroid cream or lotion can be applied to help relieve the itching, but this must be done sparingly to avoid any further contribution to the occlusive process.

> **THERAPY FOR MILIARIA**
>
> **Initial**
> - Cooling measures
> - Air exposure
> - Topical steroid (hydrocortisone 2.5% or triamcinolone 0.1% cream)

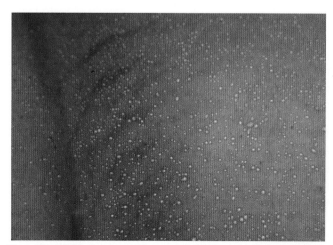

Fig. 11.19 Miliaria crystallina—superficial, noninflamed vesicles (dewdrops).

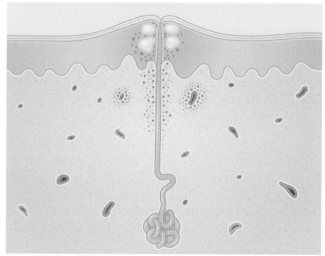

Fig. 11.20 Miliaria. Epidermis—occluded sweat duct with underlying intraepidermal edema and inflammation. Dermis—superficial inflammatory cell infiltrate.

Course and Complications

With decreasing heat and increasing air exposure, the condition resolves spontaneously within days. Complications are uncommon. Conditions that predispose to miliaria, however, can also contribute to coexisting infections with bacterial and candidal organisms.

Pathogenesis

Occlusion of the sweat duct is the primary event in the pathogenesis of miliaria. In miliaria rubra, this occurs within the epidermis at the level of the granular cell layer. Increased hydration appears to play the major role, resulting in swelling of the stratum corneum and compromise of the ductal lumina. After occlusion, sweat extravasates into the epidermis, where it produces an irritant reaction. In miliaria crystallina, sweat duct obstruction occurs in the stratum corneum. Experimentally, stripping of the stratum corneum with adhesive tape restores sweat flow, providing evidence that the occlusive process occurs in the stratum corneum. Bacteria and increased sweat tonicity have also been implicated pathogenetically in miliaria, but their pathogenetic roles have not been proved conclusively.

SCABIES

> **KEY POINTS**
>
> 1. This is the worst itch of the patient's life.
> 2. Burrows in characteristic locations are diagnostic.
> 3. Treat the entire body of the patient and close contacts with a topical agent.

Definition

Scabies is an infestation of the epidermis with the "itch" mite, *Sarcoptes scabiei* var. *hominis*. Clinically, a few burrows are usually found and are diagnostic. Inflammatory papules resulting from host hypersensitivity, however, constitute the more frequent and obvious findings (Fig. 11.21).

Incidence

Scabies is a common disease. It can occur endemically among school-aged children and may be hyperendemic among rural populations in less-developed countries. Immobilized geriatric patients in nursing homes, patients with HIV/AIDS, and medically compromised patients (e.g., Down syndrome) are predisposed to infestation with high mite counts.

History

Generalized pruritus is the major complaint. Scabies causes the worst itch of the patient's life—often severe enough to interrupt sleep. Frequently, a history of itching can be elicited in family members and other close personal contacts. The incubation time from inoculation to the onset of pruritus is usually approximately 1 month, so in early cases, other contacts may not yet be symptomatic. Because scabies also occurs in pets (canine scabies or mange), a pet history should be elicited, particularly in patients with recurrent disease.

> Itching is often severe enough to interrupt sleep.
> Family members and friends often also itch.

Physical Examination

Small inflammatory papules predominate. They are often excoriated. Scabies has a characteristic distribution with favored locations including the finger webs, wrists, elbows, axillae, girdle area, and feet. In addition, the male genitalia are usually involved (Fig. 11.22). Scabies can present in a generalized distribution. Itching papules and small nodules on the penis should be considered the result of scabies unless proved otherwise. In temperate climates, the head is almost always spared in adults but may be involved in children. In infants, vesicles may also be present, particularly on the palms and soles (Fig. 11.23).

The diagnostic finding is a burrow, which appears as a 2- to 5-mm, delicate, white, serpiginous, superficial, thread-like line (Fig. 11.24). The most common location for burrows is on the hands. With close inspection, a tiny black speck can often be

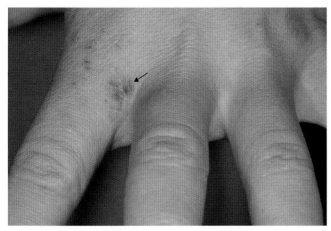

Fig. 11.21 Scabies—inflammatory crusted papules in a characteristic location.

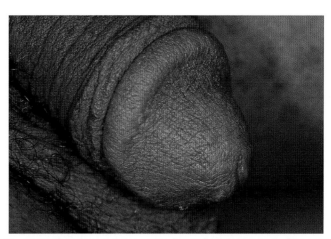

Fig. 11.22 Scabies—papules on the head of penis. This is scabies until proven otherwise!

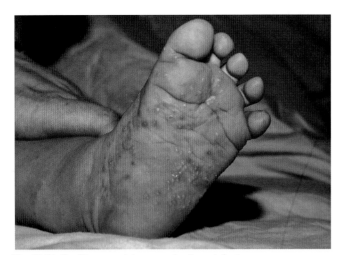

Fig. 11.23 **Scabies**—vesicles on soles in an infant.

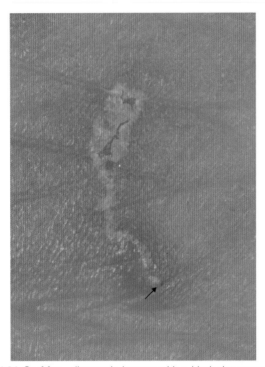

Fig. 11.24 **Scabies**—diagnostic burrow with a black dot representing an adult mite.

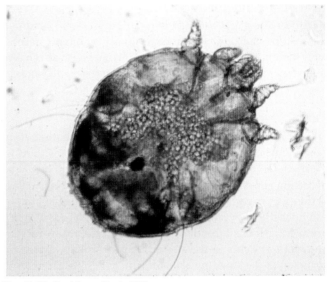

Fig. 11.25 **Scabies mite** (×400).

DIFFERENTIAL DIAGNOSIS OF SCABIES

- Neurotic excoriation (e.g., delusions of parasitosis)
- Dermatitis
  - Atopic
  - Allergic contact
  - Nummular
- Other insect bites

Laboratory and Biopsy

The presence of mites or eggs is diagnostic (Fig. 11.25). This is accomplished by skin scraping with a No. 15 blade, as described in Chapter 3. The highest yield is from a black dot at the burrow, but mites and eggs can also be recovered from papules and nodules.

A biopsy is usually not necessary but may provide the diagnosis when it previously had not been suspected. Microscopically, one sees edema in the epidermis, which may be sufficient to result in a microvesicle. An inflammatory reaction occurs in the superficial dermis with lymphocytes and eosinophils. A fortuitous but diagnostic finding is the presence of a mite in the stratum corneum (Fig. 11.26).

Therapy

Permethrin cream (Elimite) is considered the drug of choice. The topical agent must be applied to the *entire body surface*, including under fingernails. A *single application* of 5% permethrin cream is applied at bedtime from the head to the toes and is washed off in the morning. Some physicians recommend a single reapplication after 1 week, but no controlled studies have documented that two applications are better than one. Permethrin cream is preferred for infants older than 2 months of age and for pregnant females. Treatment at the same time is recommended for household contacts; those who are asymptomatic require only one application. Clothes and bed linens can be decontaminated by machine washing at a hot temperature.

seen at the end of the burrow. This black dot represents the adult mite, which is best visualized under the microscope. In some patients with scabies, particularly when the condition has been long-standing, scattered nodules may also be found.

Differential Diagnosis

Because of the intense pruritus, in some patients, only excoriations are seen. In these patients, a misdiagnosis of neurotic excoriations could be made. Widespread disease may be misdiagnosed as other causes of dermatitis, including atopic dermatitis, allergic contact dermatitis, nummular dermatitis, and insect bites. The presence of burrows or mites and eggs under microscopy distinguishes scabies from these other diseases.

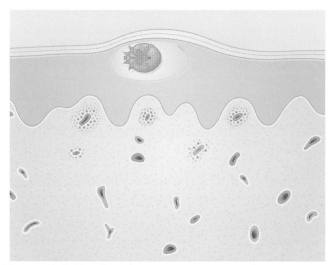

Fig. 11.26 **Epidermis**—mite burrowed in superficial epidermis. Dermis—inflammation.

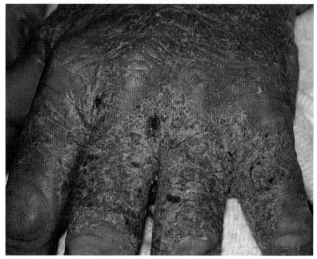

Fig. 11.27 **Crusted scabies**. Crusted plaque with a high mite load.

> The entire body is treated.

Oral ivermectin has been used successfully for treating scabies and has the advantage of ease of administration. A single oral dose of 0.1–0.2 mg/kg is sufficient for cure in most patients, although residual itching may persist for up to 1 month after this systemic treatment. Ivermectin may require repeated treatment in 1 week. Ivermectin is often used in outbreaks in institutions such as a nursing home. Oral ivermectin is not recommended for pregnant individuals and children weighing less than 15 kg; topical sulfur (compounded in petrolatum to 10% concentration) can be safely applied for 3 consecutive days in a similar fashion to topical permethrin and repeated in 7 days.

THERAPY FOR SCABIES

Initial
- Permethrin cream 5%

Alternative
- Ivermectin: 0.1–0.2 mg/kg
- Topical sulfur in neonates and pregnant individuals

Course and Complications

When untreated, itching progresses and may become unbearable. After treatment, many patients continue to itch for 1–2 weeks. This possibility must be explained so that the patient avoids overusing the medication. Residual itching can be treated symptomatically with topical steroids and oral antihistamines. Nodules, if present, may last for 1 month or longer.

> Itching may persist for 1–2 weeks after treatment.

Complications are uncommon. Secondary bacterial infection may occur in excoriated skin. In immunocompromised patients (such as those with AIDS or lymphoma), patients with Down syndrome, and debilitated patients with neurologic disorders,

scabies may appear as a widespread, crusted eruption that often *does not* itch. This uncommon variant is called *crusted scabies* (Norwegian scabies) and is easily misdiagnosed as eczema or psoriasis (Fig. 11.27). On close inspection, however, burrows and mites are usually numerous, and their presence confirms the diagnosis.

> Crusted scabies occurs in immunocompromised and debilitated patients.

Pathogenesis

The discovery in 1687 of the "itch mite" made this parasite one of the first causes of human disease to be identified. The *S. scabiei* mite lives in and on human skin, where it completes its life cycle in approximately 2 weeks. The impregnated female burrows into the stratum corneum, where she lays two or three eggs daily for as long as 30 days. Each egg produces a larva, which leaves the burrow and molts to produce a nymph. Several further moltings result in a mature mite, which then mates. After mating, the male dies, and the female completes the life cycle by burrowing back into the stratum corneum. Secretions from the burrowing female mite cause intraepidermal edema fluid, on which she feeds.

The itching and inflammation are thought to be a result of a hypersensitivity reaction by the host to the foreign material (i.e., mites, eggs, and feces) in the skin. This may account for the persistence of the itching for 1–2 weeks after successful treatment; it may take that long for the stratum corneum to turn over and shed the foreign material, and for the hypersensitivity reaction to subside. Here are a few practical tips:

1. It is difficult to transmit scabies through fomites such as bedding and clothing (human-to-human transmission is most common).
2. The incubation time from inoculation to itching usually is approximately 1 month.
3. If left untreated, the disease course is one of progressively worsening itch.
4. Previously infested individuals are more difficult to reinfest, possibly because the hypersensitivity reaction is partially protective.

UNCOMMON INFLAMMATORY PAPULES

LICHEN NITIDUS

Lichen nitidus is an uncommon eruption of minute, flat-topped papules with a shiny appearance (Fig. 11.28). Common areas of involvement include the upper extremities, dorsal hands, genitalia, and trunk. Unlike lichen planus, oral involvement is rarely appreciated and the lesions rarely itch. Skin biopsy shows the characteristic finding of the "ball and claw" configuration: inflammatory cells (the ball) held between elongated rete ridges of the epidermis (the claw). Treatment is directed at the symptoms, with spontaneous resolution occurring within several years.

LICHEN SPINULOSUS

Lichen spinulosus is characterized by the sudden onset of symmetrically distributed, often grouped patches of follicular papules that are topped by a centrally located keratotic spine (Fig. 11.29). It affects mainly children and young adults. Lichen spinulosus can occur on the abdomen, extensor arms, knees, and neck. No cure exists, but most cases remit spontaneously in 1–2 years.

LYMPHOMATOID PAPULOSIS

This uncommon, chronic disorder occurs mostly in adults but can affect children. It is similar to pityriasis lichenoides et varioliformis acuta (PLEVA, see below), but the lesions tend to be larger and fewer in number. The primary lesion is an inflammatory papule that commonly develops with a necrotic center (Fig. 11.30). Spontaneous healing often occurs with a relapsing course of crops of lesions. Histologic examination confirms the diagnosis, revealing a typical "wedge-shaped" dermal infiltrate with CD30+ cells. Approximately 10%–20% of patients develop lymphoma, most commonly cutaneous T-cell lymphoma.

PITYRIASIS LICHENOIDES ET VARIOLIFORMIS ACUTA (MUCHA–HABERMANN DISEASE)

This rare condition is characterized by recurrent crops of crusted, reddish papules (Fig. 11.31) that regress spontaneously within weeks. PLEVA is seen most commonly in children and is rarely associated with fever and malaise. The skin lesions can be in various stages: vesicular, pustular, and crusted. Skin biopsy can confirm the diagnosis. When the lesions persist for months and appear as reddish brown papules with scale, the condition is referred to as *pityriasis lichenoides chronica*. Rare cases eventuate into cutaneous T-cell lymphoma. Treatment includes topical steroids and oral antibiotics for their antiinflammatory effects (e.g., tetracycline or erythromycin).

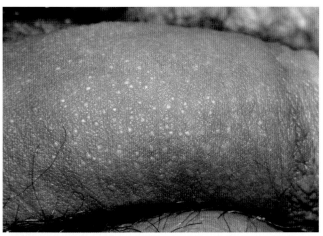

Fig. 11.28 **Lichen nitidus**—minute, flat-topped papules with a shiny appearance.

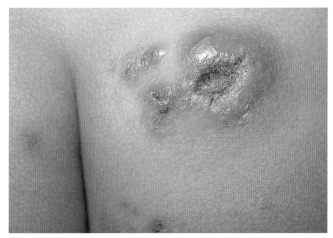

Fig. 11.30 **Lymphomatoid papulosis**—papules and nodules with necrotic centers on the buttocks.

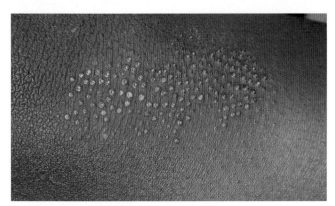

Fig. 11.29 **Lichen spinulosus**—grouped follicular papules with central keratosis spine located on the knee.

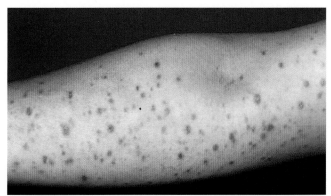

Fig. 11.31 **Pityriasis lichenoides et varioliformis acuta (PLEVA)**—papules with hemorrhagic crust.

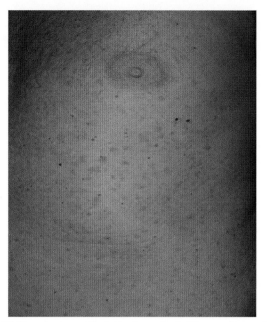

Fig. 11.32 **Transient acantholytic dermatosis (Grover disease)**—reddish brown, crusted papules with characteristic truncal location.

TRANSIENT ACANTHOLYTIC DERMATOSIS (GROVER DISEASE)

Grover disease is a pruritic eruption of truncal, reddish brown, keratotic papules (Fig. 11.32), most commonly affecting middle-aged to elderly White males. Pruritus is the hallmark of this disease. Heat tends to exacerbate the condition. Biopsy shows the characteristic finding of focal separation of keratinocytes (e.g., acantholysis) in the epidermis. Potent topical steroids can diminish the pruritus, but the disease is hardly "transient." Consider Grover disease in a middle-aged male who presents with pruritic, keratotic papules limited to the trunk.

SELF-ASSESSMENT

Case 1—Generalized Itching Papules (Fig. 11.33)
What Do You See?

Physical examination revealed discrete papules, many of which were excoriated.

What Is the Most Likely Diagnosis?

The most likely diagnosis is scabies. Scabies should be suspected for any generalized pruritic process. For pruritic papules on the penis, the diagnosis is scabies until proven otherwise.

How Would You Confirm It?

The diagnosis is secured if a mite can be found. For this, a careful examination of the entire cutaneous surface should be carried out in the search for burrows. The patient's hands, particularly the finger webs, should be scrutinized. Even if a burrow is not found, scraping of several of the papules may reveal a mite or mite products. In this patient, scraping of the penile papules was positive.

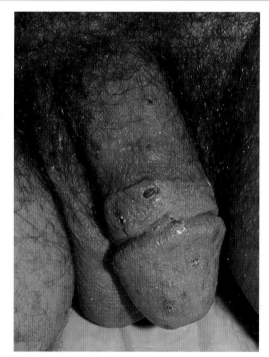

Fig. 11.33 This 30-year-old man presented with a 2-month history of itching that had become progressively more severe. The itching spared the head but was otherwise generalized, including involvement of the genitalia.

CHAPTER CONTENTS

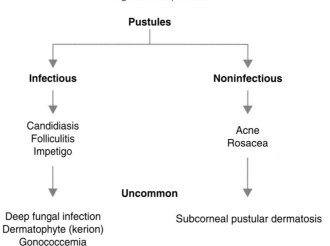

Algorithm of pustules

ABSTRACT

Pustules are collections of neutrophils that are situated superficially, usually in a hair follicle (e.g., acne and folliculitis) or just below the stratum corneum (e.g., impetigo and candidiasis). Diseases are organized based on two categories: infectious and noninfectious. Although pustules represent the unifying clinical feature of these disorders, they may not always be the predominant finding; sometimes, they might not even be present. For example, in some patients with acne, only comedones or papules are found. In impetigo, often only crusts are found because the pustules have been broken and dried. Pus often indicates an infection. For pustules (and crusts) in the skin, infection is an appropriate diagnostic consideration, but, as can be seen from Table 12.1, not all pustular dermatoses are caused by pathogenic microorganisms. However, if an infection is suspected, simple laboratory tests can be performed for confirmation.

The most common pustular diseases are listed in Table 12.1. Other rare causes of pustules are mentioned briefly at the end of the chapter.

KEY POINTS

1. Pustules represent collections of neutrophils.
2. Always rule out infection when you see pustules.
3. Pustules can be sterile.

ACNE

KEY POINTS

1. Acne is the most common dermatologic disease with negative psychosocial ramifications.
2. Comedones are the hallmark of the disease.
3. Treatment targets multifactorial causes of acne: androgens, follicular obstruction, and *Cutibacterium* (formerly *Propionibacterium*) *acnes*.

Definition

Acne vulgaris (common acne) is a disorder affecting pilosebaceous units in the skin (Fig. 12.1). The cause is multifactorial.

TABLE 12.1 Common Pustular Diseases

	Frequency (%)[a]	Etiology	Physical Examination		Differential Diagnosis	Laboratory Test
			Appearance of Lesions	Distribution		
Acne	13	Multifactorial	Pustules, papules, nodules, and *comedones*	Face and upper trunk	Folliculitis Rosacea	None
Candidiasis	0.3	Infection (*Candida albicans*)	Satellite pustules around a "*beefy red*" erythematous area	Moist areas, particularly the groin	Tinea cruris Intertrigo Miliaria Folliculitis Contact dermatitis	Potassium hydroxide preparation
Folliculitis	1.1	Infection (*Staphylococcus aureus*)	Scattered pustules, many with *centrally placed hairs*	Buttocks and thighs, beard area, scalp	Acne Fungal infection Keratosis pilaris Pseudofolliculitis	Gram stain Culture
Impetigo	0.6	Infection (*S. aureus*)	Crusts (often honey-colored) predominant	Most common nares, axillae, and groin	Ecthyma Herpes simplex	Gram stain Culture
Rosacea	1.3	Unknown	Papules and pustules on a background of *erythema* and *telangiectasia*	Central portion of face	Acne Lupus erythematosus Seborrheic dermatitis	None

[a]Percentage of new dermatology patients with this diagnosis seen in the Hershey Medical Center Dermatology Clinic, Hershey, Pennsylvania.

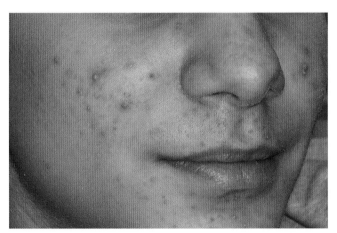

Fig. 12.1 **Acne**—characteristic papules and pustules in a teenager.

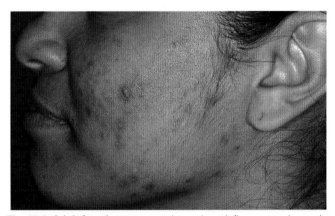

Fig. 12.2 **Adult female acne**—papules and postinflammatory hyperpigmented macules along the jawline. Note hirsutism indicating possible androgen excess.

Clinical lesions range from noninflamed *comedones* to *inflammatory papules*, *pustules*, and *nodules*.

Incidence

Acne is the most common disease seen by a dermatologist. It begins at a surprisingly young age; comedones can be found on examination in 50% of boys aged 9–11 years. Acne is a physically and psychologically devastating condition and must be treated aggressively. The incidence and severity of the disease increase during the teenage years and early adulthood, affecting approximately 85% of young people between the ages of 12 and 24 years. Contrary to popular belief, acne is not confined to teenagers. It may continue into the third and fourth decades of life, especially in women; in some patients, it does not begin until then. Adult female acne is an increasingly recognized condition, defined as a type of acne in women aged 25 years or older, and the acne can persist even after 50 years of age.

History

The patient usually makes the diagnosis and often has attempted therapy with over-the-counter medication. A history of hirsutism, hair thinning usually localized to the top of the scalp, or irregular menses in a woman with acne should lead to the consideration of possible androgen excess. Adult women often complain of acne along the jawline that worsens around the time of menstruation (Fig. 12.2). In ethnicities with darker skin, acne can often lead to marks of postinflammatory hyperpigmentation, which can take many months to resolve without treatment.

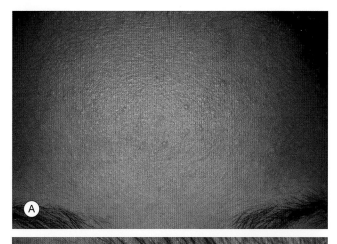

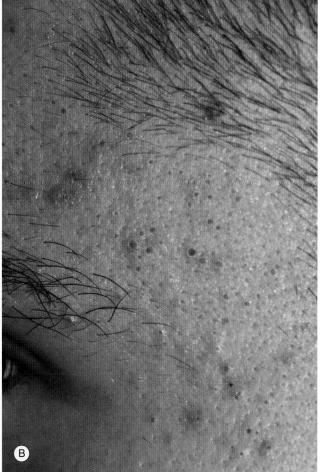

Fig. 12.3 (A) Closed comedones or "whiteheads." (B) Open comedones or "blackheads."

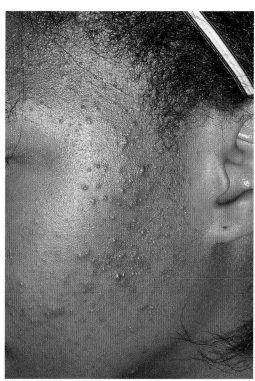

Fig. 12.4 Acne—papules and pustules. Note postinflammatory hyperpigmented macules.

associated with inflammation. Inflammatory acne lesions are seen more easily by both the patient and the physician. They appear as papules, pustules, or nodules, depending on the magnitude of the inflammatory response (Fig. 12.4). Acne is found in areas with numerous sebaceous glands, usually the face and upper trunk. The lower trunk is less often involved, and the distal extremities are always spared. Adult female acne, which has a hormonal component, affects the periphery of the face, mainly the jawline, chin, and upper neck.

Less-inflammatory lesions:
1. Open comedones
2. Closed comedones

Inflammatory lesions:
1. Papules
2. Pustules
3. Nodules

Topical or systemic corticosteroids can also cause an acneiform eruption.

Physical Examination

The less-inflamed lesions in acne are called comedones and are of two types: (1) the *open comedone* or "blackhead," which appears as a dilated pore filled with black keratinous material (not dirt) and (2) the *closed comedone* or "whitehead," which is a small, flesh-colored, dome-shaped papule that is often difficult to see (Fig. 12.3). It is now recognized that comedones are

Differential Diagnosis

The diagnosis of acne is rarely difficult, particularly in teenagers. Occasionally, acne comedones may be confused with *flat warts*, which are small, flesh-colored, flat-topped papules usually located on the face. On close inspection, the flat wart is seen to have a sharp right-angled edge and a finely textured surface, whereas a closed comedone has a dome-shaped, smooth surface (Fig. 12.5).

Steroid acne is caused by the use of corticosteroids and is distinguished from acne vulgaris by its sudden onset (usually within 2 weeks of starting high-dose systemic or potent topical corticosteroid therapy) and appearance (uniform, 2- to 3-mm,

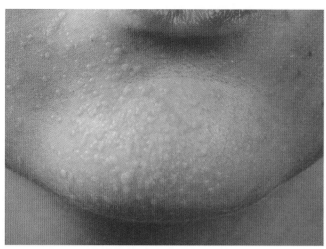

Fig. 12.5 **Flat warts**—flesh-colored papules often mistaken for acne. (Courtesy O. Fred Miller, MD.)

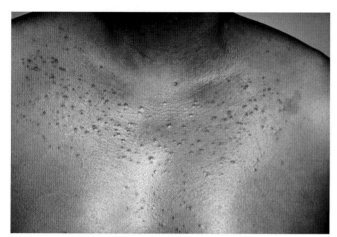

Fig. 12.6 **Steroid acne**—uniform, red papules in a kidney transplant patient on high doses of systemic steroids.

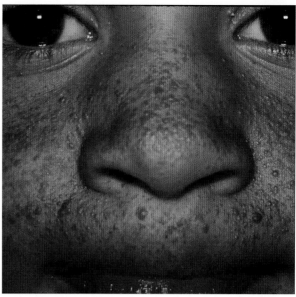

Fig. 12.7 **Tuberous sclerosis**—multiple reddish, brown papules on central face in a Black child—often confused for acne.

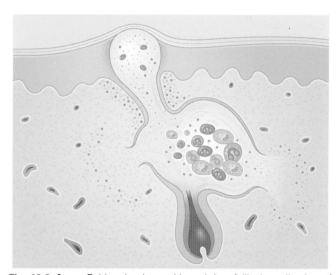

Fig. 12.8 **Acne**. Epidermis—intraepidermal, intrafollicular collection of neutrophils. Dermis—occluded pilosebaceous unit with the accumulation of keratin, sebum, and inflammatory cells. Extravasation of material through the ruptured wall leads to further dermal inflammation.

red, firm papules and pustules) (Fig. 12.6). Steroid acne caused by topically applied agents occurs most often on the face. With systemic corticosteroids, the eruption is most prominent on the upper trunk.

Pustular acne vulgaris can be confused with bacterial folliculitis or rosacea. In *bacterial folliculitis*, hairs are visible in the center of some of the pustules, and a bacterial culture is positive, usually for *Staphylococcus aureus* or, less often, for a gram-negative organism. *Rosacea* is distinguished from acne vulgaris by the presence of a background blush of erythema and telangiectasia and the absence of comedones. Rosacea also usually occurs later in life.

> Papular acne is occasionally confused with angiofibromas and keratosis pilaris.

Angiofibromas, a skin manifestation of tuberous sclerosis, are often incorrectly diagnosed as acne. Clinically, the lesions appear as firm, pink papules that are clustered primarily in the center of the face, are persistent, and are, of course, resistant to acne therapy (Fig. 12.7). Keratosis pilaris, when it affects the facial cheeks, is distinguished from acne by its minute, rough, uniform papules on the background of "red" (i.e., prominent skin vasculature) skin and by its lack of comedones. Keratosis pilaris is a chronic condition and is relatively unresponsive to acne treatments.

DIFFERENTIAL DIAGNOSIS OF ACNE

- Flat warts
- Steroid acne
- Folliculitis
- Rosacea
- Angiofibromas in tuberous sclerosis
- Keratosis pilaris

Laboratory and Biopsy

The diagnosis is almost always made clinically. Occasionally, a bacterial culture is indicated to rule out infection. A biopsy is not indicated but would show an occluded pilosebaceous unit along with inflammation (Fig. 12.8).

Therapy

Four categories of medication have proved efficacious in the treatment of acne: topical agents, systemic antibiotics, systemic retinoids, and hormonal agents. The type of acne guides the choice of treatment. For the majority of patients, systemic retinoids and hormonal therapy are not required.

THERAPY FOR ACNE

Initial

Comedone
- Topical retinoids (tretinoin 0.025% cream in p.m.)
- Over-the-counter adapalene (Differin) gel 0.1%

Papules and Pustules
- Topical: retinoid in p.m. and over-the-counter 5% or 10% benzoyl peroxide wash/bar (alone or in combination with topical clindamycin) in a.m.
- Systemic: tetracyclines (add if topicals fail)

Nodules
- Topical and systemic therapy in combination as outlined for papules and pustules

Alternative

Comedone
- Topical adapalene (Differin) gel 0.3% (prescription for sensitive skin)
- Topical tazarotene (for resistant comedones)

Papules and Pustules
- Oral isotretinoin if severe, scars, or patient fails initial treatment

Nodules
- Oral isotretinoin

Hormonal Treatment for Females
- Spironolactone
- Oral contraceptives (combination of estrogen and progesterone)

Topical agents

Topical agents are most effective for superficial lesions. For comedones, the mainstay of treatment remains topical retinoids: tretinoin (Retin-A Micro cream), adapalene (Differin cream 0.3% prescription or over-the-counter adapalene gel 0.1%), and tazarotene (Tazorac). Benzoyl peroxide has mild comedolytic activity and also exerts an antibacterial effect. Topical antibiotics (erythromycin and clindamycin) should be used in combination with topical benzoyl peroxide to prevent bacterial resistance. Newer medications have emerged for topical therapy. Clascoterone 1% cream (Winlevi), a topical androgen receptor inhibitor and the first of its kind, can be applied to affected areas twice daily. It is approved by the US Food and Drug Administration (FDA) for patients aged 12 years and older. Another newer medication is the topical antibiotic, 4% minocycline foam (Amzeeq), applied once daily. It is FDA-approved only for patients with moderate-to-severe acne. The most common side-effects of the topical antibiotic include headaches and increased creatinine phosphokinase levels.

The authors usually start treatment with a topical retinoid at bedtime and a benzoyl peroxide cream or wash (available over the counter) in the morning. The patient should apply these medications to the *entire affected area* (e.g., the entire face) rather than just to the individual lesions. In addition, patients must be advised that retinoids and benzoyl peroxide preparations can cause skin irritation, which is usually worst during the first 1–2 weeks of use and afterward diminishes. In part because of the irritation, the patient may notice that the condition appears worse rather than better after the first several weeks of use.

Systemic antibiotics

Systemic antibiotics are indicated in patients with inflammatory papules or pustules, especially if there is truncal involvement. Doxycycline (50–100 mg twice daily) is the most commonly prescribed oral antibiotic because of its efficacy and relative safety. Minocycline (100 mg twice daily) is used mostly in people who cannot tolerate doxycycline. A newer tetracycline, sarecycline, is an oral weight-based pill given once daily, is more specific to *C. acnes*, and has the potential for less disruption of the gut microbiome. Tetracycline (500 mg twice daily) is less commonly prescribed. The authors try to limit systemic antibiotic use to no more than 3 months; if there is no improvement, then consider referral to a dermatologist. To promote compliance, the authors recommend taking tetracyclines with food and even dairy products, despite package insert recommendations.

Systemic retinoids

The oral retinoid isotretinoin became available commercially in September 1982 for use in the treatment of patients with severe acne (Fig. 12.9). This potent vitamin A analog decreases inflammation, follicular keratinization, sebum production, and intrafollicular bacterial counts. Side-effects are common. Almost all patients experience chapped lips and dry skin, and extracutaneous complications also occur; for example, increased levels of liver enzymes and plasma lipids. Most importantly, systemic retinoids are *teratogenic*. It is mandatory that patients who can get pregnant should not become so when taking isotretinoin. Special consent forms, strict birth control measures, and monthly pregnancy tests are required for patients who can get pregnant taking isotretinoin. A consent form acknowledging the risk of depression and suicide while on isotretinoin is required for all patients. There is also a controversial link between isotretinoin and inflammatory bowel disease. Because of these restrictions, the drug is recommended mainly for the treatment of selected patients with severe, therapy-resistant papular/pustular acne or scarring nodular acne (Fig. 12.10). The authors have a low threshold to use isotretinoin in patients with skin of color who have persistent, inflammatory acne unresponsive to first-line therapies to prevent the unpleasant and persistent side-effects of postinflammatory hyperpigmentation. Isotretinoin should be prescribed only by physicians who are familiar with its use and participate in a national risk management program (https://www.ipledgeprogram.com).

Isotretinoin is teratogenic.

Hormonal therapy

This class of treatment can help females who have acne that fails to respond to initial treatment outlined above and that flares

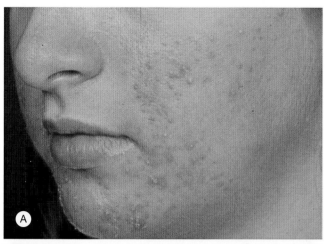

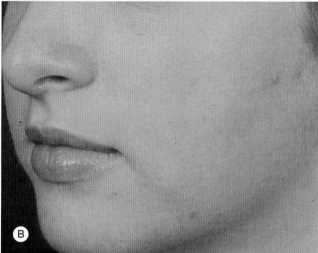

Fig. 12.9 Acne. (A) Before isotretinoin application. Severe nodular "cystic" acne with scarring. (B) After isotretinoin application.

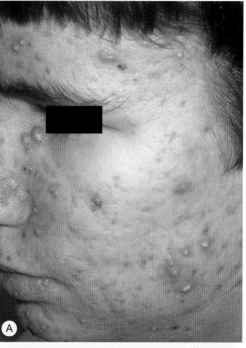

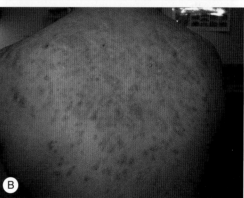

Fig. 12.10 Acne. (A) Severe nodular acne with papules, pustules, and scarring. (B) Note postinflammatory hyperpigmentation from the scarring acne in a patient with darker skin type.

with their menstrual cycle. Spironolactone 50–100 mg twice daily has become a first-line therapy for adult female acne. In healthy females, it is not necessary to monitor labwork, mainly potassium levels. Side-effects of spironolactone include breast tenderness and menstrual irregularity; these can be prevented by also prescribing oral contraceptive pills.

Birth control pills with low androgenicity improve acne in many patients. Several products are available, including Ortho Tri-Cyclen and Estrostep, for which the FDA has approved acne as an indicated use.

Hormonal therapy should be prescribed only by physicians who are fully aware of its potential side-effects.

Patient education

The most important aspect of a successful acne treatment program is patient compliance. Instructions should be given both verbally at the time of the patient's initial visit and on a written take-home sheet that reinforces what was said. Patients are best able to comply if medications are used only twice daily, so that the medication schedule can be centered on an already established daily habit such as teeth brushing. At the time of the initial visit, answers can also be given to several common

questions (often unasked) that patients with acne or their parents frequently have regarding the following:

1. *Diet.* Some evidence indicates that a "Western" diet may have an adverse effect on acne, but specific foods have not been implicated. For most patients, a sensible diet is all that is suggested.
2. *Cleanliness.* Acne is not a function of poor hygiene. In general, acne cleansing agents are also not recommended because they cause irritation that unnecessarily compounds the irritation from the recommended topical comedolytics. Instruct patients to wash their face with their hands and not with a washcloth.
3. *Cosmetics.* If cosmetics are used, they should be water-based and used sparingly. Most cosmetic products are noncomedogenic.
4. *Picking.* In many patients with acne, much of the skin damage is self-inflicted. Although the temptation to squeeze a fresh pustule is often overwhelming, it should be vigorously discouraged because it can produce more tissue damage, sometimes resulting in postinflammatory hyperpigmentation and scars.

Course and Complications

With therapy, the prognosis for acne is good, if not excellent. The patient should understand that most therapies provide control of the disease rather than cure, and that improvement does not occur overnight. The only potential cure, other than time, for acne is isotretinoin. The authors recommend aggressive, up-front treatment that is tailored to the type and distribution of acne. Improvement is typically seen after 2–3 months of therapy, so managing the patient's expectation is critically important. Systemic antibiotics are recommended for 3 months and then should be discontinued; bacterial resistance to antibiotics is becoming more frequent, thereby limiting the usefulness of long-term antibiotic therapy for acne. Most patients require prolonged (often lasting for years) maintenance therapy with topical agents. If acne is not responding to systemic antibiotics and topical therapies, then referral to a dermatologist is warranted. Isotretinoin induces prolonged remissions, if not "cures," in many patients.

Acne remits spontaneously with time, to a degree that varies widely. For individual patients, there is no way to predict in advance when they will "outgrow" their acne. The goal of therapy is to keep the condition under control for as long as it is active.

The major complication of acne is its psychosocial ramifications, which can be devastating for some patients. Patients with severe cystic acne may even be socially ostracized. In an ironic quirk of timing, acne occurs at a time in life when personal appearance is a prime concern and self-consciousness may be at its peak. Regardless of the severity of the acne, for patients seeking help (even those with apparently mild disease), the disease is important and deserves serious attention. Patients are not impressed with soothing advice that trivializes their disease and reassures them that they will eventually "outgrow" it.

In addition to the cosmetic liability of active lesions, scars further compound and perpetuate a poor self-image in some patients long after the acne has remitted. Scars are difficult to treat. Dermabrasion, laser "resurfacing," chemical peels, and surgery have all been employed, with varying results. Because scars are more easily prevented than treated, the emphasis on acne is on early and aggressive medical therapy.

Pathogenesis

Multiple factors are involved in the pathogenesis of acne. The three most significant are as follows:

Factors involved in acne pathogenesis:
1. Androgens
2. Follicular obstruction
3. *C. acnes*

1. *Androgenic hormones.* Under androgen stimulation, sebaceous glands enlarge and increase their sebum production. Before puberty, the responsible androgens are secreted by the adrenal gland. During puberty, the addition of gonadal androgens provides further sebaceous gland stimulation.
2. *Follicular obstruction.* For acne to occur, outlet obstruction of the follicular canal is required. All acne lesions begin with a microcomedone. This obstruction occurs because of the accumulation of adherent keratinized cells within the canal, forming an impaction. The cause of follicular obstruction is not known but may also be influenced by androgens.
3. *Bacteria.* Proximal to the follicular outlet obstruction, sebum and keratinous debris accumulate. This provides an attractive environment for the growth of anaerobic bacteria, specifically *C. acnes*. These bacteria produce lipase enzymes that hydrolyze the sebaceous lipids, resulting in the release of free fatty acids, which are presumed to cause inflammation, another important factor in acne. *C. acnes* play other roles in the pathogenesis of acne (e.g., these bacteria are chemotactic for neutrophils). Regardless of the mechanism, the therapeutic benefit of antibiotics supports the notion that bacteria play a pathogenetic role in acne.

CANDIDIASIS

KEY POINTS
1. "Beefy red" erythema with satellite papules and pustules.
2. Common in the setting of diaper dermatitis.
3. Moisture is the major predisposing factor.

Definition

Candidiasis represents an inflammatory reaction in the skin resulting from infection of the epidermis with *Candida albicans*. Clinically, the infection appears as a "beefy red" erythematous area with surrounding satellite papules and pustules (Fig. 12.11). The pustules, when present, help in the diagnosis. In this section, candidiasis of the skin is discussed. Mucous membrane infection is discussed in Chapter 22.

Incidence

Candidiasis can affect people of all ages. Although only 0.3% of the authors' new patient visits are for candidiasis, in some situations this disease is much more common. It is particularly common in diaper-clad infants and hospitalized patients. Some 2% of the authors' in-hospital consultations are for candidiasis.

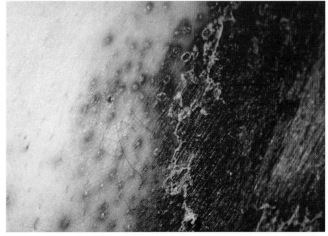

Fig. 12.11 Candidiasis—"beefy red" erythema with satellite papules and pustules.

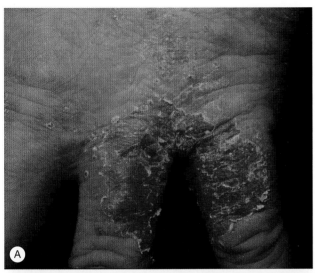

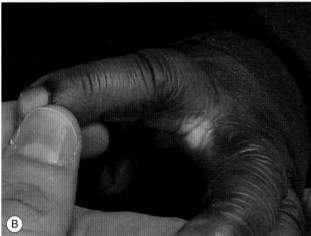

Fig. 12.12 Candidiasis between finger webs. (A) "Beefy red" erythema with desquamation. (B) Macerated or moist skin presenting as a white patch.

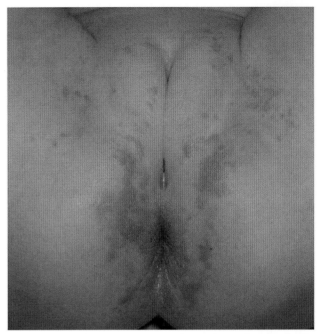

Fig. 12.13 Candidiasis—perineal location with satellite papules in a diapered infant.

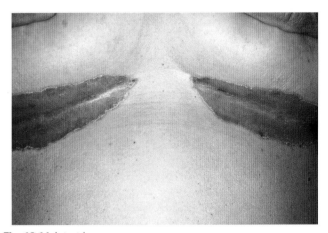

Fig. 12.14 Intertrigo.

History

Patients usually complain of itching and burning of the skin. A moist environment is the most important local predisposing factor for the development of this disease. For infections in the perineal area, diapers and excessive skin folds help to provide this moist environment. Wet surgical dressings can do the same in other locations. On the hands, *C. albicans* infection between the fingers occurs in patients who frequently have their hands in water, such as bartenders and dishwashers (Fig. 12.12). In women with recurrent candidal vulvovaginitis, a history should be taken for predisposing factors, such as pregnancy, diabetes mellitus, birth control pills, and antibiotics.

Moisture predisposes to candidiasis.

Physical Examination

The most consistent finding in cutaneous candidiasis is bright red erythema of the affected skin, characteristically surrounded by satellite pustules and papules. Pustules are not always present but often their residua are noted. These appear as small, 2- to 3-mm, erythematous macules rimmed with a collarette of scale that represents the remnant of the pustule roof. As noted, the distribution of candidiasis favors moist areas. Perineal infection is most common in diapered infants (Fig. 12.13) and in women, in whom it is often accompanied by candidal vaginitis. In bedridden patients, especially those taking antibiotics, perianal involvement occurs and often extends up the back with multiple papules and pustules. Other favored locations are the intertriginous areas under the breasts, in the axillae, between the fingers, and under wet dressings.

Cutaneous candidiasis is "beefy red" with satellite papules and pustules.

Differential Diagnosis

The differential diagnosis depends in part on the location of the infection. In the groin area, candidiasis may be confused with *tinea cruris* or *intertrigo*, an irritant dermatitis caused by maceration and rubbing in intertriginous folds, usually the inguinal or submammary folds in obese patients (Fig. 12.14). Compared with candidiasis, tinea cruris is much more sharply demarcated, and intertrigo is less likely to be so brightly erythematous. Neither exhibits the satellite papules and pustules of candidiasis.

On the back of a bedridden patient, candidal infection may be confused with *miliaria* (heat rash) or *folliculitis*. In candidiasis, however, the papular and pustular lesions are usually accompanied by confluent erythematous involvement in the perianal and, often, perineal areas from which the infection spreads. A potassium hydroxide (KOH) preparation is negative for miliaria and folliculitis. Candidiasis developing under wet dressings can be confused with contact dermatitis. The finding of pustules favors candidiasis. The KOH preparation confirms the diagnosis.

DIFFERENTIAL DIAGNOSIS OF CANDIDIASIS

- Tinea cruris
- Intertrigo
- Miliaria
- Folliculitis
- Contact dermatitis

Laboratory and Biopsy

The important laboratory test is the KOH examination of scrapings from pustules or peripheral scale. If a pustule is present, scraping of its roof and contents has a high positive yield. The finding of hyphae and pseudohyphae is diagnostic for infection (Fig. 12.15). Spores alone are not diagnostic, because *C. albicans* and other yeast organisms can colonize skin without causing infection. For this reason, a skin culture for *C. albicans* is less helpful than a positive KOH scraping; a positive culture from skin does not distinguish between colonization and infection, whereas the KOH preparation does, because the KOH examination detects the infectious filamentous form of the organism. It can be difficult, if not impossible, to distinguish between the hyphae and pseudohyphae of candidiasis and the hyphae of dermatophytic infections. Usually, however, the clinical picture is sufficient to distinguish between the two. A biopsy is not needed.

Hyphae and pseudohyphae are found on KOH examination.

Therapy

Candidiasis is best treated with one of the topical imidazole creams. Over-the-counter creams include clotrimazole (Lotrimin) and miconazole (Micatin). Creams containing econazole (Spectazole) and ketoconazole (Nizoral) require a prescription. The imidazole cream should be applied twice daily. The clinician should instruct the patient to apply the medication *sparingly*, because excessive application of creams to already moist areas can contribute to maceration and may cause further irritation.

Topical medication should be applied sparingly.

Widespread candidiasis is treated with systemic therapy. Fluconazole (Diflucan, 150 mg once weekly for 4 weeks) is an effective oral agent but is seldom needed for local cutaneous infection. This oral agent is more often indicated for severe, persistent, or recurrent mucous membrane candidiasis. Oral ketoconazole is not to be used for candidiasis due to the risk of hepatotoxicity and adrenal insufficiency.

Widespread candidiasis is treated systemically.

Attention should also be given to predisposing factors, especially moisture. Drying measures depend on the situation. For example, an infant with candidal diaper dermatitis should have more frequent diaper changes, and a bedridden patient should be turned more frequently to increase air exposure to the back and buttocks.

THERAPY FOR CANDIDIASIS

Initial
- Topical creams twice daily
  - Clotrimazole
  - Miconazole
  - Ketoconazole

Alternative
- Systemic
  - Fluconazole 150 mg once weekly for up to 4 weeks

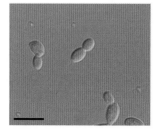 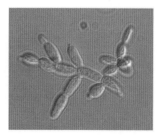 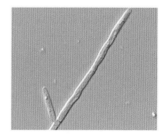

Yeast   **Pseudohyphae**   **Hyphae**

Fig. 12.15 Candidiasis. Epidermis—subcorneal pustules; note associated hyphae and spores. Dermis—perivascular inflammation. Inset—spores and pseudohyphae.

Course and Complications

In most instances, response to topical therapy is prompt and, if the predisposing factors have been corrected, recurrence is unlikely. In patients with recurrent disease, both local (e.g., occlusion, moisture) and systemic (e.g., diabetes, immunosuppression from systemic corticosteroids) predisposing factors should be considered. Most patients with local candidiasis are not immunologically deficient, and the disease resolves with treatment of the infection and correction of the predisposing factors. *Systemic candidiasis* occurs exclusively in severely immunocompromised patients, particularly in those with hematologic malignant diseases. In such patients, the mucous membrane or cutaneous candidal infection may serve as the portal of entry for the systemic infection. *Chronic mucocutaneous candidiasis* is another rare disorder and represents chronic infection of the skin and mucous membranes in patients who are deficient in cellular immunity against *C. albicans*.

Pathogenesis

No special pathogenic strains of *C. albicans* exist. The organism commonly colonizes the skin and bowel, particularly the colon. Pathogenicity in tissue is associated with the conversion of the organism from its yeast to its filamentous form. The most important local factor that encourages this conversion is moisture. Accordingly, skin folds are most commonly involved, as are areas occluded with wet dressings, including diapers. After penetrating the stratum corneum barrier, the organism elicits a complement-mediated acute inflammatory response that causes the dermatitis and prevents deeper tissue invasion.

FOLLICULITIS

KEY POINTS
1. Bacterial infection of hair follicle.
2. *S. aureus* is the most common cause.
3. Colonization of *S. aureus* can occur in the nose, axillae, and groin.

Definition

Folliculitis is an inflammatory reaction in the hair follicle caused by bacteria, usually *S. aureus*. Clinically, the lesion appears as a pustule, often with a central hair (Fig. 12.16).

Incidence

Folliculitis is relatively common, representing approximately 1% of the authors' new patients. The disorder affects primarily young adults but can occur at any age.

History

Folliculitis is usually asymptomatic; occasionally, patients complain of mild discomfort or pruritus associated with the lesions. The process may be chronic or recurrent.

Physical Examination

A pustule is the predominant lesion, although papules may be found. The lesions are individual and do not become confluent. They are usually distributed on the buttocks and thighs (Fig. 12.17) but may also occur in the beard area and sometimes on the scalp.

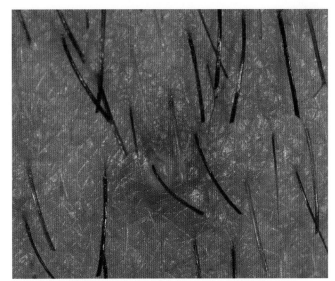
Fig. 12.16 **Folliculitis**—pustule with centrally placed hair.

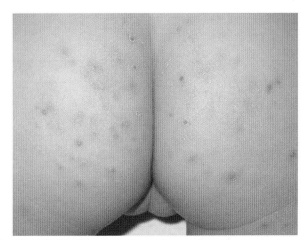
Fig. 12.17 **Folliculitis**—pustules and crusted papules on the buttocks of an infant that cultured positive for *Staphylococcus aureus*.

The key to the diagnosis is appreciated only on close inspection, whereby hairs can be seen in the exact center of many of the lesions.

Differential Diagnosis

The distribution, absence of comedones, and presence of a hair growing from the pustules help to differentiate folliculitis from *acne*. Gram-negative organisms can cause *Gram-negative folliculitis*, mainly in two settings: patients with acne who are receiving antibiotic therapy in whom gram-negative pathogens are selected out, and individuals exposed to hot tubs and swimming pools contaminated with *Pseudomonas aeruginosa* (Fig. 12.18). Both types are uncommon. *Pseudofolliculitis barbae* is a disorder of the neck and jaw of men whose beard hairs are sharply curved. This configuration causes the hairs to reenter the skin, where they induce an inflammatory reaction, resulting in papules and pustules (Fig. 12.19). The ingrowing hairs can often be visualized. *Keratosis pilaris* is a common follicular disorder that presents as tiny, rough, scaling, and follicular papules (*no pustules*) on the backs of the upper arms, buttocks, thighs, and facial cheeks. Rarely, *fungal infections* can result in follicular

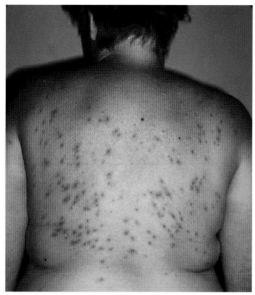

Fig. 12.18 Hot-tub folliculitis—originally pustules that became hemorrhagic centrally with characteristic red flare; often appear under the area of bathing suit occlusion.

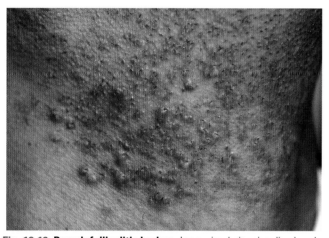

Fig. 12.19 Pseudofolliculitis barbae. Ingrowing hairs visualized under erythematous papules and pustules.

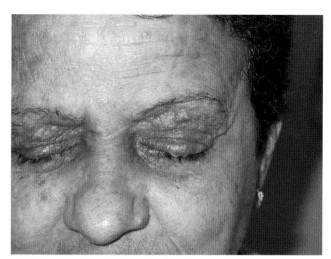

Fig. 12.20 Majocchi granuloma. Red papules and pustules in periorbital distribution. Note fine scale and hint on annular arrangement of papules.

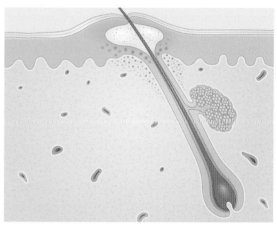

Fig. 12.21 Folliculitis. Epidermis—subcorneal pustule at the opening of a hair follicle. Dermis—inflammation in the upper dermis.

pustules, referred to as *Majocchi granuloma*. These are usually associated with an annular, scaling plaque, which can be hard to detect, and therefore can be distinguished from the individual pustules of bacterial folliculitis (Fig. 12.20).

DIFFERENTIAL DIAGNOSIS OF FOLLICULITIS
• Acne
• Gram-negative folliculitis
• Pseudofolliculitis barbae
• Keratosis pilaris
• Fungal infection

Laboratory and Biopsy

In staphylococcal folliculitis, Gram staining of the pus reveals gram-positive cocci, and bacterial culture confirms the diagnosis. A biopsy is not necessary but, if done, would reveal a collection of neutrophils in the superficial portion of the hair follicle (Fig. 12.21). It is important to send a culture and sensitivity test to check for methicillin-resistant *S. aureus* (MRSA), a not uncommon hospital and community problem.

Therapy

Most cases of staphylococcal folliculitis are mild and can be managed with an antiseptic cleanser such as povidone-iodine (Betadine), chlorhexidine (Hibiclens), or benzoyl peroxide used daily or every other day for at least several weeks. Antibiotic ointments may be used for localized disease (bacitracin or mupirocin 2%). For more extensive involvement, a 10-day course of a systemic antibiotic such as dicloxacillin (250 mg four times daily) is suggested in addition to the cleansers. If a bacterial culture reveals MRSA, then therapy should be directed by antibiotic sensitivities. The authors use doxycycline or trimethoprim–sulfamethoxazole most frequently for MRSA.

THERAPY FOR FOLLICULITIS

Initial
Topical
- Antiseptic cleansers:
  - Betadine
  - Hibiclens
  - Benzoyl peroxide
- Topical antibiotics
  - Mupirocin
  - Bacitracin

Oral
- Dicloxacillin 250 mg q.i.d.

Alternative
- Doxycycline or minocycline (MRSA)
- Trimethoprim–sulfamethoxazole (MRSA)
- Mupirocin to nares for chronic carriers

Course and Complications

Response to therapy is usually good, but recurrences are common. Such patients may be carriers of *S. aureus*, and more prolonged use of antiseptic cleansers is recommended. In addition, the authors often ask these patients to apply an antibiotic ointment (e.g., mupirocin) twice daily in their nares, because this is a common site for *S. aureus*. Other sites of colonization include the axillae and groin. Complications are uncommon and local. Occasionally, the follicular infection can extend more deeply, resulting in a furuncle that requires incision and drainage.

> Patients with recurrent folliculitis may be chronic "carriers" of *S. aureus*.

Pathogenesis

In folliculitis, the bacteria gain entry into the skin through the follicular orifice and establish low-grade infection within the epidermis surrounding the follicular canal. Patients who carry *S. aureus* on their skin are more susceptible to this disorder. Remember that patients with atopic dermatitis are prone to bacterial infections due to lower levels of innate peptides in the epidermis that have antimicrobial properties. Occlusion and maceration are sometimes also predisposing factors.

IMPETIGO

KEY POINTS
1. Characterized by honey-colored crust.
2. *S. aureus* is the most common cause.
3. Treat with oral or topical antibiotics.

Definition

Impetigo represents a superficial skin infection caused by gram-positive bacteria, usually *S. aureus*, and less commonly *Streptococcus pyogenes*. The early lesions are pustules, which quickly break to form crusts (Fig. 12.22). Crusts are the most commonly encountered clinical lesions. Some strains of

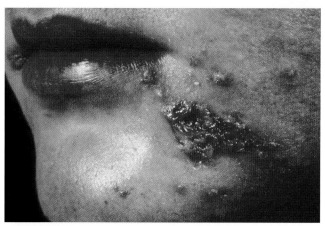

Fig. 12.22 Impetigo—pustules and crusted plaque with surrounding erythema. (Courtesy O. Fred Miller, MD.)

S. aureus can also cause blisters (bullous impetigo), as discussed in Chapter 10.

> Most impetigo is caused by *S. aureus*.

Incidence

Impetigo occurs most often in children and is the most common bacterial infection in children. Although less than 1% of the authors' new patients present with impetigo, this rate would be higher in a general medical practice, particularly a pediatric practice. Nasal carriage of *S. aureus* leads to a higher risk of occurrence in children.

History

The eruption often starts as a single lesion, but patients and parents often do not seek medical help until multiple new lesions develop. Other family members are sometimes affected. Staphylococcal bacterial infection also occurs secondarily (impetiginization) in association with certain skin diseases, especially atopic dermatitis.

Physical Examination

The most commonly encountered clinical finding is a honey-colored crust. Intact pustules are usually not found. When the crust is removed, a superficial glistening base is revealed. Impetigo does not extend deeply, so ulcerations are not present. Lesions can be found anywhere but are most often located on the face around the nose and mouth. Brown or honey-colored crusts are also the hallmark of secondary bacterial infections.

Differential Diagnosis

Different from the staphylococcal impetigo described above, *ecthyma* is caused by group A streptococci but much confusion exists regarding these two types of bacterial skin infection. In both types, the presenting lesion is usually a crust, but the more important clinical difference is the depth of the infection. With staphylococcal impetigo, the process is superficial (just below the stratum corneum), so when the crust is removed, only a shallow, glistening erosion is seen (Fig. 12.23). In streptococcal pyoderma, the infection is usually deeper, extending through the epidermis, so when

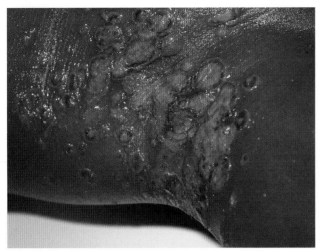

Fig. 12.23 **Impetigo in the axilla**—annular plaques with central erosion. Petrolatum ointment hides the scale.

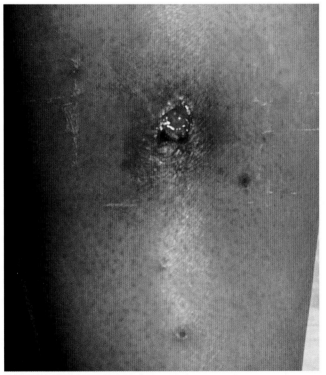

Fig. 12.24 **Ecthyma on the lower leg**—streptococcal skin infection extends more deeply, often forming an ulcer (ecthyma).

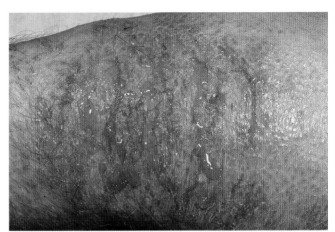

Fig. 12.25 **Eczematous dermatitis**—crusted plaque in elbow crease in the setting of atopic dermatitis.

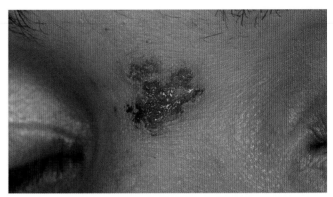

Fig. 12.26 **Herpes simplex**. Note erosions with scalloped borders. Honey-colored crusts represent secondary impetiginization.

recognition (by patient or physician) of clear vesicles present at the start, a history of recurrence in the same location, and the presence of erosions with scalloped borders (Fig. 12.26). Inflammatory *fungal infections* can cause pustules and are in the differential diagnosis for "sterile" pustular processes. KOH examination and fungal cultures are indicated in patients with negative Gram stains and bacterial cultures or in patients with a poor response to antibiotic therapy.

DIFFERENTIAL DIAGNOSIS OF IMPETIGO

- Ecthyma
- Eczematous dermatitis
- Herpes simplex infection
- Fungal infection (e.g., candidiasis)

Laboratory

A Gram stain reveals gram-positive cocci. Bacterial culture typically grows *S. aureus*. In obtaining material for Gram staining and culture, the clinician should first remove the crust so that the specimen can be obtained from the weeping, glistening erosion. Biopsy is rarely performed but would show a subcorneal pustule (Fig. 12.27).

Therapy

Both topical and systemic antibiotics have been advocated for treating impetigo. Uncomplicated impetigo resolves on its own

the crust is removed, a deeper defect (i.e., an ulcer) is noted (Fig. 12.24). In addition, with staphylococcal impetigo, there is usually little or no surrounding erythema, whereas with streptococcal infection, erythema is moderate to marked. Finally, staphylococcal impetigo is most common on the face, whereas ecthyma is usually found on the lower extremities, occurring after a scratch or insect bite. Eczematous (Greek—"to boil") dermatitis, including nummular and atopic dermatitis, can be confused with impetigo. The oozing from the inflamed skin leads to crust, and history and physical examination findings help distinguish impetigo from eczematous dermatitis (Fig. 12.25).

When the vesicles in *herpes simplex* age, they become cloudy and eventually form crusts. At this stage, herpes is often misdiagnosed as impetigo. Features favoring herpes include the

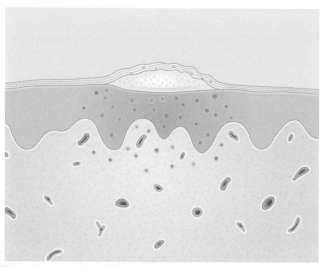

Fig. 12.27 Impetigo. Epidermis—subcorneal pustules. Dermis—mild inflammatory reaction in the upper dermis.

after approximately 2 weeks. Topical preparations such as over-the-counter bacitracin and triple antibiotic (neomycin, bacitracin, and polymyxin) ointments and prescription mupirocin (Bactroban) and retapamulin (Altabax) ointments are used for localized impetigo. General hygiene measures are also recommended to prevent its spread and recurrence. For more extensive lesions, systemic antibiotic therapy is preferred. Most *S. aureus* strains, including those encountered in outpatients, produce penicillinase, so penicillin is not an appropriate treatment. The preferred antibiotics are oral cefalexin or penicillinase-resistant penicillins such as dicloxacillin used over a 7- to 10-day course. The increasing resistance of *S. aureus* to erythromycin may limit the usefulness of this agent in impetigo. MRSA has also been encountered and requires a tailored antibiotic regimen based on sensitivities, with doxycycline and trimethoprim–sulfamethoxazole double strength commonly prescribed.

> Resistance patterns of causative bacteria guide treatment decisions.

THERAPY FOR IMPETIGO

Initial
- General hygiene
  - Antibacterial soaps—chlorhexidine gluconate
  - Changing of towel, washcloth, shaver, etc., daily
  - Bleach bathers: ¼–½ cup of bleach in ½ tub of water
- Antibiotics
  - Triple antibiotic, mupirocin, or retapamulin ointment—applied t.i.d.

Alternative
- Systemic antibiotics—for more wider spread infection
  - Dicloxacillin
  - Cefalexin
- Systemic antibiotics—for MRSA—based on its bacterial resistant patterns
  - Doxycycline 100 g b.i.d. (for older than 8 years of age)
  - Trimethoprim–sulfamethoxazole double strength b.i.d. or 4–6 mg/kg b.i.d.

Course and Complications

With appropriate antibiotic therapy, prompt healing is to be expected, with marked improvement within several days in most patients. Bacteriologic cure is achieved in 7–10 days in nearly all cases. If a rapid response to therapy does not occur, the physician should consider the possibility that the infection is caused by an antibiotic-resistant strain. In such instances, the result of the initial culture, if obtained, serves as a guide in selecting an alternative antibiotic.

The bacteria can colonize the skin without causing actual infection. This is particularly true in patients with chronic dermatoses such as atopic dermatitis. More than 10% of patients with atopic dermatitis have *S. aureus* colonizing their eczematous skin. Impetiginization, characterized by honey-colored crusts, occurs more often in these patients than in those with psoriasis. Naturally occurring antimicrobial peptides in the skin are deficient in patients with atopic dermatitis, thereby leading to increased susceptibility to bacterial infections.

> Honey-colored crusts indicate that the skin is secondarily infected, which can be difficult to differentiate from the "oozing" of inflamed skin in atopic dermatitis and nummular dermatitis.

Complications are rare. Acute glomerulonephritis may occur as a sequela to skin infection from streptococcal but not from staphylococcal infections. This emphasizes the importance of discriminating between these two types of skin infections.

Pathogenesis

S. aureus is ubiquitous in the environment. With staphylococcal infection, "trauma" to the skin is often subclinical, and most patients cannot recall obvious trauma to their skin. Once bacteria have gained entry, they establish infection in the uppermost layer of the viable epidermis, just below the stratum corneum. Inflammatory cells, primarily neutrophils, respond and are responsible for the pus that is clinically evident and eventuates into the characteristic crusts.

Infection with group A streptococci is more difficult to establish. These organisms do not colonize normal skin but must be inoculated through a damaged surface, such as a scratch or insect bite. Once established, the organism produces proteolytic enzymes, which are in part responsible for the surrounding inflammation.

ROSACEA

KEY POINTS

1. Papules and pustules with a background of erythema affect the central third of the face.
2. Eye involvement is common.
3. Treat with topical and oral antibiotics.
4. Disease of adults.

Definition

Rosacea is a chronic inflammatory disorder affecting the blood vessels and pilosebaceous units of the face (Fig. 12.28). The

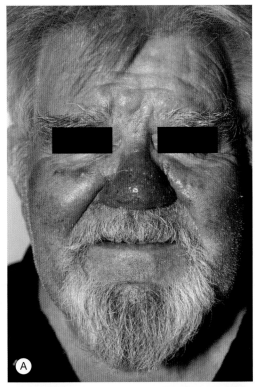

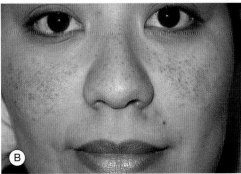

Fig. 12.28 Rosacea. (A) papules and pustules superimposed on the background of erythema in a typical, fair-skinned patient. (B) Rosacea seen in a patient with a darker skin type.

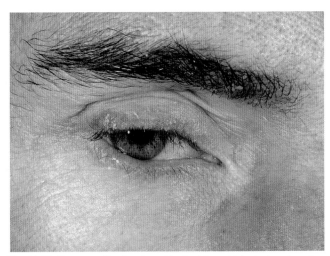

Fig. 12.29 Rosacea. Ocular sign—blepharitis and injected conjunctiva.

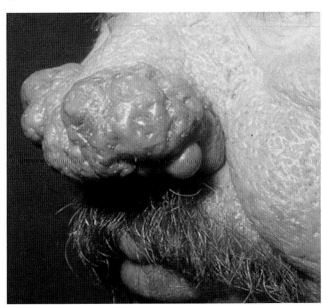

Fig. 12.30 Rosacea. Extreme phymatous change leading to bulbous thickening.

etiology is not well understood. Clinically, papules and pustules are superimposed on the background of erythema and telangiectasia.

Incidence

Rosacea is a relatively common disorder that affects primarily middle-aged adults. Approximately 1% of the authors' new patients are seen for this disease.

History

The disorder often has a gradual onset. Usually, the patient first notices erythema; with time, telangiectasia appears. The development of papules and pustules is usually sufficient for the patient to bring the problem to a physician's attention. Trigger factors, such as exercise and alcohol, can cause a flare of the redness. Most, but not all, patients have a fair complexion and light-colored irises. Rosacea can affect the eyes, known as ocular rosacea. Eye symptoms include redness, burning, itching, or a foreign body sensation; always ask a patient with rosacea if they have eye symptoms.

Physical Examination

The four major clinical subtypes of rosacea are as follows: (1) vascular, (2) papulopustular, (3) rhinophyma, and (4) ocular. Each type may occur independently, and there is no typical progression from one to the other. Usually a patient with rosacea presents with a combination of vascular, papulopustular, and ocular findings. Typically, papules and pustules are superimposed on a background of erythema and telangiectasia. Sometimes, only the erythema and telangiectasia are present. Characteristically, comedones are not found. The disease affects the central third of the face and spares the lateral aspects of the forehead and cheeks. Blepharitis and conjunctivitis are common (Fig. 12.29). Bulbous thickening of the nose is rare and occurs most commonly in men (Fig. 12.30). Rarely, inflammation from rosacea can lead to facial edema (Fig. 12.31).

> Papules and pustules are superimposed on a background of erythema and telangiectasia.

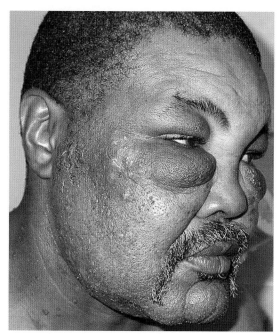

Fig. 12.31 Rosacea. Chronic inflammation causing periorbital edema—note the papules on cheeks.

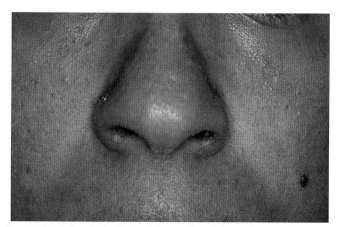

Fig. 12.32 Seborrheic dermatitis—scaly red, hypopigmented patches affecting nasolabial (convex surface) folds.

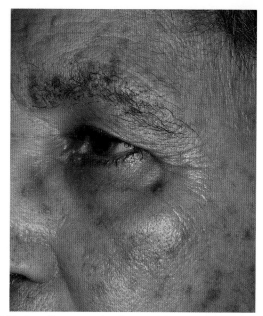

Fig. 12.33 Acneiform eruption from epidermal growth factor—papules and pustules on the face.

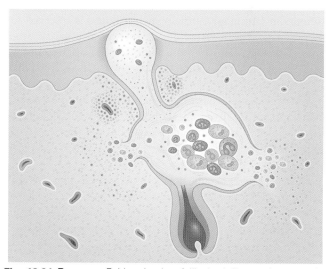

Fig. 12.34 Rosacea. Epidermis—intrafollicular inflammation; granulomatous reaction to the contents of a ruptured pilosebaceous unit.

Differential Diagnosis

Rosacea is distinguished from *acne vulgaris* by the absence of comedones, the background of erythema and telangiectasia, the onset in middle life, and the distribution in the central third of the face. Rashes that may be confused with the vascular element in rosacea occur in lupus erythematosus, dermatomyositis, photodermatitis, and, most commonly, seborrheic dermatitis (Fig. 12.32), but none of these exhibit pustules. Interestingly, seborrheic dermatitis is often seen in conjunction with rosacea. Seborrheic dermatitis affects the concave surfaces (nasolabial folds), whereas rosacea affects the convex surfaces. In patients with rosacea with a prominent flushing component, *carcinoid syndrome* sometimes enters the differential diagnosis. Epidermal growth factor inhibitors, used to treat a variety of malignancies, can lead to a facial acneiform eruption, which can be confused with rosacea (Fig. 12.33).

DIFFERENTIAL DIAGNOSIS OF ROSACEA
• Acne
• Lupus/dermatomyositis
• Seborrheic dermatitis
• Carcinoid syndrome
• Acneiform eruption from epidermal growth factor

Laboratory and Biopsy

The diagnosis is almost always made clinically. A biopsy is rarely needed, but if performed, shows vascular dilation, often with degenerative changes in the collagen and elastic fibers in the upper dermis (Fig. 12.34). The papules and pustules in rosacea are similar histologically to those found in acne vulgaris, but in rosacea, the inflammatory infiltrate is more likely to have a granulomatous component. This represents a foreign body reaction in the dermis to the extravasated contents of affected pilosebaceous units. The granulomatous response can be impressive and has been occasionally confused with granulomatous disorders, such as sarcoidosis and tuberculosis.

> Histologically, a granulomatous reaction is often present and may be confused with sarcoidosis or tuberculosis.

Therapy

Topical metronidazole 0.75% (MetroGel, MetroCream) or topical azelaic acid 15% (Finacea) applied twice daily are both effective in treating the papules, pustules, and erythema of rosacea. The mechanisms of action are unknown. Systemic antibiotics are used frequently for the papular and pustular components and are especially beneficial in treating ocular rosacea (Do not forget to ask each patient with rosacea if they have eye symptoms!). Sometimes, the erythema is also improved. Low-dose doxycycline (20 mg twice daily) exerts an antiinflammatory effect and is the usual treatment. Most patients respond within 1 month, after which the drug can often be tapered, but some patients require long-term maintenance treatment. Systemic isotretinoin (Accutane), usually in low doses, is reserved for the rare patient with severe disease that has resisted all other types of therapy, but it does not lead to a lasting response as seen in acne. Laser treatment (e.g., pulsed dye laser) is the only effective and definitive therapy for the erythema of rosacea, and treatment typically needs to be repeated every several years to maintain response. Two topical, alpha-adrenergic receptor agonist therapies, brimonidine tartrate 0.33% gel (Mirvaso) and oxymetazoline 1% cream (Rhofade), are FDA-approved to treat persistent facial erythema from rosacea.

Topical steroids should not be used because they are well known to aggravate the disease. Sun exposure can also be an aggravating factor, and sun-protective measures should be recommended. Avoidance of "triggers" like alcohol prevents flushing.

> Strong topical steroids are contraindicated.

THERAPY FOR ROSACEA

Initial
- Metronidazole gel or cream b.i.d.
- Azelaic acid gel b.i.d.
- Daily moisturizer containing sunscreen

Alternative
- Doxycycline 20 mg b.i.d. for papulopustular and ocular rosacea
- Isotretinoin
- Pulsed dye laser (vascular rosacea) or topical brimonidine 0.33% gel/oxymetazoline 1% cream for persistent facial erythema

Course and Complications

The disease is usually chronic, but most patients respond well to therapy. In many patients, however, therapy must be continued for months to years. The erythematous component may be improved by therapy but telangiectasia persists.

Rhinophyma sometimes develops in patients with rosacea. As the name suggests, this disease involves hyperplasia of the sebaceous glands, connective tissue, and vascular bed of the nose. The hyperplasia can be striking, resulting in a bulbous nose. Contrary to popular belief, rosacea is not a sign of excessive alcohol intake. Rhinophyma requires referral for surgical treatment of anatomic resculpturing of the nose (e.g., dermabrasion, Shaw scalpel excision). Alternatively, lasers can be used for sculpting (e.g., ablative carbon dioxide). Ocular complications occur in some patients with rosacea. Eye findings range from blepharitis to conjunctivitis and even keratitis. The latter can be severe and has been known to result in visual impairment. Oral doxycycline is helpful for ocular complications.

Pathogenesis

The pathogenetic mechanisms in this disease are not well understood. For the vascular component, investigators have suggested that sun exposure damages the collagen support of the vascular network, thereby resulting in vasodilation. Other aggravating factors that have been incriminated, but not well proven, include the ingestion of foods that cause vasodilation (e.g., hot liquids, alcohol, and spicy foods) and psychologic stress. Immune mechanisms have also been implicated, with immunoglobulin deposition occurring at the dermal–epidermal interface. The pathogenetic significance of this finding remains unclear. Clearly, genetics play a role as the family history of rosacea is often positive in a patient with rosacea.

UNCOMMON CAUSES OF PUSTULES

DEEP FUNGAL INFECTION—COCCIDIOIDOMYCOSIS

Coccidioidomycosis is a rare deep fungal infection presenting with skin manifestations. It is caused by the dimorphic fungus, *Coccidioides immitis*. Most cases result from the inhalation of

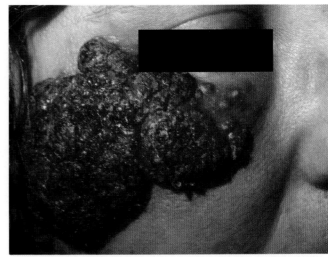

Fig. 12.35 Coccidioidomycosis—large verrucous plaque with pustules.

spores with subsequent dissemination to the skin and other organs. Immunocompromised patients, especially HIV-infected individuals, are at highest risk. Clinical features of most deep fungal infections, including blastomycosis, are initial formation of pustules, plaques, and nodules evolving into verrucous plaques (Fig. 12.35). Biopsy and tissue culture confirm the diagnosis.

DERMATOPHYTE (KERION)

Dermatophytes can infect hair follicles and may result in pustules (Fig. 12.36). This condition is sometimes confused with bacterial folliculitis. A *kerion* is a dermatophytic infection, frequently of the scalp, that appears as an indurated, boggy, inflammatory

plaque studded with pustules. Kerions are frequently confused with bacterial pyodermas. The most common organism causing a kerion is *Trichophyton rubrum*. Systemic antifungal therapy is necessary.

GONOCOCCEMIA

Gonococcemia (gonococcal arthritis–dermatitis syndrome) represents a systemic infection characterized by fever, arthralgia, tenosynovitis, septic arthritis, and hemorrhagic (or purpuric) pustules. The hemorrhagic pustules appear in an acral distribution and are few in number (Fig. 12.37). The disease results from the dissemination of gonococci from an infected mucosal site. Diagnosis is confirmed by a bacterial culture of the affected mucosal site. Treatment is with intravenous or intramuscular antibiotics, most commonly ceftriaxone.

> Pustules in bacteremia often have a purpuric or hemorrhagic quality.

SUBCORNEAL PUSTULAR DERMATOSIS

Sterile pustules are the hallmark of subcorneal pustular dermatosis. The disease is characterized by annular or expanding, polycyclic collections of pustules on a red base (Fig. 12.38). Flexural accentuation is common. The disease has a waxing and waning course. Monoclonal gammopathies have been reported with this condition. Skin biopsy confirms clinical suspicion of the disease. Dapsone is the treatment of choice.

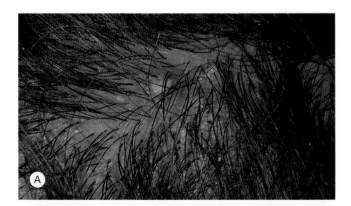
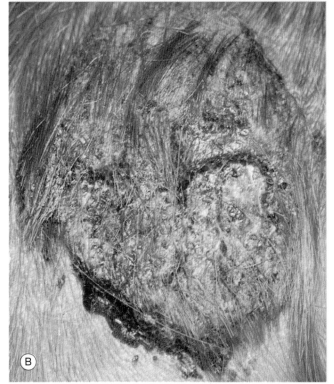

Fig. 12.36 Dermatophyte. (A) Pustules infecting hair follicle (culture necessary for the diagnosis). (B) Kerion—a boggy plaque representing severe immunologic reaction to dermatophytes infecting hair follicles.

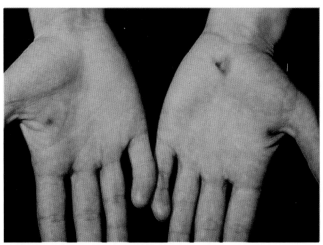

Fig. 12.37 Gonococcemia—few hemorrhagic pustules in characteristic acral distribution.

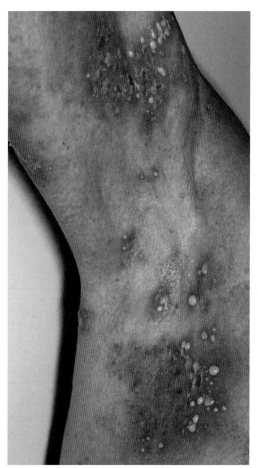

Fig. 12.38 **Subcorneal pustular dermatosis**—annular plaques studded with pustules in the axilla; flexural location is characteristic.

SELF-ASSESSMENT

Case 1—Pustules and Papules Surrounding an Ulcer
(Fig. 12.39)

Describe What You See

Surrounding the ulcer is a pink, slightly scaling patch with satellite pustules and papules.

What Is Your Differential Diagnosis?

The differential diagnosis includes contact dermatitis from the medications used in the dressings. However, with the satellite pustules and papules, candidiasis also needs to be considered.

What Is the First Diagnostic Test You Would Do?

The first diagnostic test should be a KOH examination of a scraping from the border of the lesion. In this patient's case, it was positive for hyphae. It is difficult to distinguish microscopically between candidal and dermatophytic hyphae, but the clinical picture favors candidiasis.

How Would You Treat It?

Local therapy with a topical imidazole cream, applied sparingly twice daily, and discontinuation of the wet dressings resulted in prompt clearing of the eruption.

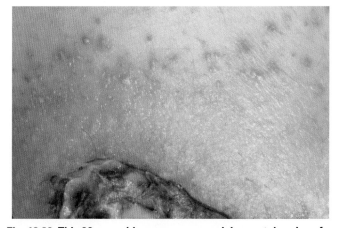

Fig. 12.39 **This 38-year-old woman was receiving wet dressings for her leg ulcer**. After 1 week, a rash developed around the ulcer.

CHAPTER CONTENTS

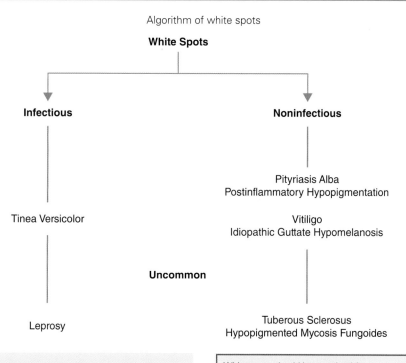

Algorithm of white spots

ABSTRACT

White spots in the skin result from decreased melanin pigmentation. This can be caused by a reduction in the number of melanocytes or a decrease in their melanin production. Inflammatory events are frequently responsible for a condition called postinflammatory hypopigmentation, even though the inflammation may not be clinically appreciated. Table 13.1 lists the four most common causes of white spots. Determination of the degree (partial versus complete) of pigment loss and identification of the presence or absence of scale are helpful in distinguishing clinical features.

KEY POINTS

1. Examine for partial versus complete pigment loss and the presence or absence of scale.
2. A Wood's light examination accentuates white spots, especially in fair-skinned individuals.
3. Vitiligo is a common cause of depigmentation.

> White spots should be examined for:
> 1. Partial versus complete pigment loss
> 2. Presence or absence of scale

The degree of pigment loss can be assessed roughly with a Wood's light examination, which helps to accentuate pigment contrast. In a darkened room with a Wood's light, lesions that are completely depigmented appear almost chalk white. This finding is characteristic of vitiligo. The Wood's light examination is also helpful in identifying white spots in lightly pigmented individuals; in patients with extremely fair complexions, white spots may not be evident under bright illumination (Fig. 13.1).

> White spots are seen more easily by Wood's light examination.

The admonition, "If it scales, scrape it!" also pertains to white spots. The two common hypopigmentary conditions that scale (i.e., tinea versicolor and pityriasis alba) can be distinguished with a potassium hydroxide (KOH) preparation.

PITYRIASIS ALBA

KEY POINTS

1. Characterized by hypopigmented, white patches
2. More commonly seen in darkly pigmented children
3. Probably a low-grade "eczematous" reaction

Definition

Pityriasis alba is an idiopathic hypopigmentary condition that appears clinically as white (alba) patches with overlying fine, "bran-like" (*pityron*, Greek for bran) scales (Fig. 13.2).

Incidence

The disease is extremely common but usually not sufficiently disturbing for most patients to seek medical attention. It affects mainly children between the ages of 3 and 16 years and is most common (or most noticeable) in darker-skinned individuals. It is a chronic condition, with periods of flares and resolution. Individuals with atopic dermatitis have a predilection for pityriasis alba.

> Pityriasis alba is most commonly recognized and appreciated in darkly pigmented children but affects children of all skin tones.

History

Pityriasis alba is usually asymptomatic, although an occasional patient may complain of mild itching. Patients or parents are most concerned about the appearance of the lesions. It may worsen in the summer months with increased ultraviolet (UV) exposure.

TABLE 13.1	**White Spots**						
	Frequency (%)[a]	**Etiology**	**Physical Examination**			**Differential Diagnosis**	**Laboratory Test**
			Degree of Pigment Loss[b]	Presence of Scale	Distribution		
Pityriasis alba	0.4	Unknown	Partial	+	Face, upper arms	Tinea versicolor	–
Postinflammatory hypopigmentation		Nonspecific sequelae of skin inflammation	Partial	–	Anywhere (sites of prior inflammation)	Vitiligo	–
Tinea versicolor	1.4	Fungus	Partial	+	Trunk	Vitiligo	KOH preparation
Vitiligo	0.6	Unknown	Complete	–	Anywhere		–

KOH, Potassium hydroxide.
[a]Percentage of new dermatology patients with this diagnosis seen in the Hershey Medical Center Dermatology Clinic, Hershey, Pennsylvania.
[b]As assessed by Wood's light examination.

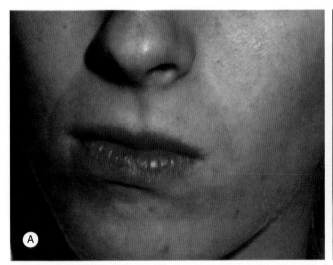
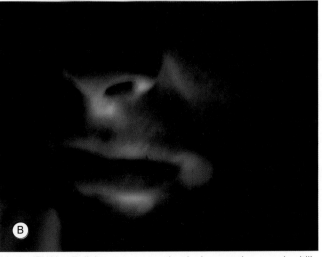

Fig. 13.1 (A) Periorificial vitiligo is difficult to appreciate in fair-skinned individuals. (B) Wood's light accentuates the depigmentation seen in vitiligo.

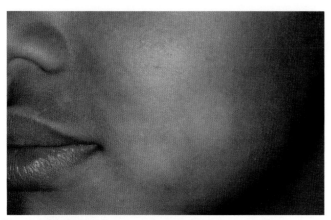

Fig. 13.2 **Pityriasis alba**—hypopigmented patches in a child.

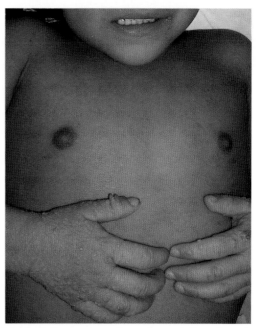

Fig. 13.4 **Postinflammatory hypopigmentation**—hypopigmented patches on the chest in a child with atopic dermatitis. Note multiple warts on hands and around the mouth.

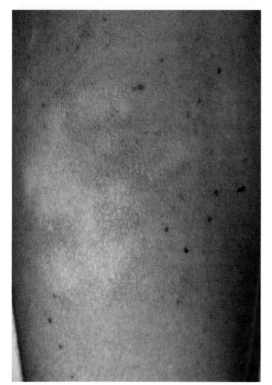

Fig. 13.3 **Pityriasis alba**—hypopigmented patches on upper arms in an adult.

Physical Examination

The early lesion is a mildly erythematous, slightly scaling patch with an irregular but defined margin. Most often, only the subsequent lesion is seen—a 1- to 4-cm white patch with a fine, powdery scale. In children, the face is the most common area of involvement, and they may have one to several lesions. Pityriasis alba can occur in other locations. Another common area of involvement is the upper arms, especially in children with atopic dermatitis (Fig. 13.3). Rarely, widespread involvement occurs.

Differential Diagnosis

The disease is most often misdiagnosed as *tinea versicolor*. In temperate climates, adults with tinea versicolor seldom have facial involvement, but in children (in whom the disease is

much less common) the face is affected in approximately one-third of cases. Accordingly, a KOH preparation should be performed on all scaling white spots to rule out tinea versicolor. The white spots in *vitiligo* are distinguished by sharp demarcation, complete depigmentation, and a lack of scale. Postinflammatory hypopigmentation from inflammatory dermatoses (e.g., atopic dermatitis or psoriasis) is distinguished by the history and extrafacial distribution of skin lesions (Fig. 13.4).

DIFFERENTIAL DIAGNOSIS OF PITYRIASIS ALBA

- Tinea versicolor
- Vitiligo
- Postinflammatory hypopigmentation

Laboratory and Biopsy

No specific laboratory test is available to establish the diagnosis, and it is typically recognized clinically. The KOH preparation is negative. The histologic picture is nonspecific, showing slight hyperkeratosis, decreased pigmentation in the basal cell layer, and a mild inflammatory reaction in the upper dermis (Fig. 13.5).

Therapy

Treatment is not often necessary as spontaneous resolution occurs. Moisturizers can be used for the dry scaling, and 1% hydrocortisone cream is used for the inflammatory reaction. Studies have shown that twice daily application of tacrolimus 0.1% ointment or twice daily pimecrolimus 1% cream can also be effective. For more severe diseases, a trial of triamcinolone 0.1% cream twice daily for several weeks may be beneficial for involvement on the trunk.

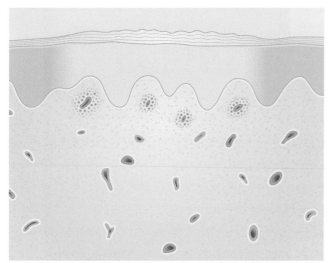

Fig. 13.5 Pityriasis alba. Epidermis—hyperkeratosis; decreased pigmentation. Dermis—mild inflammation around superficial blood vessels.

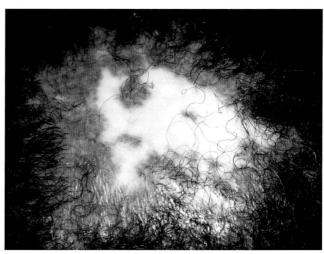

Fig. 13.6 Postinflammatory hypopigmentation—white macules on scalp secondary to "burned out" discoid lupus erythematosus.

THERAPY FOR PITYRIASIS ALBA

Initial
- Moisturizers
- 1% Hydrocortisone cream

Alternative
- Tacrolimus 0.1% ointment twice daily
- Pimecrolimus 1% cream twice daily
- Triamcinolone 0.1% twice daily (avoid chronic, continuous application)

Course and Complications

The patient must understand that repigmentation will be slow. In most patients, the disease resolves spontaneously but can take months to years. For affected children, the disease rarely persists into adulthood. The disorder has no complications.

Pathogenesis

The origin of this common disorder is unknown. Most investigators believe that the decreased pigment is a postinflammatory phenomenon and that the initial event is a low-grade eczematous reaction. It may be a manifestation of inflammation related to decreased barrier protection from dry skin. The fact that the condition is commonly seen in children with atopic dermatitis lends credence to this dry skin association.

> Pityriasis alba may be a low-grade eczema.

POSTINFLAMMATORY HYPOPIGMENTATION

KEY POINTS
1. Inflammation suppresses or destroys melanocytes
2. Characterized by white macules with or without scale
3. Repigmentation takes months to years

Definition

Postinflammatory hypopigmentation is the result of melanocyte destruction or suppressed melanin production secondary to inflammation of the skin (Fig. 13.6). It appears as a hypopigmented or, in severe cases, a depigmented macule. The inflammation may be due to physical trauma, a chemical agent, or a primary inflammatory skin disease.

> Causes of postinflammatory hypopigmentation:
> 1. Physical trauma
> 2. Chemicals
> 3. Inflammatory skin diseases

Incidence

Inflammation-induced white spots are common incidental findings. Occasionally, they are the patient's primary complaint.

History

The inflammatory event responsible for the white spots is almost always remembered by the patient. Physical agents that may induce white spots include X-irradiation, frostbite, intralesional triamcinolone injections, and skin resurfacing lasers. Industrial exposure to chemicals such as phenolic and sulfhydryl compounds can also produce hypopigmentation. Some inflammatory skin diseases can leave residual hypopigmentation. Common examples are discoid lupus erythematosus, psoriasis, and dermatitis, particularly atopic dermatitis and seborrheic dermatitis in a darker-skinned individual (Fig. 13.7). Uncommon causes are cutaneous sarcoidosis and mycosis fungoides (MF), a form of cutaneous T-cell lymphoma.

Physical Examination

Whitish macules (no scale) or patches (with scale) conform to areas of prior inflammation. In the case of intralesional triamcinolone injection, medication can spread into the surrounding skin, causing hypopigmentation outside the original lesion (Fig. 13.8).

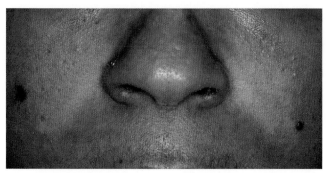

Fig. 13.7 Postinflammatory hypopigmentation—irregular white patch surrounding a hypertrophic scar after intralesional triamcinolone leaked into surrounding skin. Note the scar is also hypopigmented.

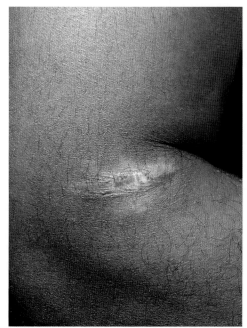

Fig. 13.8 Postinflammatory hypopigmentation—subtle white patches secondary to seborrheic dermatitis, more commonly seen in darker-skinned individuals. Note characteristic nasolabial involvement.

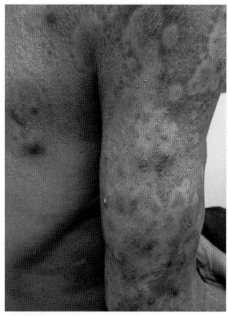

Fig. 13.9 Postinflammatory hypopigmentation—hypopigmented patches and plaques in a patient with cutaneous T-cell lymphoma.

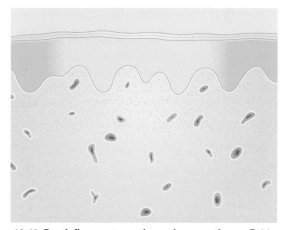

Fig. 13.10 Postinflammatory hypopigmentation. Epidermis—hypopigmented. Dermis—may show some residual inflammation.

Differential Diagnosis

Postinflammatory hypopigmentation may be confused with *vitiligo*, particularly when hypopigmentation is profound. However, the pigment loss is rarely complete, as it is in vitiligo. Moreover, in vitiligo, the depigmentation is only rarely preceded by recognizable inflammation. It is important to determine the cause of postinflammatory diagnosis, ruling out inflammatory conditions, like atopic dermatitis or psoriasis, and neoplastic conditions, like cutaneous T-cell lymphoma (Fig. 13.9).

Laboratory and Biopsy

No specific laboratory test is available. The biopsy is not specific, showing decreased pigmentation in the epidermis and occasional mild residual inflammation in the dermis (Fig. 13.10).

Therapy

Treatment is not usually required. No effective agent for repigmenting skin is available. Cosmetically troublesome areas can be disguised with opaque cosmetics such as Dermablend and Covermark. To avoid future hypopigmentation, patients are advised to avoid contact with any responsible physical or chemical agents and to treat primary skin disease promptly.

DIFFERENTIAL DIAGNOSIS OF POSTINFLAMMATORY HYPOPIGMENTATION

- Vitiligo
- Determine primary skin condition
  - Inflammatory (e.g., atopic dermatitis)
  - Neoplastic (e.g., cutaneous T-cell lymphoma)

THERAPY FOR POSTINFLAMMATORY HYPOPIGMENTATION

- None
- Cosmetic covering
- Treat primary skin disease

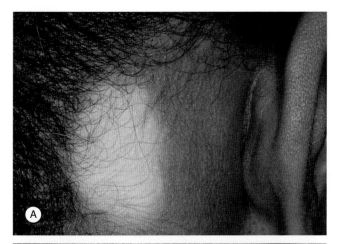

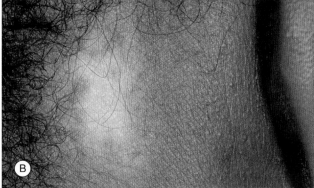

Fig. 13.11 (A). Postinflammatory hypopigmentation secondary to the chemical squaric acid used to treat alopecia areata. (B) Postinflammatory hypopigmentation improved after 8 months of observation.

Course and Complications

Usually, pigmentation returns gradually. Patients need to understand that this process takes months, and sometimes longer (Fig. 13.11). However, if the damage has been severe, the hypopigmentation may be permanent.

> Repigmentation, if it occurs, takes months and, sometimes, years.

TINEA VERSICOLOR

KEY POINTS

1. Common superficial fungal infection caused by *Malassezia* organisms
2. KOH preparation of subtle scale confirms the diagnosis
3. Appears on neck, trunk, and upper arms

Definition

Tinea versicolor, also called pityriasis versicolor, is a superficial fungal infection of the stratum corneum that results in altered pigment in the epidermis. Clinically, the lesions appear as finely scaling patches, which, as the name "versicolor" implies, can be pink, tan, brown, or white (Figs. 13.12 and 13.13). Of these, white is the most common.

> Lesions in tinea versicolor can be of varying colors, the most common being white.

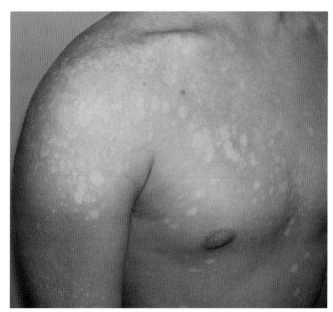

Fig. 13.12 Tinea versicolor—hypopigmented patches.

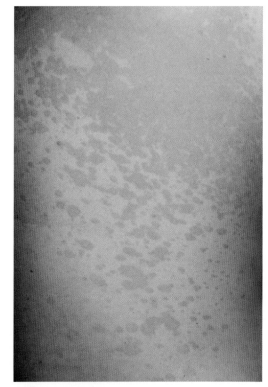

Fig. 13.13 Tinea versicolor—pink, tan patches.

Incidence

Tinea versicolor is a common disease, affecting nearly 1% of the general population. In the authors' clinic, 1.4% of new patients are seen for tinea versicolor. The incidence is higher in tropical climates. Any age group may be affected, but the disease is most common in young adults. Immunosuppression, including that from systemic corticosteroids (either endogenous or exogenous), can be a predisposing factor, but most patients are healthy.

History

Tinea versicolor is occasionally associated with mild pruritus but more often it is asymptomatic. Most patients seek medical attention because of its cosmetic appearance. Because the affected areas do not tan, the patient often first becomes aware of the condition after sun exposure. The surrounding normal skin tans, providing a contrast to the "white spots." During the winter months and in persons with darker complexions, the lesions appear more deeply pigmented than the normal skin (Fig. 13.14).

Physical Examination

The usual lesion is a round, hypopigmented, slightly scaling patch. It often starts as multiple small follicular macules, which subsequently become confluent. The scale is usually subtle and sometimes appreciated only with gentle scraping of the skin, which reveals a fine, crumbly scale. If a Wood's light examination is performed, the lesions will appear hypopigmented but not chalk white, as in vitiligo. With Wood's light examination, sometimes the scale fluoresces pale yellow or orange, but this finding is not universal and should not be relied on for diagnosis.

> In tinea versicolor, the scaling may be subtle.

The usual distribution for tinea versicolor is the neck, trunk, and upper arms, that is, the distribution of a "short-sleeved" turtleneck sweater. Distal extremity involvement is uncommon, except in tropical climates. Facial involvement is more common in people of African descent, particularly in children.

Differential Diagnosis

In adults, the white spots of tinea versicolor are most often misdiagnosed as *vitiligo*. In vitiligo, the absence of scale and complete depigmentation are distinguishing factors from tinea versicolor. Tinea versicolor appearing as pink or tan scaling patches on the chest may be misdiagnosed as *seborrheic dermatitis*. The distribution of seborrheic dermatitis involves the hairline, eyebrows, nasolabial folds, and middle chest.

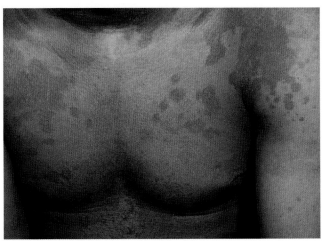

Fig. 13.14 **Tinea versicolor**—darker brown patches.

DIFFERENTIAL DIAGNOSIS OF TINEA VERSICOLOR

- Vitiligo
- Seborrheic dermatitis

Laboratory Examination

The organism cannot be grown on routine fungal culture; therefore the diagnosis rests with the KOH examination. Examination of the scale with a KOH preparation reveals short hyphae, which are often mixed with spores, giving the appearance of spaghetti (hyphae) and meatballs (spores) (Fig. 13.15). Biopsy, seldom performed, shows abundant fungal organisms in a hyperkeratotic stratum corneum (Fig. 13.16).

Therapy

Topical selenium sulfide, zinc pyrithione (Head & Shoulders), and ketoconazole (Nizoral) shampoos are commonly used as body washes for the affected skin. These agents are effective,

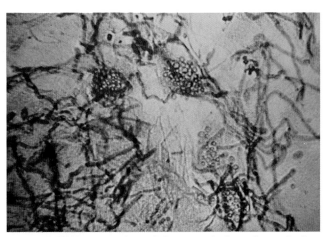

Fig. 13.15 **KOH preparation of tinea versicolor**—diagnostic "spaghetti (short hyphae) and meatballs (spores)."

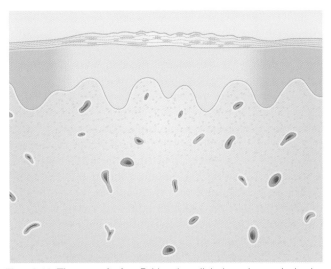

Fig. 13.16 **Tinea versicolor**. Epidermis—slight hyperkeratosis; hyphae and spores, decreased pigmentation. Dermis—normal.

easy to apply to a widespread area, and relatively inexpensive. Topical imidazole antifungal creams are effective against the organism, but this approach is expensive when the eruption is widespread—which it often is. Terbinafine (Lamisil) spray is also effective but expensive.

Oral fluconazole (Diflucan) is the simplest and most effective therapy. In most adult patients, the fungus is eradicated with a single 200-mg dose, which may be repeated in 2 weeks. Efficacy is enhanced if the patient works up a sweat 2 hours after ingesting the fluconazole, thereby delivering the drug, which is concentrated in sweat, to the stratum corneum. For patients with recurrent disease, this regimen can be repeated every 3 months for 1 year.

THERAPY FOR TINEA VERSICOLOR

Initial
- Lather selenium sulfide, zinc pyrithione, or ketoconazole shampoo in a "turtleneck sweater" distribution, preferably with a "mesh puff"
- Rinse after 10 minutes
- Repeat this for 3 days in a row, then once weekly for 4 weeks, then once monthly to prevent recurrence. Alternatively, can use it daily for 1–4 weeks.
- Apply over-the-counter terbinafine (Lamisil) cream daily if just a few spots

Alternative
- Fluconazole (Diflucan) one 200-mg tablet repeated again in 1–2 weeks

---

Course and complications

The fungus is killed rapidly with therapy, but it takes 1–2 months or much longer for the pigmentation to return to its normal color. It is important to explain this so that the patient will not view the treatment as a failure. After topical therapy, the recurrence rate is more than 50%, but this rate can be reduced to less than 15% with a monthly retreatment program using any of the recommended treatment shampoos.

> After the initial therapy, it takes months for the white spots to regain pigment.

Pathogenesis

Tinea versicolor is caused by infection with the fungus *Malassezia* species (*globosa*, *sympodialis*, and *furfur*). This organism is frequently present in its yeast form as a colonizer of normal skin. In tinea versicolor, the spores proliferate in the outer layers of the stratum corneum, often beginning in the areas of follicular openings. When the spore forms are transformed into hyphae, infection occurs as the hyphal structures invade more deeply into the stratum corneum, but they do not penetrate the viable epidermis. They cause thickening and disruption of the stratum corneum, expressed clinically as a fine scale. Fungal enzymes act on surface lipids and produce dicarboxylic acids that diffuse into the epidermis. These acids inhibit tyrosinase, the enzyme in melanocytes that is responsible for melanin production.

Not all patients exposed to this ubiquitous organism develop an infection. In fact, conjugal cases are uncommon. Some individuals may be more susceptible by virtue of a genetic predisposition, the nature of which is not known.

VITILIGO

KEY POINTS

1. A Wood's light examination accentuates completely depigmented macules without scale.
2. Commonly seen in periorificial and dorsal hands, elbows, and knees.
3. Vitiligo is a common cause of depigmentation.

Definition

Vitiligo is an acquired, autoimmune condition in which functional melanocytes disappear from affected skin. The cause is unknown. Lesions clinically appear as totally white, nonscaling, sharply demarcated macules (Fig. 13.17).

Incidence

The reported incidence of vitiligo varies with the population studied, but it is thought that about 1 in 100 people are affected worldwide. In the past, higher incidence rates were thought to occur in dark-skinned individuals, but actually this reflected the observation that vitiligo is more noticeable in more darkly pigmented skin. It is now known to occur equally across all ethnicities, genders, and ages. The peak incidence is in the 10- to 30-year age group. In the United States, vitiligo is estimated to occur in around 1% of the general population. Vitiligo represents the presenting complaint in 0.6% of the authors' new patients.

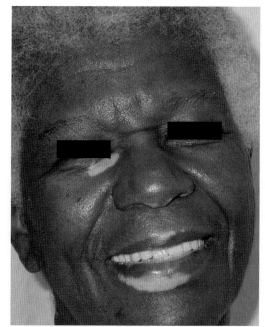

Fig. 13.17 Vitiligo—depigmented macules in common periorificial distribution.

History

Vitiligo is usually asymptomatic. It begins as one or more small spots that gradually enlarge. The affected areas sunburn easily. Most patients seek medical help because of cosmetic and cultural concerns.

Physical Examination

The primary lesion is a white macule that is usually totally depigmented. This feature can be appreciated best by Wood's light examination, which accentuates the pigment contrast and may also make evident previously undetected areas in lightly pigmented skin. The skin otherwise is normal; specifically, no scale is present. Macules of vitiligo are round or oval. They may become confluent as they enlarge, resulting in a large macule that has an irregular border but remains sharply demarcated from the surrounding normal skin.

> In vitiligo, depigmentation is complete; this is best seen by Wood's light examination.

Vitiligo can affect any area of the skin and mucous membranes, but the most common areas are the extensor bony surfaces (backs of the hands, elbows, and knees) and the periorificial areas (around the mouth, eyes, rectum, and genitalia) (Fig. 13.18). Involvement of hairy areas often results in depigmentation of the hair (Fig. 13.19). Vitiligo often presents in a symmetric distribution, underscoring the autoimmune nature of the condition.

Differential Diagnosis

Vitiligo is more often overdiagnosed than underdiagnosed. Any of the conditions listed in Table 13.1 may be misdiagnosed as vitiligo. Less often, vitiligo is misdiagnosed as one of these conditions. However, vitiligo is the only one of the common white spot diseases that results in total depigmentation. In addition, it can be differentiated clinically from *tinea versicolor* and *pityriasis alba* by the absence of scale. Finally, vitiligo lies flush with the skin, so note the absence of elevation to also aid in differentiation.

DIFFERENTIAL DIAGNOSIS OF VITILIGO

- Tinea versicolor
- Pityriasis alba
- Postinflammatory hypopigmentation

Laboratory and Biopsy

The laboratory is not helpful for diagnosing vitiligo. Serum thyroid tests, blood glucose or hemoglobin A1C, and a complete blood count with differential may be ordered to screen for occasionally associated thyroid disease, diabetes, and the rarely associated pernicious anemia. Biopsy is not usually necessary. If performed, it will show an absence of melanocytes, sometimes with accompanying inflammation (Fig. 13.20). The presence or absence of melanocytes may be difficult to appreciate with routine hematoxylin and eosin staining. Special stains and techniques are required for definitive identification. Clinicians can consider taking a biopsy with a portion of normal skin included to evaluate for the absence and presence of melanocytes in affected and unaffected skin, respectively.

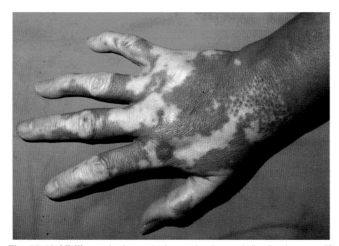

Fig. 13.18 **Vitiligo**—depigmented macules in acral distribution are difficult to treat.

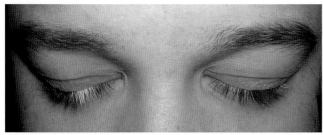

Fig. 13.19 **Vitiligo**—hair turns white with follicular involvement.

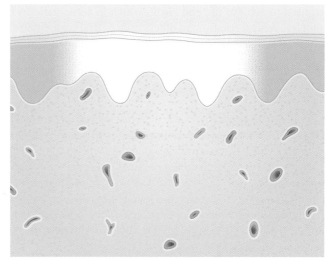

Fig. 13.20 **Vitiligo**. Epidermis—complete absence of pigment and melanocytes. Dermis—normal.

Therapy

There is no cure for vitiligo. Emotional support is a top priority. The goal of therapy is to manage the cosmetic disfigurement caused by the disease. Therapy for repigmentation is prolonged, and the results are often suboptimal. For limited disease, the topical Janus kinase inhibitor, ruxolitinib 1.5% cream, is the first treatment approved by the US Food and Drug Administration (FDA) for repigmentation in patients aged 12 years and older and is applied twice daily. Topical high-potency steroids (e.g., clobetasol) have been successful in some patients. To avoid skin atrophy, the authors like to use the treatment at intervals (e.g., alternating twice daily for 1 week and then 1 week off). Topical macrolides (Protopic or Elidel) are popular for use in facial and genital vitiligo. These agents do not cause skin atrophy. Small studies have demonstrated efficacy using mometasone steroid topically with bimatoprost 0.03% (Latisse) daily for 12 weeks. Facial and truncal vitiligo respond more favorably to medical therapy than vitiligo located on the extremities. For rapidly progressing vitiligo, a short course of systemic corticosteroids can be considered; however, dosing guidelines and length of treatment have not been delineated, and this treatment should be used thoughtfully, weighing the risks and benefits. For extensive involvement, the administration of UV light is recommended. The current treatment of choice is narrow-band UVB, which can be used in adults, children, and pregnant patients. The excimer laser, which emits light at 308 nm (close to narrow-band UVB wavelength), is another form of phototherapy with the added advantage of delivering laser light to affected skin only, usually done twice weekly for up to 6 months. Long-term effects are unknown. Another phototherapy, which is more difficult for the patient and reserved for the most severe and recalcitrant cases, is the administration of a psoralen medication (trimethylpsoralen or 8-methoxypsoralen) followed by exposure to long-wave ultraviolet A light (PUVA). The psoralens can be administered topically or systemically (more frequently the latter), especially for widespread disease. Some 100 or more treatments are often required to achieve the end result, which in some patients is complete repigmentation; in others only partial pigmentation occurs, and in the remainder, treatment fails.

> Initial therapy: topical ruxolitinib, topical steroids, narrow-band UVB.

Surgical therapies have also been employed occasionally. Normally pigmented skin is harvested (by suction blisters or punch biopsies) and transplanted into vitiliginous areas. Experimental transplantation of cultured melanocytes has also been reported.

An alternative is to cover the lesions with a cosmetic that is blended to match the color of the patient's normal skin. The products most frequently used for this are Covermark and Dermablend.

> Cosmetic covering agents may be helpful.

In selected patients with extensive disease, the best cosmetic result may be obtained by depigmenting the remaining normal skin. Topical application of 20% monobenzyl ether of hydroquinone (Benoquin) is used for this, but the patient must be aware that the resulting depigmentation is irreversible and treatment can take up to a year. This option is FDA approved for depigmentation.

THERAPY FOR VITILIGO

Initial
- Emotional support and covering cosmetics:
  - Covermark
  - Dermablend
- Topicals:
  - Ruxolitinib 1.5% cream applied twice daily
  - Clobetasol cream twice daily alternating 1 week on/off
  - Topical macrolides twice daily (especially facial and genital vitiligo)
- Narrow-band UVB or 308-nm excimer laser

Alternative
- PUVA, topical or systemic
- Surgical: epidermal grafting or autologous minigrafting
- Depigmentation of normal skin in recalcitrant, widespread disease

Course and Complications

The course of vitiligo is unpredictable. In most patients, it is chronic and often slowly progressive but can be rapid in others. Occasionally, it involves the total body surface, resulting in complete depigmentation. Spontaneous repigmentation occurs in a minority of patients but is usually incomplete. Repigmentation begins around the hair follicles, so it appears as freckles that become confluent as they enlarge. Approximately 40% of patients will relapse within the first year after successful repigmentation.

Associated systemic disorders occur in some patients with vitiligo. Thyroid abnormalities, including Graves disease and thyroiditis, are the most common, with a frequency ranging from 1% to 30%, depending on the series. Addison disease, pernicious anemia, diabetes mellitus, and alopecia areata are other "autoimmune" disorders uncommonly found in association with vitiligo. Experiments indicate polymorphisms located in the gene *NALP1*, which is involved in the regulation of innate immune responses, play a role in these other disease susceptibilities in a subset of patients with vitiligo.

Many patients with vitiligo, particularly deeply pigmented patients, may experience social stigmatization. In some cultures, vitiligo has been confused with the white spots of leprosy and has resulted in social ostracism. Advocates, social media movements, and the arts have made efforts to destigmatize vitiligo in recent years. Whether or not to manage and treat this condition ultimately lies with the patient.

Pathogenesis

Melanocytes are absent in vitiligo. The mechanism for their disappearance is not known, but multiple theories exist. Four proposed theories, not necessarily mutually exclusive, are highlighted:

> Proposed pathologic mechanisms:
> 1. Autoimmune
> 2. Oxidative stress
> 3. Neural
> 4. Self-destruction

1. *Autoimmune.* Investigators have proposed that melanocytes are destroyed by an immune mechanism. Antibodies against melanocyte antigens have been detected in patients with vitiligo. These may be the primary cause of the disease, or they may occur secondary to an initial injury to the melanocytes that results in the production of antigens with subsequent antibody formation. Cellular immune mechanisms have also been implicated in melanocyte destruction, such as activated cytotoxic CD8+ T lymphocytes and numerous cytokines.
2. *Oxidative stress.* This theory posits that oxidative stress promotes vitiligo by the activation of the innate immune response. It is thought that reactive oxygen species act as signals which activate pattern recognition receptors which then trigger inflammation leading to the recruitment of cells in the innate immune system such as macrophages and natural killer cells, with the end result being the destruction of melanocytes.
3. *Neural.* This theory proposes that a neurochemical mediator is responsible for the destruction of the melanocytes. Some animal models have clear-cut neural control mechanisms for pigment formation.
4. *Self-destruction.* The intermediate compounds in melanin synthesis are cytotoxic when present in sufficient concentrations. The self-destruction theory holds that, in vitiligo, these compounds accumulate in melanocytes and eventually destroy them.

UNCOMMON CAUSES OF WHITE SPOTS

Tuberous Sclerosis

Tuberous sclerosis, or tuberous sclerosis complex, is a rare, autosomal dominantly inherited, neurocutaneous disorder that can affect multiple organ systems. Expression of this disease varies widely; however, the classic triad consists of seizures, intellectual disability, and angiofibromas (also called fibroadenomas, previously called by the misnomer adenoma sebaceum). Classic skin manifestations include white macules, angiofibromas, shagreen patches, and periungual fibromas. White macules are important diagnostically because they are usually present at birth (Fig. 13.21). They appear as hypopigmented macules, ranging in size from 1 to 3 cm. They are often shaped like a "thumbprint" or an "ash leaf" on an ash tree—oval at one end and pointed at the other. They are most often found on the trunk and less often on the face and extremities. Patients may have as few as 3 or as many as 100 lesions. The spots are most easily seen with Wood's light examination; sometimes, particularly in infants with extremely fair skin, this is the only method of detection. Therefore all infants with a seizure disorder should be screened for white spots with a Wood's light examination. Tuberous sclerosis

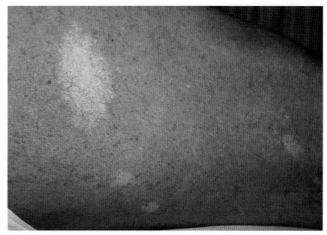

Fig. 13.21 Tuberous sclerosis—white "ash leaf" macule.

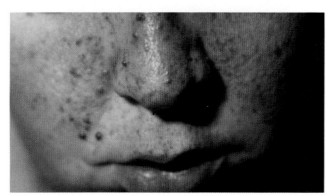

Fig. 13.22 Tuberous sclerosis—angiofibromas of the face.

is strongly suspected if more than three white spots are detected. Angiofibromas typically begin in childhood and appear clinically as red papules on the face, often confused with "acne" (Fig. 13.22). Definitive diagnosis is hard to achieve given the variation in age and severity of the various manifestations. The disorder is caused by mutations in tuberous sclerosis complex genes (*TSC1* or *TSC2*), which code for the proteins harmartin and tuberin, respectively. These gene products are involved in cellular signaling mediated by the mammalian target of rapamycin (mTOR), and aberrant mTOR activity leads to tumor formation. Therefore topical sirolimus, an mTOR inhibitor, can be used to treat the angiofibromas that are associated with this disorder.

Hypopigmented Mycosis Fungoides

MF is the most common type of cutaneous T-cell lymphoma. Hypopigmented MF is more common in patients with darkly pigmented skin and those of Asian descent, and is the most common variant of MF in children. Patients often present with patches that have been diagnosed as "nonspecific eczema." Although the patches of MF are characteristically erythematous with fine scale, they can appear as hypopigmented patches. The skin lesions have a predilection for sun-protected skin, like on the buttocks, hips, and trunk (Fig. 13.23), and can evolve into plaques or tumors. If a dermatitis fails to respond to topical steroids, especially when located on the trunk, a skin biopsy should be performed to confirm the suspicion of MF.

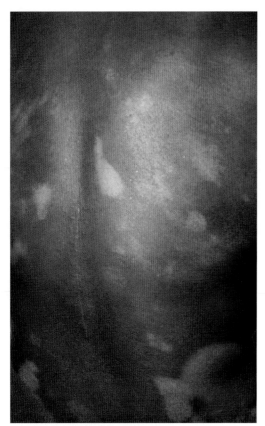

Fig. 13.23 **Hypopigmented mycosis fungoides**—hypopigmented patches located on the trunk.

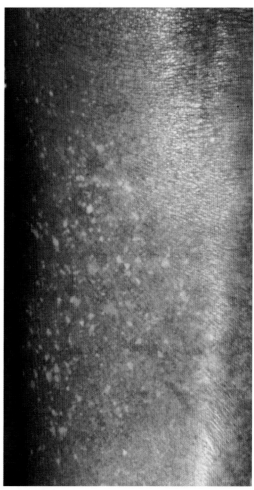

Fig. 13.24 **Idiopathic guttate hypomelanosis**—"confetti-like" white macules on anterior shin.

Idiopathic Guttate Hypomelanosis

Although this is a relatively common condition, it is underrecognized by physicians. The lesions appear as well-demarcated, small macules, like "sprinkled confetti" (Fig. 13.24). They appear most commonly on the shins but may also be found on the forearms. In rare instances, the face is affected. There is no effective treatment and unlike vitiligo, spontaneous repigmentation is not observed. It is considered a normal part of the aging process and is hypothesized to be in part from chronic UV exposure.

Leprosy

Leprosy is endemic in the southeastern United States and Hawaii. It is caused by the acid-fast organism *Mycobacterium leprae*. The diagnosis is frequently delayed by 1 year in the United States. Often the earliest sign is a solitary hypopigmented macule (Fig. 13.25). The earliest sensory change is loss of feeling to light touch and cold in the hands and feet. Nerve involvement is a disease hallmark. A biopsy with special stains (Fite stain) for the organism confirms the diagnosis. When skin biopsies are inconclusive, a polymerase chain reaction test can be performed to identify *M. leprae* DNA in tissue.

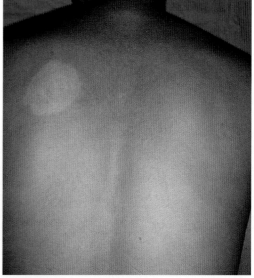

Fig. 13.25 **Leprosy**—hypopigmented patch. (Courtesy Shyam B. Verma, MBBS, DVD, PhD. Vadodara, India.)

SELF-ASSESSMENT

Case 1—White Spots (Fig. 13.26)

What Is the Most Likely Diagnosis?

This patient has a typical history for tinea versicolor. Scratching the affected areas elicited a fine, crumbly scale, further heightening the uspicion of tinea versicolor.

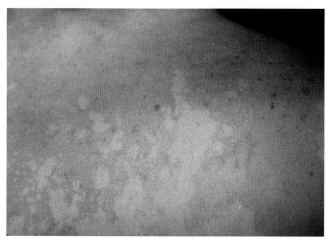

Fig. 13.26 This 25-year-old woman was seen in the dermatology clinic in October, with a 4-month history of white spots on her upper trunk. With sun exposure over the summer, the spots had become more noticeable. They had not been red or symptomatic.

What Test Would You Do?

The potassium hydroxide (KOH) preparation is diagnostic, revealing numerous short hyphae and spores.

How Would You Treat This Patient?

Fluconazole was prescribed in a single 200 mg dose and repeated again in 2 weeks. The skin gradually repigmented over the following 3 months. Prevention of recurrence can be achieved with periodic washing of the affected areas with zinc pyrithione or selenium sulfide shampoo. Localized areas may be treated with Micatin cream.

IMPORTANT POINTS

1. If it scales, scrape it.
2. It takes months for repigmentation to occur.

14

Generalized Erythema

CHAPTER CONTENTS

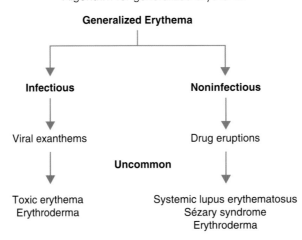

Algorithm for generalized erythema

ABSTRACT

The rashes discussed in this chapter are composed of erythematous macules and papules that are widespread and sometimes confluent. Various terms have been used to describe this type of eruption, including maculopapular, exanthematous, and morbilliform (measles-like). To correctly diagnose generalized erythema, one must focus primarily on a complete history and physical examination, with special attention to sites of skin involvement. Skin biopsies tend to show nonspecific findings and fail to distinguish the causes of generalized erythema, except in the cases of systemic lupus erythematosus (SLE) and Sézary syndrome. Most causes of generalized erythematous eruptions are listed in Table 14.1 in the order of relative frequency.

KEY POINTS

1. Drug reactions and viral exanthems are the most common causes of a generalized erythema.
2. Rule out infection first in a patient with generalized erythema.
3. A correct diagnosis requires a complete history, physical examination with attention to sites of skin involvement, skin biopsy consideration, and appropriate laboratory workup.

DRUG ERUPTIONS

KEY POINTS

1. Appear suddenly and with symmetry.
2. Antibiotics, especially penicillins and sulfonamides, are common culprits.
3. Discontinuation of offending drugs leads to quick resolution.

TABLE 14.1 Generalized Erythema

	Frequency[a]	Etiology	History	Physical Examination	Differential Diagnosis	Laboratory Test
Drug eruption	0.6[b]	Drug	Recent new drug Pruritus Usually no fever	Rash bright red and confluent	Exfoliative erythroderma (chronic)	–
Viral exanthem	0.2	Rubeola (measles) Rubella Enteroviruses, etc.	Associated "viral" symptoms	Erythema mild to moderate Mucous membranes occasionally involved	Drug reaction	Acute and convalescent viral titers
"Toxic" erythema	<0.1	Group A streptococci *Staphylococcus aureus* Unknown	Patient feels extremely ill (toxic) No pruritus	Rash accentuated in flexural folds and often feels like sandpaper Mucous membranes often involved	Drug reaction	Bacterial cultures
Systemic lupus erythematosus (SLE)	<0.1	Autoimmune	Other symptoms of SLE	"Butterfly" distribution on face Sun-exposed areas favored Rarely total body	Drug reaction	Antinuclear antibody Anti-DNA antibodies Complete blood count Urinalysis

[a]Percentage of new dermatology patients with this diagnosis seen in the Hershey Medical Center Dermatology Clinic, Hershey, Pennsylvania.
[b]Frequency in outpatients. For an inpatient, a drug eruption is the most common dermatologic problem acquired in the hospital.

Definition

The expression: "For any rash, think drug!" reflects the finding that drug eruptions can appear similar to many inflammatory skin diseases. The skin is the most common target of adverse drug reactions. Think drug reaction for any symmetric rash of sudden onset. The two most common eruptions for drug reactions are hives (discussed in Chapter 16) and morbilliform rashes. Of these two, morbilliform rashes are more common. A morbilliform drug rash appears as a generalized eruption of erythematous macules and papules, often confluent in large areas (Fig. 14.1).

Incidence

Only 0.6% of the authors' new outpatients are seen for a drug eruption. The frequency, however, is much higher among hospitalized patients, most of whom are elderly and who receive an average of nine drugs. Drug rashes head the list for our hospital consultations and account for 7% of all dermatology consultations. It is estimated that 7% of inpatients experience an adverse drug reaction and that 2.3% of inpatients have skin reactions related to medications. Common offenders are as follows:

- Antibiotics:
  - β-Lactam antibiotics—penicillins, cephalosporins
  - Sulfonamides–trimethoprim–sulfamethoxazole (be aware of cross-reactivity with sulfonamide derivatives, especially in the following drug classes: diuretics, hypoglycemic, and antiinflammatories)
- Diuretics:
  - Furosemide (contains sulfonamide)
  - Hydrochlorothiazide (contains sulfonamide)
- Nonsteroidal antiinflammatory drugs
- Anticonvulsants:
  - Carbamazepine
  - Phenytoin

Approximately 2% of all medical inpatients experience drug-induced skin reactions.

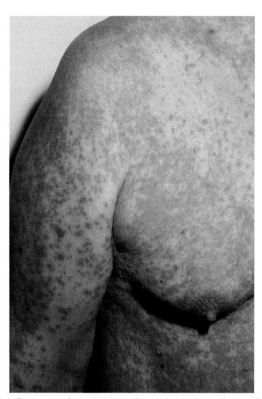

Fig. 14.1 **Drug eruption**—bright red macules and papules confluent in large areas.

History

The onset of a drug-induced morbilliform eruption is usually not immediate but rather begins within several days of the initiation of the drug. Onset is sometimes delayed for as long as 1 week but seldom longer. Because no laboratory tests are available to identify the responsible drug, reliance is placed on the history. For patients receiving multiple drugs, this presents

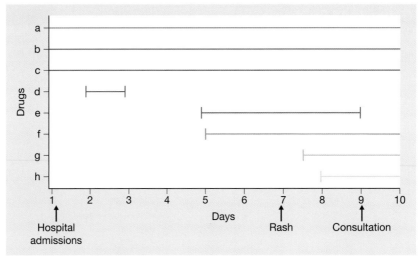

Fig. 14.2 Graphic depiction of drug history (see the text for the discussion of drugs "a–h").

a problem. In selecting a single drug from a list of many, the two variables to be considered are (1) the temporal relationship between the initiation of the drug and the onset of the rash and (2) the likelihood that a given drug is likely to cause a drug eruption. In selecting a putative drug, it is helpful to construct a graph that depicts the patient's drug history (Fig. 14.2). In the example in Fig. 14.2, drugs "a," "b," and "c" are unlikely to be implicated because the patient had been receiving these agents for months. Drug "d" was stopped 4 days before the rash began, thus making it a less likely cause. Drug "g" was started 6 hours *after* the rash appeared, and drug "h" was started the following day. Drugs "e" and "f" were started 2 days before the rash and therefore have the best temporal relationship. Drug "e" is a cephalosporin, a well-known cause of rash, and drug "f" is codeine, a rare cause of morbilliform eruptions. Therefore drug "e" is the probable cause and is the first to be discontinued. Remember to include over-the-counter medications such as vitamins in your exposure list as well as PRN medications for inpatients, such as furosemide, which contains sulfonamide, a common cause of inpatient drug reactions.

> Suspect drugs that are:
> 1. New (started within 1 week of the rash)
> 2. Frequent offenders

In patients with drug rashes, itching is usually present but is not helpful as a diagnostic marker. Fever is rarely found.

Most drug eruptions do not cause major morbidity, and the signs and symptoms are mild to moderate, resolving in 1–2 weeks.

Physical Examination

The eruption is generalized and composed of brightly erythematous macules and papules that tend to be confluent in large areas. Characteristically, the erythema is intense or "drug red." Drug rashes usually start proximally (e.g., affects the upper chest and back first) and proceed distally to the arms and legs, with the legs being the last to be involved as well as the last to

TABLE 14.2	**Other Patterns of Drug Reactions**
Type of Reaction	**Drugs**
Acneiform	Lithium, epidermal growth factor inhibitors, steroids, isoniazid
Pustules (acute generalized exanthematous pustulosis)	β-Lactam antibiotics, macrolides, calcium channel blockers
Erythroderma	Allopurinol
Erythema multiforme, Stevens–Johnson syndrome, toxic epidermal necrolysis	Anticonvulsants, allopurinol, nonsteroidal antiinflammatory drugs (NSAIDs), sulfonamides
Vasculitis	NSAIDs
Psoriasiform dermatitis	Interferon and granulocyte colony–stimulating factor, tumor necrosis factor inhibitors, lithium, beta-blockers, antimalarials
Angioedema	Angiotensin-converting enzyme inhibitors
Acneiform eruptions	Epidermal growth factor inhibitors
Skin cancer—squamous cell skin cancer	BRAF inhibitor
Morbilliform eruptions/lichenoid eruptions/vitiligo	Immune checkpoint inhibitors
Bullous pemphigoid	Furosemide, dipeptidyl peptidase-4 inhibitor
Drug-induced hypersensitivity syndrome	Anticonvulsants, lamotrigine, sulfonamides, allopurinol, minocycline

clear. See Table 14.2 for typical medications associated with other drug reaction patterns that are important to recognize clinically (Fig. 14.3). It is important for the physician to recognize two life-threatening drug reactions: (1) toxic epidermal necrolysis and (2) Stevens–Johnson syndrome. Toxic epidermal necrolysis is characterized by widespread erythema (>30% body surface area) and full, epidermal thick skin separation; transfer to a burn unit is critical (Fig. 14.4). The erythema of

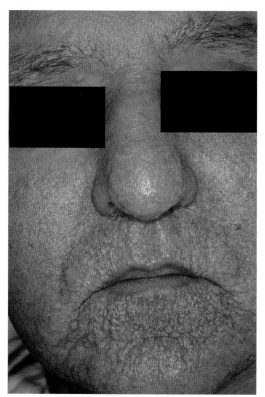

Fig. 14.3 Pustular drug eruption—note the symmetric distribution of minute pustules.

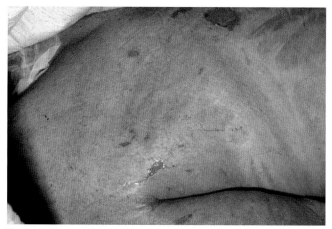

Fig. 14.4 Toxic epidermal necrolysis—note erythema and full-thickness skin separation. The patient was in the intensive care unit.

Stevens–Johnson syndrome typically involves more than 10% body surface area and involves two mucosal surfaces (e.g., conjunctiva and oral mucosa); hemorrhagic crusting of the lips is pathognomonic (Fig. 14.5). There is often an overlap of the features between these two conditions. For practical purposes, it is important to diagnose a "life-threatening drug reaction." Both potentially fatal drug reactions require prompt evaluation, recognition, discontinuation of offending medication, and intensive supportive care.

Drug rashes are usually:
1. Bright red
2. Confluent in large areas

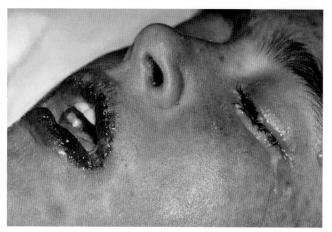

Fig. 14.5 Stevens–Johnson syndrome—note erythema and involvement of two mucosal surfaces—hemorrhagic lips and conjunctiva.

Differential Diagnosis

The differential diagnosis includes viral exanthem, toxic erythema, and chronic exfoliative erythroderma.

DIFFERENTIAL DIAGNOSIS FOR ACUTE MORBILLIFORM ERUPTIONS:

1. Drug
2. Viral
3. Toxic

A *viral exanthem* and a drug eruption can be indistinguishable clinically. Often, a drug eruption is much more erythematous, more confluent, and more *pruritic*. The presence of viral signs and symptoms favors a diagnosis of a viral exanthem.

Toxic erythemas include scarlet fever, staphylococcal scalded skin syndrome eruptions, and Kawasaki syndrome (mucocutaneous lymph node syndrome). Features that help to distinguish these rashes from drug eruptions include a sandpaper-like texture of the "toxic" rash, mucous membrane involvement (scarlet fever and Kawasaki syndrome), the presence of fever, and a focus of infection or the presence of lymphadenopathy (Fig. 14.6).

When a generalized erythema becomes chronic, it is called an *exfoliative* erythroderma—exfoliative because of the prominent desquamation (Fig. 14.7). Long-term administration of an offending drug is one cause. The other three causes are generalization of a primary skin disease (most often, psoriasis or atopic dermatitis), malignancy (most often, the Sézary variant of cutaneous T-cell lymphoma; see Chapter 9), or an idiopathic disorder.

DIFFERENTIAL DIAGNOSIS FOR DRUG ERUPTIONS

- Viral exanthema—identify cause
- Toxic erythemas—identify cause
- Exfoliative erythroderma

Laboratory and Biopsy

No laboratory tests can determine the diagnosis of a drug eruption or the incrimination of a specific drug. Peripheral blood eosinophilia is sometimes present and may heighten the suspicion of a drug reaction. Skin biopsy is most often performed

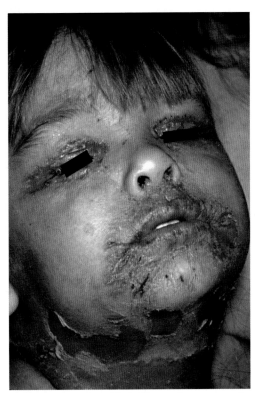

Fig. 14.6 Staphylococcal scalded skin syndrome—a toxin-mediated eruption characterized by erythema, skin separation (split is at granular layer and not full-thickness epidermis), and focus of infection—nares.

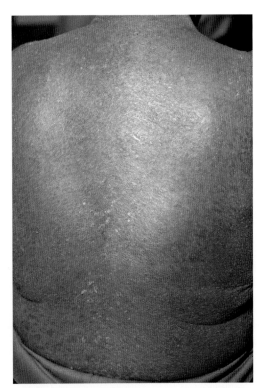

Fig. 14.7 Exfoliative erythroderma.

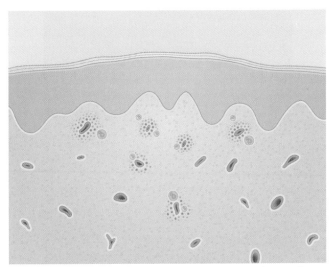

Fig. 14.8 Epidermis—normal. Dermis—superficial and deep perivascular inflammatory cell infiltrate that includes eosinophils.

important clue suggesting a drug-related cause. Skin tests for penicillin may be useful for the diagnosis of immediate hypersensitivity reactions (hives and anaphylaxis) but not for morbilliform eruptions. Skin biopsies can also help distinguish the level of epidermal separation for toxic epidermal necrolysis (full thickness) versus staphylococcal scalded skin syndrome (granular layer).

Therapy

When the offending drug is identified, it should be discontinued. If the patient is taking multiple drugs and it is not possible to be certain of the offending drug, the number of administered drugs should be reduced to an absolute minimum, and any remaining possible offenders should be changed to alternative agents when possible.

- Therapy otherwise is symptomatic, with antihistamines (e.g., hydroxyzine 10–25 mg four times daily) most often used for the pruritus. Moisturizing creams are helpful during the late desquamative phase of the reaction. Topical steroids are of little value. Systemic steroids are rarely required but are helpful for the patient experiencing intense pruritus. Intensive care therapy is necessary for life-threatening drug reactions. Immediate transfer to a burn unit is important for toxic epidermal necrolysis.

THERAPY FOR DRUG ERUPTIONS

Initial
- Discontinuation of the offending drug
- Antihistamines:
  - Hydroxyzine (Atarax) 10–25 mg q.i.d.
  - Diphenhydramine (Benadryl) 25–50 mg q.i.d.
- Moisturizers:
  - Eucerin cream b.i.d.

Alternative
- Systemic steroids: prednisone 1 mg/kg then taper dose over 7–10 days
- Intensive care therapy for life-threatening reactions

in patients with chronic exfoliative erythrodermas, especially to rule out cutaneous T-cell lymphoma. A drug eruption shows a superficial and deep perivascular inflammatory cell infiltrate (Fig. 14.8). The presence of eosinophils in the infiltrate is an

Course and Complications

Drug eruptions clear slowly with *time* after discontinuation of the responsible agent. The time required for total clearing is usually 1–2 weeks. For several days after the offending drug has been stopped, the eruption may actually worsen.

> Drug eruptions take 1–2 weeks to clear.

Complications are uncommon and primarily cutaneous. When large areas of skin are inflamed, increased body heat and water loss occur. For a patient who is already seriously ill, this could be a problem, but for most patients, it is not.

One main risk of continuing an offending agent in the presence of a drug eruption involves progressive worsening of the rash, possibly eventuating in toxic epidermal necrolysis, which is characterized by the loss of large sheets of epidermis. Fortunately, this complication rarely occurs; the mortality rate for Stevens–Johnson syndrome approaches 5% and for toxic epidermal necrolysis 35%. Sometimes a drug eruption clears despite continued treatment with the offending agent, although this approach is not desirable if an alternative drug is available. If the responsible drug has been identified, the patient should be advised to avoid the drug in the future, and the medical record should be clearly labeled.

One unique adverse drug reaction is drug-induced hypersensitivity syndrome (aka drug reaction with eosinophilia and systemic symptoms [DRESS]). A morbilliform eruption often develops 2–3 weeks after exposure to a limited number of medications. Facial swelling is a unique physical examination finding. The syndrome is characterized by fever, elevated liver function tests, eosinophilia and lymphadenopathy. Prompt discontinuation of the offending drug and a course of systemic steroids typically leads to a quick recovery of laboratory abnormalities and clinical findings; however, all patients should be monitored long term to be evaluated for potential autoimmune sequelae.

> Potential consequences of continuing the offending drug—worsening rash.

Pathogenesis

Although specific immunologic and nonimmunologic mechanisms have been documented for some types of drug-induced cutaneous reaction (e.g., hives and vasculitis), the mechanism for the morbilliform eruption remains unclear. Increasing experimental evidence points to a major role for cellular immune (type IV) processes. The clinical course with delayed-onset and prolonged duration of the rash also favors this mechanism.

VIRAL EXANTHEMS

KEY POINTS

1. Caused by hematogenous dissemination of virus to the skin.
2. Preceded by a prodrome of fever and constitutional symptoms.
3. Treatment is symptomatic.

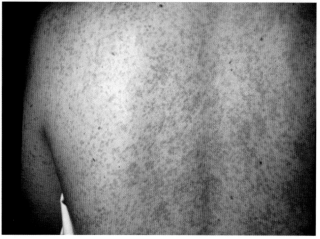

Fig. 14.9 **Viral exanthema**—symmetric red macules and papules.

Definition

Viral exanthems are caused by hematogenous dissemination of virus to the skin, in which a vascular response is elicited (Fig. 14.9). The clinical appearance of a virus-induced generalized erythema is not specific to a given virus; other signs and symptoms, however, may indicate a particular etiologic agent. The viruses that are most often associated with exanthems are rubeola (measles), rubella (German measles), herpesvirus type 6 (roseola), parvovirus B19 (erythema infectiosum), and the enteroviruses (enteric cytopathic human orphan [ECHO] and coxsackievirus). Viral infection with severe acute respiratory syndrome coronavirus 2 and the subsequent illness it causes, coronavirus disease 2019 (COVID-19), can lead to a variety of cutaneous reactions, including a generalized morbilliform eruption.

> Major viruses producing exanthems:
> 1. Measles (rubeola)
> 2. German measles (rubella)
> 3. Herpesvirus type 6 (roseola)
> 4. Parvovirus B19 (erythema infectiosum)
> 5. Enteroviruses (ECHO and coxsackievirus)

Incidence

Exanthem-producing viral infections rank high among the classic "common childhood diseases." Widespread immunization for rubella and rubeola has significantly reduced the incidence of these diseases. Vaccine hesitancy and misinformation, which worsened during the COVID-19 pandemic, have led to a fall in measles vaccination rates and subsequent outbreaks of this highly contagious virus.

Viral exanthems occur in adults but much less often than in children. In children younger than 2 years, roseola is the most common viral exanthem. Erythema infectiosum ("fifth" disease) occurs in young school-aged children, often in epidemics. Enteroviral infections are most common in the summer and fall.

History

Most viral exanthems are preceded by a prodrome of fever and constitutional symptoms. In *measles*, the prodrome is characterized by the three Cs: cough, coryza, and conjunctivitis. A history of previous exposure to infected individuals may be elicited. Incubation times vary from days to weeks, depending on the virus. *Mononucleosis* alone is associated with rash only about 3% of the time, but with the administration of ampicillin the frequency of rash approaches 100%.

> In patients with infectious mononucleosis, ampicillin increases the likelihood of rash from 3% to nearly 100%.

Physical Examination

The generalized eruption is composed of erythematous macules and papules. In *measles* (rubeola) and German measles, the rash typically begins on the head (characteristically behind the ears in measles) and proceeds to involve the trunk and extremities. In measles, individual lesions tend to become confluent on the face and trunk but remain discrete on the extremities. The macules and papules in *rubella* are discrete, even on the trunk, and have a cephalocaudal spread of exanthema, like measles. In *roseola* (exanthem subitem or sixth disease), rose-red macules and papules develop primarily on the trunk and proximal extremities. *Erythema infectiosum* characteristically begins with red cheeks that have a "slapped" appearance, followed by a reticulated (net-like) erythema on the trunk and proximal extremities (Fig. 14.10). The rashes associated with *enterovirus infections* are most often rubella-like but occasionally purpuric. Vesicular eruptions also occur with some types of enterovirus infections (e.g., hand, foot, and mouth disease from coxsackievirus A16 infection) (Fig. 14.11).

Mucous membranes are sometimes involved. In rubella, red spots occur on the soft palate. In measles, Koplik spots are characteristic and often precede the rash. *Koplik spots* are found on the buccal mucosa and appear as tiny gray-white papules on an erythematous base. In roseola, erythematous macules develop on the soft palate 48 hours before the exanthem.

Fever is almost always present. In patients with roseola caused by human herpesvirus type 6, the fever characteristically subsides abruptly just before the rash appears. The rash lasts 24–48 hours and appears as discrete rose-red macules or maculopapules, similar to rubella and measles (Fig. 14.12). In rubella, the most strikingly enlarged lymph nodes are found in the head and neck; in measles, lymphadenopathy is often generalized. Aseptic meningitis occasionally occurs in enterovirus infections. COVID-19 infection is most commonly associated with a morbilliform rash; another unique cutaneous manifestation is "COVID toes," which is theorized to be due to vascular injury and seen most commonly in children. COVID toes is similar in appearance to an uncommon skin condition called pernio (Fig. 14.13). Symptoms tend to be mild, and the rash resolves in 2–8 weeks.

> In roseola, fever subsides just before the rash appears.

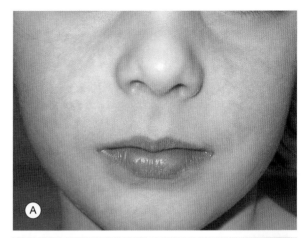
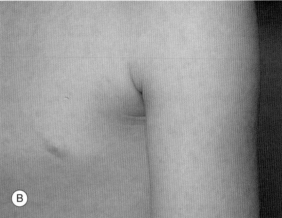

Fig. 14.10 Erythema infectiosum. (A) Characteristic "slapped" cheeks. (B) Reticulated (net-like) erythema on the upper arm.

Differential Diagnosis

Drug rashes are usually pruritic and are redder and more confluent than viral exanthems. *Toxic erythemas* favor flexural folds, may feel like sandpaper, and often have more extensive mucous membrane involvement. The rash in *Rocky Mountain spotted fever* begins as erythematous macules and papules but typically starts distally (hands and feet) and becomes *purpuric* as it progresses (see Chapter 17).

DIFFERENTIAL DIAGNOSIS FOR VIRAL EXANTHEMS

- Drug eruption
- Toxic erythemas
- Rocky mountain spotted fever

Laboratory and Biopsy

Routine laboratory tests are of no help. Usually, no tests are ordered; however, serologic tests can confirm the diagnosis by detecting a rise in antibody titer in convalescent compared with acute serum samples. Viral cultures are available but are not often obtained.

A skin biopsy is not indicated; histologic examination usually shows a nonspecific lymphocytic perivascular infiltrate. In

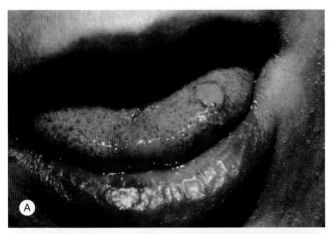

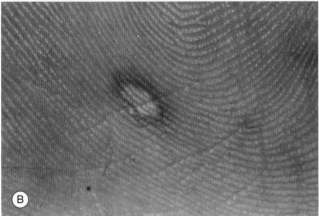

Fig. 14.11 Hand–foot–mouth disease. (A) Erosion with fibrinous base on the tongue. (B) Pustule with peripheral erythema oriented along skin lines on the palm.

measles, the infection also involves the epidermal cells, resulting in intranuclear inclusions, multinucleated giant cells, and individual cell necrosis.

Therapy

Treatment of acute disease is symptomatic. Measles, mumps, and rubella can be prevented through vaccination with a combined attenuated live virus vaccine, administered in two doses.

THERAPY FOR VIRAL EXANTHEMS

Initial
- Antipyretics and analgesics: acetaminophen or ibuprofen
- Hydration
- Vaccine

Course and Complications

Spontaneous, complete resolution usually occurs over several days to a week. Systemic complications are uncommon. Encephalitis is the most serious, occurring in patients with measles at a rate of approximately 1 in 1000; it results in death in 10%–20% of affected patients. The rate is much higher in some developing countries, where encephalitis remains a leading cause of death in children. Worldwide, measles continues to cause about 1 million deaths per year among children younger than 5 years of age.

> Encephalitis is the most serious complication of measles.

Rubella and erythema infectiosum are frequently complicated by arthritis in adults. Infection with parvovirus B19 has also been associated with acute aplastic crises in patients with a history of chronic hemolytic anemia, such as sickle cell disease. The most important complication of rubella is *congenital rubella syndrome*, which occurs in babies born to mothers who were infected during the first trimester of pregnancy. With rubella vaccination in widespread use, this condition is rare. Herpesvirus type 6 is a major precipitant of febrile seizures in infants.

Pathogenesis

In all the viral exanthems, the virus gains entry through the upper respiratory (e.g., rubella and rubeola) or gastrointestinal (enteroviruses) route, incubates "silently" for a period of days to weeks, and then enters a viremic phase that causes the febrile prodrome and results in the dissemination of viruses to other tissues, including the skin.

UNCOMMON CAUSES OF GENERALIZED ERYTHEMA

SYSTEMIC LUPUS ERYTHEMATOSUS AND CUTANEOUS LUPUS ERYTHEMATOSUS

KEY POINTS
1. An "autoimmune" disorder
2. Malar rash is characteristic
3. Screen for systemic involvement
4. Stress sun protection

Definition

SLE is an "autoimmune" disorder that affects many different organ systems. Cutaneous lupus erythematosus (CLE) is a disease state distinct from SLE and can occur either alongside systemic disease or without any internal organ involvement. Stated another way, most patients with SLE have CLE, but many patients with CLE do not have SLE. CLE may manifest with virtually any kind of skin lesion, including macules, papules, plaques, bullae, purpura, subcutaneous nodules, and ulcers (Fig. 14.14). The face is frequently involved. Different types of skin involvement have discrete rates of systemic involvement. The most important types are acute cutaneous lupus erythematosus (ACLE), discoid lupus erythematosus (DLE), and subacute cutaneous lupus erythematosus (SCLE). Nearly all patients with ACLE have SLE. DLE and SCLE are scaling disorders, discussed in Chapter 9, and most patients with these types of CLE do not have systemic disease. For generalized erythematous eruptions, SLE should be

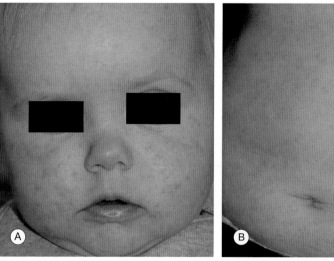

Fig. 14.12 Roseola. (A) Discrete rose-red macules and papules on the face. (B) Discrete rose-red macules and papules on the trunk of the same infant.

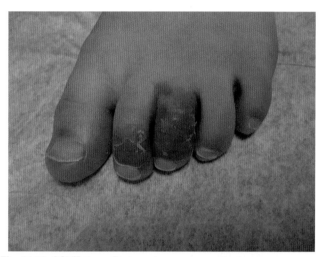

Fig. 14.13 COVID toes. Red-purple macules on the toes.

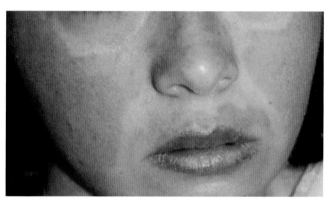

Fig. 14.14 Systemic lupus erythematosus—"butterfly" rash characterized by erythema with or without telangiectasia.

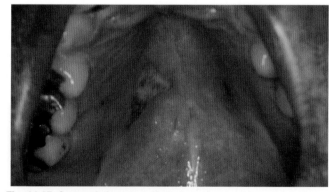

Fig. 14.15 Systemic lupus erythematosus—erosion on hard palate.

considered a possible (although uncommon) cause, particularly when other signs and symptoms of the disease are present.

Incidence

In the United States, the number of women with SLE outnumbers men with the condition by approximately 9:1. SLE occurs more commonly in certain racial and ethnic groups, in particular Black, Asian, and Hispanic populations compared with White populations. Women of childbearing age are most commonly affected.

History

With active SLE, fatigue, fever, arthralgia, and weight change are the most common constitutional symptoms. Mucocutaneous symptoms of SLE include nasal and oral ulcerations, photosensitivity, CLE, alopecia, and Raynaud phenomenon (Fig. 14.15). Arthritis is common. Serositis (with pleuritis or pericarditis) and neurologic manifestations (e.g., headache and seizures) may also occur.

Because both SLE and CLE can be drug induced, a careful drug history is important. The drugs most often implicated in SLE are procainamide, hydralazine, quinidine, and isoniazid. These patients tend to develop skin changes of vasculitis. Drug-induced lupus tends to occur in patients over 50 years of age, has a male-to-female ratio of 1:1, and symptoms resolve after drug discontinuation. Drug-induced CLE is most commonly caused by tumor necrosis factor inhibitors, antihypertensive agents, proton pump inhibitors, and antifungal medications.

Physical Examination

CLE often has a violaceous hue. All types are frequently accentuated in sun-exposed areas, but in some patients, they are generalized. The most classic form of ACLE appears on the malar area of the face, where it produces the "butterfly rash." The malar rash in lupus tends to spare the nasolabial folds and is frequently accompanied by telangiectasia. This rash strongly suggests the presence of SLE. When present, DLE causes destructive erythematous and scaly plaques with pigment and hair loss in affected areas. SCLE causes ring-shaped erythema in the sun-exposed areas. Recall that DLE and SCLE are less commonly associated with SLE.

Differential Diagnosis

The diagnosis of SLE is complex and is established by a combination of historic, physical, and laboratory findings. Several classification schema exist for identifying SLE, but they exceed the scope of this text (see the 2019 European League Against Rheumatism/American College of Rheumatology [EULAR/ACR] criteria and the Systemic Lupus International Collaborating Clinics [SLICC] criteria). The key takeaway is that *the presence of CLE should prompt evaluation for SLE*. This evaluation should include historical and laboratory evaluation for the presence of protein or cellular casts in the urine (which would suggest nephritis, a serious complication of SLE); cytopenias (red cell, white cell, or platelets); neurologic manifestations like seizure or psychosis; history of thrombotic episodes or miscarriage (indicative of antiphospholipid syndrome, confirmed with laboratory testing); historical evidence of pleuritis or pericarditis; history consistent with inflammatory joint disease; and other immunologic phenomena like the presence of antinuclear antibodies (ANAs), anti-double-stranded DNA (anti-dsDNA) or anti-Smith (Sm) antibodies, or depressed complement 3 and 4 levels. Historical or laboratory abnormalities prompt referral to rheumatology for further workup.

American College of Rheumatology criteria for SLE*:
1. Malar rash
2. Discoid rash
3. Photosensitivity
4. Oral ulcers
5. Arthritis
6. Serositis
7. Renal disorder
8. Neurologic disorder
9. Hematologic disorder
10. Immunologic disorders
11. Antinuclear antibody

* SLE is diagnosed if four or more are present.

Other *collagen vascular diseases* may be considered in the differential diagnosis, and sometimes an overlap occurs among several of these disorders; mixed connective tissue disease is an example. In *dermatomyositis*, the characteristic skin findings are violaceous (heliotrope) edema of the eyelids and erythema

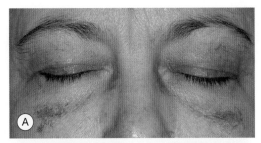
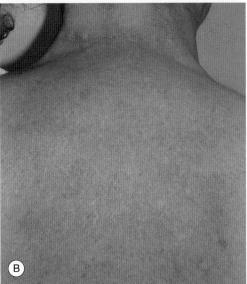

Fig. 14.16 (A) **Dermatomyositis**—violaceous (heliotrope) macules of eyelids. (B) Dermatomyositis—erythema in "shawl" distribution.

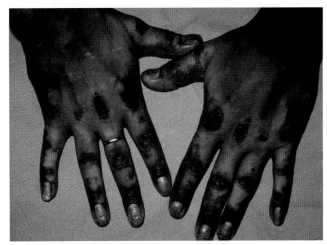

Fig. 14.17 Dermatomyositis—Gottron papules; hyperpigmented papules over the knuckles.

of the upper trunk (e.g., shawl distribution), upper arms and thighs (Fig. 14.16), flat-topped papules over the knuckles (Gottron papules) (Fig. 14.17), and reticulated patches of pigment, erythema, and telangiectasia (poikiloderma) often in systemic distribution. Periungual erythema with telangiectasia, along with "ragged" cuticles, is virtually diagnostic of a collagen vascular disease, most often dermatomyositis (Fig. 14.18). A key finding of the facial rash in dermatomyositis is involvement of

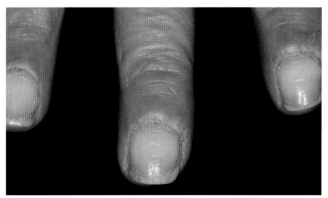

Fig. 14.18 Periungual telangiectasia and ragged cuticles in a patient with dermatomyositis.

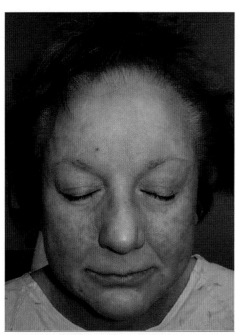

Fig. 14.19 **Dermatomyositis**. Note the involvement of nasolabial fold.

> **DIFFERENTIAL DIAGNOSIS FOR SYSTEMIC LUPUS ERYTHEMATOSUS**
>
> - Other collagen vascular disease
>   - Dermatomyositis
>   - Scleroderma
> - Photosensitive disorders
>   - Drug
>   - Porphyria
>   - Polymorphous light eruption
> - Seborrheic dermatitis
> - Rosacea

Laboratory and Biopsy

The screening tests for SLE are complete blood count, platelet count, urinalysis, and ANA test. If the ANA test is positive, an anti-DNA antibody test is ordered because it is more specific for SLE. Antibodies to the Sm antigen are also highly specific for SLE but are found less frequently than the antibodies to dsDNA. Serum complement is often depressed in patients with active SLE. Antibodies to DNA histones are historically associated with drug-induced lupus from hydralazine and procainamide, but many modern cases are anti-histone negative. A number of other autoantibodies are associated with CLE and SLE but are not specific, including Sjogren syndrome A (SSA), Sjogren syndrome B (SSB), and ribonucleoprotein (RNP), as examples.

> SLE initial screen:
> 1. Complete blood count with platelet count
> 2. Urinalysis
> 3. Antinuclear antibody test

> Autoantibody tests specific for lupus:
> 1. Double-stranded DNA
> 2. Smith

the nasolabial fold, which is often spared in lupus (Fig. 14.19). *Scleroderma* is less likely to be confused with SLE, but Raynaud phenomenon, although less common in SLE, occurs in both conditions, and some patients have features that overlap the two diseases.

In patients with *photosensitivity*, causes other than lupus should be considered. The major causes are drugs, porphyria, and polymorphous light eruption (see Chapter 23).

The most common cause of a butterfly rash is not SLE but rather *seborrheic dermatitis*. Seborrheic dermatitis can be usually distinguished by the presence of the fine, yellowish scale, involvement of the nasolabial folds, and coexistence of a similar scaling rash on the scalp, behind the ears, on the eyebrows, and, often, in the presternal area. Also, rosacea is commonly mistaken for lupus. Like lupus, rosacea flares with sun exposure. The presence of papules and pustules on convex surfaces of the face and the lack of systemic symptoms in rosacea distinguish it from lupus.

Findings of a skin biopsy in lupus include vacuolar degeneration of the basal cell layer with a perivascular and periappendageal lymphocytic infiltrate (Fig. 14.20).

Therapy

Cutaneous involvement can be treated with moderate- to high-potency topical steroids or topical macrolides (tacrolimus) and sunscreens that filter out both short- and long-wave ultraviolet light (e.g., sunscreens that contain zinc oxide or titanium dioxide). An antimalarial such as hydroxychloroquine (Plaquenil) at a dosage of 5 mg/kg maximum is used for more severe cutaneous disease that is unresponsive to topical therapy. Antimalarials are also helpful for fatigue and arthritis. In patients with systemic diseases including renal involvement, systemic steroids and other disease-modifying antirheumatic drugs (DMARDs) are used. Anifrolumab, a monoclonal antibody to type 1 interferon, received US Food and Drug Administration approval for the treatment of moderate-to-severe SLE.

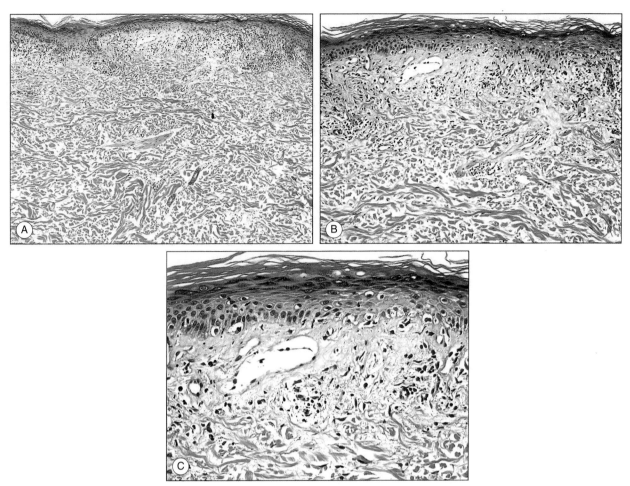

Fig. 14.20 **Graphic for a skin biopsy**.

THERAPY FOR CUTANEOUS LUPUS

Initial
- Sunscreens and protective clothing
- Topical steroids:
  - Triamcinolone cream 0.1% (medium)
  - Fluocinonide cream 0.05% (strong)
- Topical macrolides:
  - Tacrolimus
  - Pimecrolimus
- Antimalarials (for more severe disease):
  - Hydroxychloroquine 200 mg b.i.d.

Alternative
- DMARDs:
  - Mycophenolate mofetil
  - Azathioprine
  - Methotrexate
- Systemic steroids
- Anifrolumab

Course and Complications

In patients with SLE, the 5-year survival rate is now greater than 90%, and more than 80% of patients survive for at least 10 years. Patients with nephritis have a worse prognosis than those without the complication. Men do worse than women. Patients younger than 16 years of age who have no renal involvement have an excellent prognosis. In one large series, the most common causes of death were renal disease and sepsis, often secondary to iatrogenic immunosuppression.

Pathogenesis

The pathogenesis of the skin lesions in lupus is discussed in Chapter 9. In SLE, autoantibodies are formed to nuclear antigens (e.g., ANA, anti-dsDNA, Smith), but it is unclear if they are involved in clinical disease manifestations. Research on SLE pathophysiology consistently describes abnormal DNA repair following damage (such as from sunlight), increased type 1 interferon expression, increased cell death rates, abnormal clearance of apoptotic debris, and loss of immune tolerance to these exposed antigens. These processes contribute to the inflammatory response in many tissues, including the skin and kidney.

In lupus, the autoantibodies are produced by B cells, which appear to be stimulated by activated T cells (higher ratio of CD4+ to CD8+ T cells) that have escaped from the normal mechanisms of tolerance to self-antigens.

Genetic factors play a role in many patients with lupus. Familial lupus is well documented. Concordant disease is approximately 30% in monozygotic twins compared with 5% in dizygotic twins.

Environmental factors also have been implicated in lupus. Sunlight is definitely involved. Yet there is a perception that lupus is more common in African-Americans compared to Africans, suggesting environmental differences that may impact autoimmune disease progression.

TOXIC ERYTHEMA

KEY POINTS

1. Infection is usually the cause.
2. Flexural accentuation of exanthem is often present.
3. Treat underlying infection.

Definition

Toxic erythema is a cutaneous response to a circulating toxin. In scarlet fever, erythrogenic toxin is elaborated by group A streptococci (*Streptococcus pyogenes*), usually infecting the pharynx. In staphylococcal scarlatiniform eruption, staphylococcal scalded skin syndrome (SSSS), and toxic shock syndrome, the responsible toxins are elaborated by a focus of *Staphylococcus aureus* infection or colonization (Fig. 14.21). Cases of toxic shock–like syndrome have also been reported in association with severe infections with group A streptococci. In Kawasaki disease, aka mucocutaneous lymph node syndrome (Fig. 14.22), a toxin is presumed but has not been identified. For all toxic erythemas, the skin becomes generally red, often feels like sandpaper, and undergoes postinflammatory desquamation. Mucous membrane involvement is also common.

Toxic erythemas:
1. Scarlet fever
2. SSSS
3. Toxic shock syndrome
4. Kawasaki disease

Incidence

Toxic erythemas are still uncommon, although they have been increasing in frequency in recent years. Children are affected most often, except for toxic shock syndrome, which usually occurs in adults. After the advent of antibiotics, scarlet fever became a less common and generally less serious disease, although this trend has been reversing in recent years. Neonates are at the highest risk for SSSS because of the decreased toxin clearance by the kidneys and a lack of antibody to the toxin.

Except for toxic shock syndrome, toxic erythemas occur most often in children.

History

Fever is common to all toxic erythemas. Patients with scarlet fever have a history of a sore throat preceding the rash by 1–2 days. In SSSS, patients may have a history of a local

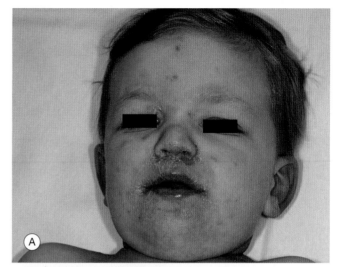

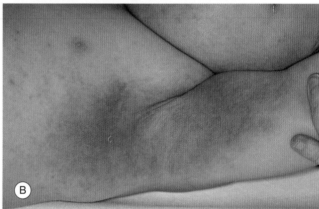

Fig. 14.21 (A) **Staphylococcal scalded skin syndrome**—note nares as focus of infection. (B) Toxin-mediated erythema from *Staphylococcal aureus* is accentuated in flexural fold.

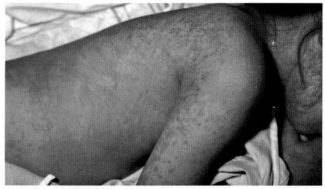

Fig. 14.22 **Kawasaki disease**—generalized erythema with sandpaper texture.

staphylococcal infection causing conjunctivitis, cutaneous abscess, or external otitis. Patients with toxic shock syndrome and Kawasaki disease look and feel the most seriously ill. Staphylococcal toxic shock syndrome was first described in menstruating women who used occlusive tampons that allowed staphylococcal organisms to proliferate in the occluded vaginal tract. This disorder is now more frequently found in postoperative patients. The focus of infection for staphylococcal toxic shock syndrome is usually the skin, most commonly an area of painful cellulitis on an extremity. The onset of toxic shock syndrome is abrupt. As the name suggests, hypotension is common, as are vomiting, diarrhea, severe myalgia, and encephalopathy with mental confusion. Patients with Kawasaki syndrome frequently experience abdominal pain, diarrhea, arthralgia, and other systemic symptoms.

Physical Examination

Toxic erythemas are characterized by a generalized, usually brightly erythematous eruption that frequently feels sandpapery and is accentuated in flexural folds (Fig. 14.23). Postinflammatory desquamation, particularly of the hands and feet, is common, especially in Kawasaki syndrome, but not pathognomonic (Fig. 14.24).

> Toxic erythemas are usually:
> 1. Sandpapery
> 2. Accentuated in flexural folds
> 3. Followed by desquamation

Mucous membrane involvement is usually striking, occurring in all toxic eruptions except SSSS. Patients with scarlet fever have acute streptococcal pharyngitis and a "strawberry tongue," which starts with a white exudate studded with prominent red papillae (white strawberry). After several days, the tongue becomes "beefy red" (red strawberry). In toxic shock syndrome, mucous membrane hyperemia frequently affects the conjunctivae, oral pharynx, or vagina. In Kawasaki syndrome, patients usually have marked erythema of the lips (cherry-red lips), tongue (strawberry tongue), and conjunctivae. In this disease, asymmetric lymphadenopathy occurs in approximately 75% of patients—hence the previous name mucocutaneous lymph node syndrome.

> Mucous membrane involvement accompanies all toxic erythemas except SSSS.

Differential Diagnosis

The differential diagnosis includes *drug eruption*, *viral exanthem*, and *toxic epidermal necrolysis*. Toxic epidermal necrolysis is a severe, generalized form of erythema multiforme (see Chapter 16) characterized by intense erythema and extensive blistering that occurs in sheets. Skin biopsy in this disease shows the blister to be subepidermal, rather than intraepidermal. In SSSS, the skin split is intraepidermal, specifically in the granular layer.

Group A streptococci are recovered from the pharynx in patients with scarlet fever. The absence of mucous membrane involvement suggests staphylococcal scalded skin eruption. Multisystem involvement, including hypotension in a menstruating female patient, strongly suggests toxic shock syndrome. Striking mucous membrane involvement and lymphadenopathy in a child who appears seriously ill are the features of Kawasaki syndrome. The diagnostic criteria for toxic shock syndrome and Kawasaki syndrome are listed in Table 14.3.

DIFFERENTIAL DIAGNOSIS FOR TOXIC ERYTHEMA

- Drug eruption
- Viral exanthem
- Toxic epidermal necrolysis

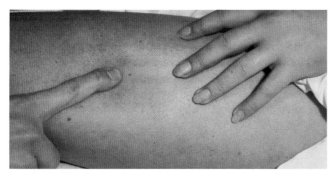

Fig. 14.23 Toxic shock syndrome—generalized erythema that blanches.

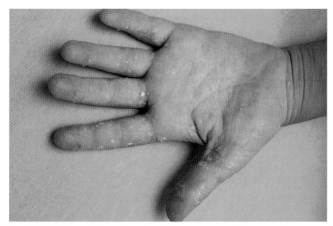

Fig. 14.24 Kawasaki syndrome—desquamation follows erythema and edema of the hands, a typical finding.

TABLE 14.3   Diagnostic Criteria for Toxic Shock Syndrome and Kawasaki Disease

Toxic Shock Syndrome	Kawasaki Disease
Fever of ≥38.9°C	Fever for ≥5 days
Scarlatiniform rash	Red palms and soles with edema, then desquamation
Desquamation of skin 1–2 weeks after the onset	Exanthem on trunk
Hypotension	Conjunctivitis
Clinical or laboratory abnormalities of at least three organ systems	Mucosal erythema (lips, tongue, or pharynx)
Absence of other causes of the illness	Cervical lymphadenopathy
(All six are required for the diagnosis)	(Fever plus four of the remaining five criteria are required for the diagnosis)

Laboratory and Biopsy

Bacterial cultures from potential foci of infection are mandatory. In suspected cases of scarlet fever, a throat culture should be taken. Less often, streptococcal impetigo serves as the focus of infection. For staphylococcal toxic erythemas, a focus of bacterial colonization or infection should be sought and cultured. For women with suspected toxic shock syndrome, vaginal cultures should be obtained. In seriously ill patients, blood cultures should also be drawn because some patients with staphylococcal toxic shock syndrome are septic. The focus of infection in patients with streptococcal toxic shock syndrome most often is a severe necrotizing cellulitis, which should be cultured. These patients often also have positive blood cultures. Laboratory evaluation of other organ systems is appropriate in toxic shock syndrome and Kawasaki disease. These include tests of hematopoietic, hepatic, cardiac, and renal functions. In toxic shock syndrome, thrombocytopenia occurs early; in Kawasaki disease, thrombocytosis occurs late.

Cultures should be obtained from potential bacterial reservoirs:
1. Throat
2. Skin
3. Vagina
4. Blood

The biopsy is nonspecific in toxic erythemas, except in SSSS, in which an intraepidermal separation is found.

Therapy

Initial management of toxic erythemas often requires inpatient hospitalization, except for scarlet fever to provide intensive supportive care. Streptococcal disease is usually treated with penicillin, although penicillin-resistant strains of streptococci are beginning to be reported. Staphylococcal infections are treated with penicillinase-resistant antibiotics such as oral dicloxacillin or intravenous nafcillin. Intravenous γ-globulin and aspirin are used to treat Kawasaki syndrome.

THERAPY FOR TOXIC ERYTHEMA

Initial treatment
- Hospitalization for supportive and ancillary care
- Antibiotics for infections
- Aspirin and γ-globulin for Kawasaki syndrome

Course and Complications

Scarlet fever follows a relatively benign course, with complete recovery usually within 5–10 days. Penicillin has dramatically altered the course of scarlet fever in both duration and severity. Complications are uncommon with scarlet fever, although post–streptococcal glomerulonephritis may occur. Death has occurred in patients with toxic shock syndrome as a result of severe hypotension, sepsis, or multisystem organ failure. The death rate for streptococcal toxic shock syndrome is higher than that for staphylococcal toxic shock syndrome (70% versus 30%, respectively).

Fever is most prolonged in Kawasaki syndrome, usually lasting for more than 5 days. Death can result from Kawasaki syndrome, usually the result of coronary artery aneurysm and thrombosis, which is striking given the young age of these patients. Cardiology consultation and follow-up are critical. This complication occurs in up to 20% of patients and can be delayed by 1 year or more after the acute episode. It can often be prevented with the acute-phase therapy mentioned above.

For all these disorders, postinflammatory desquamation usually occurs in 1–2 weeks. It is most striking on the hands and feet, where stratum corneum often sheds in large sheets.

Pathogenesis

The toxins involved in toxic erythemas act as "superantigens" that directly activate T cells, thus causing the release of massive amounts of cytokines, especially tumor necrosis factor-α, interleukin 1, and interleukin 6. These cytokines are thought to be responsible for the clinical manifestations. An erythrogenic toxin is produced by a lysogenic bacteriophage found in most strains of group A β-hemolytic streptococci. Although repeated streptococcal infections may occur, scarlet fever does not usually recur because of specific antitoxin antibodies that are formed from the first episode.

SSSS is caused by a toxin produced by phage group II *S. aureus*. This toxin binds to and disrupts the desmosomal protein, desmoglein 1, which is heavily concentrated in the granular layer of the epidermis. This is why a skin biopsy in SSSS shows separation in the granular layer of the epidermis. In toxic shock syndrome, several staphylococcal toxins have been isolated, although the one most often implicated is an exoprotein-designated toxic shock syndrome toxin 1. Other toxins (e.g., *S. pyogenes* exotoxin), as well as the host responses to the toxins, also probably play a role in the pathogenesis of toxic shock syndrome.

OTHER UNCOMMON CAUSES— GENERALIZED ERYTHEMA

ERYTHRODERMA

Erythroderma is a generalized, inflammatory skin condition involving more than 90% of the skin surface area (Fig. 14.25). Erythema is remarkable, and when significant scaling is present, the term *exfoliative erythroderma* is often used. The causes of erythroderma fall into four broad categories: (1) primary skin disease (e.g., psoriasis, atopic dermatitis), (2) medication reactions, (3) reaction to underlying malignancy, and (4) idiopathic. Workup of a patient with erythroderma requires a complete history and physical examination, with special attention to age-related malignancy screens, and appropriate laboratory and imaging evaluation. Skin biopsies rarely help distinguish the multiple causes of erythroderma. Unfortunately, a large proportion of cases of erythroderma are of unknown trigger, labeled idiopathic, and require periodic evaluation to search for the underlying causes.

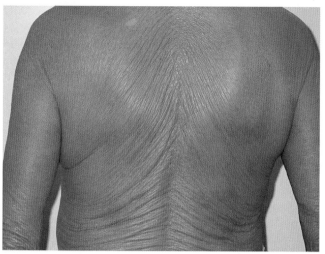

Fig. 14.25 **Erythroderma**—generalized erythema that despite intensive workup remained idiopathic in nature.

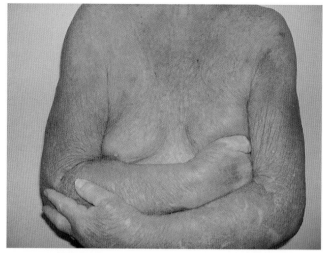

Fig. 14.26 **Sézary syndrome**—exfoliative erythroderma with palpable lymphadenopathy.

SÉZARY SYNDROME

Sézary syndrome is a specific cause of erythroderma, being labeled as a malignancy (cutaneous T-cell lymphoma) and a primary skin disease (Fig. 14.26). It is characterized by erythroderma, generalized lymphadenopathy, and circulating malignant T cells, called Sézary cells, in the blood. Immunophenotypic analysis reveals a CD4-to-CD8 ratio that exceeds 10:1 because the malignant T cells that expand are CD4 positive. Skin and lymph node biopsies show the malignant T cells infiltrating the epidermis and lymph node, respectively. Sézary syndrome has a high mortality rate, with the majority of patients dying from infection secondary to immunosuppression. Treatment is based on the staging of the disease, and experts in this disease differ in their approach.

▊ SELF-ASSESSMENT

Case 14.1—Generalized Erythema (Fig. 14.27)

The patient had been taking furosemide and diazepam on a long-term basis. On the day of surgery, he was started on cefazolin, codeine, morphine, and flurazepam.

What Is the Most Likely Diagnosis?

A drug eruption is favored by virtue of the intensity of the erythema, the confluence of the rash, the presence of pruritus, and the absence of fever or other constitutional symptoms.

If You Suspect a Drug Reaction, What Is the Most Likely Drug?

The most likely drug is one that has been recently administered. From the list of this patient's recent drugs, cefazolin, a cephalosporin antibiotic, is statistically the most likely culprit.

How Can You Prove It?

No confirmatory tests are available. The diagnosis is purely clinical. Only a rechallenge with the suspected drug (which is rarely done) could confirm your clinical suspicion.

IMPORTANT POINTS

1. For any eruption, consider a drug etiology.
2. In most cases, the history and physical examination suggest a drug eruption. There are no definitive diagnostic tests.

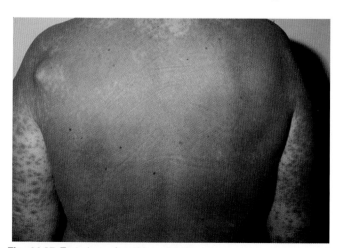

Fig. 14.27 Two days after this patient's coronary artery bypass graft, he developed a pruritic, intensely erythematous eruption that began on his face and trunk, became confluent, and subsequently involved the extremities. He was afebrile and otherwise was recovering uneventfully from the surgical procedure.

Case 14.2—Scaling Rash on Head, Neck, Trunk, and Arms (Fig. 14.28)

What Is Your Differential Diagnosis?

A widespread scaling eruption suggests a differential diagnosis of psoriasis, tinea, pityriasis rosea, secondary syphilis, lupus, T-cell cutaneous lymphoma, and dermatitis. The chronic course eliminates pityriasis rosea and syphilis.

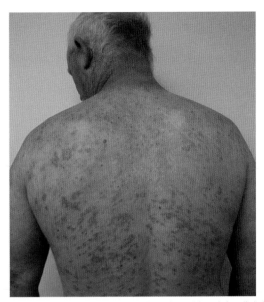

Fig. 14.28 This 48-year-old man developed pruritic, pink, slightly scaling papules and plaques 3 years ago, on the head, neck, trunk, and arms. His review of systems and previous medical history were unremarkable. It was uncertain whether the eruption was exacerbated by sunlight.

What Would You Do Now?

A KOH preparation was negative for fungal elements. A skin biopsy helped make the diagnosis, and it revealed pathological changes of lupus erythematosus. Further laboratory testing resulted in normal antinuclear antibody, dsDNA, complete blood cell count with platelet count, urinalysis, and complete metabolic profile. Testing for SSA was positive and SSB was negative. All these tests confirm the diagnosis of CLE.

How Would You Treat This Patient?

Sun protection is first and foremost, even with the patient's questionable history of sun sensitivity. Topical steroids such as triamcinolone cream 0.1% in large volumes may suppress the lupus. The next step would be an antimalarial such as hydroxychloroquine 200 mg b.i.d. If these interventions fail, then systemic immunosuppressants are warranted.

IMPORTANT POINTS

1. Scaling eruptions in a sun-exposed distribution suggest the possibility of lupus erythematosus.
2. A skin biopsy is diagnostic of lupus.
3. The medical history, general physical, and laboratory examination will separate cutaneous versus systemic involvement.

Localized Erythema

CHAPTER CONTENTS

Algorithm of localized erythema

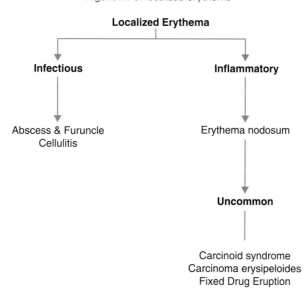

Localized Erythema

Infectious   **Inflammatory**

Abscess & Furuncle   Erythema nodosum
Cellulitis

Uncommon

Carcinoid syndrome
Carcinoma erysipeloides
Fixed Drug Eruption

ABSTRACT

In the disorders described in this chapter, the erythema is con-fined to discrete lesions and is localized to a small area of the body surface. Characteristically the epidermis is spared, but the dermal inflammation may extend into the subcutaneous fat. The three most common examples of localized erythema are as follows: *cellulitis*, an indurated plaque; *abscess* and *furuncle*, each of which is a fluctuant mass; and *erythema nodosum*, a nodule (Table 15.1).

KEY POINTS

1. Dermal inflammation often presents as localized erythema.
2. Localized erythema is most commonly owing to infection (e.g., cellulitis or abscess) or inflammation (e.g., erythema nodosum).

ABSCESS AND FURUNCLE

KEY POINTS

1. *Staphylococcus aureus* is a common pathogen.
2. Recurrent furunculosis is often associated with nasal colonization of *S. aureus*.
3. Check bacterial culture and sensitivity for methicillin-resistant *S. aureus*.

Definition

Abscesses and furuncles (boils) are pus-filled nodules in the dermis. *S. aureus* is the usual pathogen, but gram-negative organisms and anaerobic bacteria may also be causes. Abscesses often arise from the traumatic inoculation of bacteria into the skin, whereas furuncles arise from infected hair follicles. The clinical lesion is a red, tender, and fluctuant nodule (Fig. 15.1).

TABLE 15.1 Localized Erythema

	Frequency (%)[a]	Etiology	History	Physical Examination	Differential Diagnosis	Laboratory Test
Abscess and furuncle	0.4	*Staphylococcus aureus* (usually)	–	Red, tender, fluctuant mass	Nodular acne Hidradenitis suppurativa	Culture
Cellulitis	0.1	Group A streptococci (usually)	Fever	Red, warm, indurated, tender area of skin	Contact dermatitis Superficial thrombophlebitis	Culture Skin aspirate Blood
Erythema nodosum	0.3	Hypersensitivity reaction	Search for associated conditions, including drug history	Red, tender, deep nodules, usually on lower legs	Thrombophlebitis Pancreatic panniculitis	Chest radiography Throat culture Antistreptolysin-O titers PPD skin test with or without skin biopsy

PPD, Purified protein derivative.
[a]Percentage of new dermatology outpatients with this diagnosis seen in the Hershey Medical Center Dermatology Clinic, Hershey, Pennsylvania.

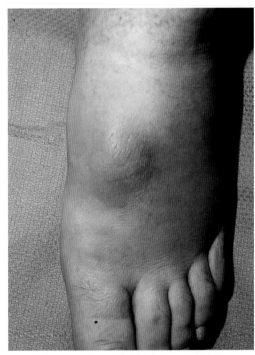

Fig. 15.1 Abscess—red, fluctuant nodule.

> *Staphylococcus aureus* is the usual pathogen.

Incidence

In one survey, cutaneous abscesses accounted for 2% of all patient visits to the emergency department of a large city hospital. Patients with recurrent furuncles are seen more often by a dermatologist.

History

Patients with abscesses may give a history of preceding trauma, including surgery. Some patients with furuncles give a history of recurrent lesions. Immunodeficiency, intravenous drug abuse, a history of atopic dermatitis, and perhaps diabetes mellitus predispose some patients to bacterial infections, but most patients with a furuncle or an abscess have no underlying medical disease.

Physical Examination

Furuncles and abscesses often begin as hard, tender, red nodules that become more fluctuant and more painful with time. Abscesses tend to be larger and deeper than furuncles. Regional lymph nodes are sometimes enlarged, but fever is rarely present.

Differential Diagnosis

Abscesses and furuncles are rarely confused with other entities. Acne and hidradenitis suppurativa can cause pus-filled nodules and cysts. In both conditions, the distribution of the lesions usually provides the diagnostic clue. In *nodular acne*, multiple lesions are distributed on the face and upper trunk, and other acne lesions (e.g., comedones, papules, pustules) are usually present. In *hidradenitis suppurativa*, draining nodules are present in the axillary, inguinal, and perineal areas (intertriginous zones). These nodules are often accompanied by open comedones, draining sinus tracts, and scars (Fig. 15.2). Hidradenitis suppurativa is predominantly an inflammatory disease associated with poral occlusion of the pilosebaceous units and secondary inflammation of the apocrine glands. The most commonly mistaken diagnosis for an abscess is a ruptured *epidermal inclusion cyst*. The intense inflammatory reaction to keratin, usually contained by the cyst lining, creates a fluctuant nodule, most commonly located on the back. Lack of fever, history of a cyst, and the presence of a punctum on top of the cyst are distinguishing factors (Fig. 15.3). Primary treatment includes incision and drainage, which often result in immediate relief (Fig. 15.4).

DIFFERENTIAL DIAGNOSIS FOR ABSCESS AND FURUNCLE

- Nodular acne
- Hidradenitis suppurativa
- Ruptured epidermal inclusion cyst

Laboratory and Biopsy

The diagnosis is usually made clinically and confirmed by routine culture of the purulent material that has been obtained from

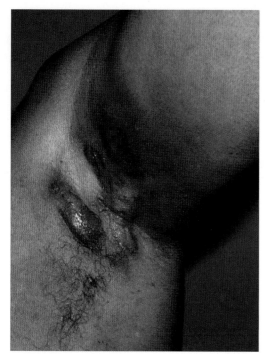

Fig. 15.2 **Hidradenitis suppurativa**—recurrent, draining nodules and scarring in the axilla.

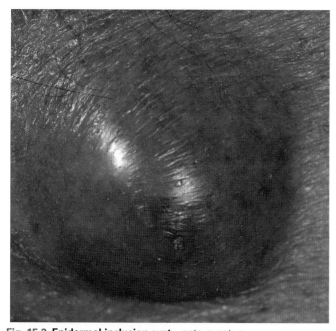

Fig. 15.3 **Epidermal inclusion cyst**—note punctum.

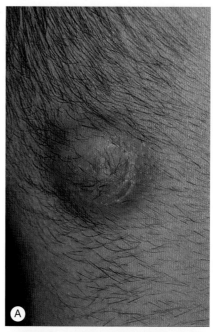

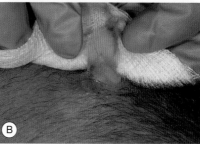

Fig. 15.4 (A) Ruptured epidermal inclusion cyst. (B) Incision and drainage provide an immediate relief.

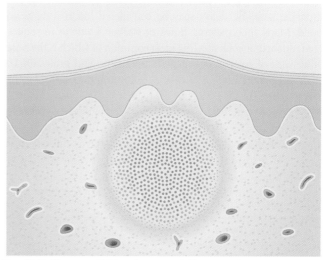

Fig. 15.5 **Abscess**. Epidermis—normal. Dermis—dense aggregate of acute inflammatory cells replacing necrotic dermis.

incision and drainage. Methicillin-resistant *S. aureus* (MRSA) is now a common pathogen in hospitals and communities and needs to be checked by obtaining a culture and sensitivity. In immunocompromised patients, anaerobic cultures may be desired. Blood cultures are rarely positive and are not indicated unless the patient has signs of sepsis.

Biopsy is rarely indicated. If a biopsy is performed, a large, dense collection of neutrophils will be found in necrotic dermis (Fig. 15.5).

Therapy

The principal therapy consists of incision and drainage. In a study of 135 patients, this approach resulted in complete healing in all patients, including those who did not receive systemic antibiotics. However, the authors recommend incision and drainage along with oral antibiotics. Systemic antibiotics may result in the involution of early lesions, may prevent the progression of nodular lesions to fluctuant ones, and may decrease contagiousness. With the emergence of MRSA and high proportion of abscesses and furuncles caused by *S. aureus*, doxycycline and trimethoprim–sulfamethoxazole are often used as first-line treatments. It is appropriate to treat with cefalexin (Keflex) or dicloxacillin in doses of 250–500 mg four times daily for 1 week in appropriate patients (children <8 years old), provided a culture and sensitivity is performed first, especially with the emergence of MRSA. If the clinical response is poor, a change in antibiotic therapy can be considered. For this, culture results are helpful. Parenteral antibiotics are indicated for patients with surrounding cellulitis.

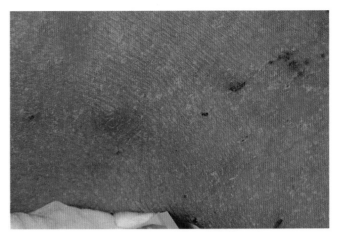

Fig. 15.6 Abscess. Note nodule in the popliteal fossa on the inflamed skin of a patient with atopic dermatitis.

THERAPY FOR ABSCESSES

Initial
- Incision and drainage
- Antibiotics:
  - Doxycycline
  - Trimethoprim–sulfamethoxazole
  - Beta-lactamase-resistant penicillin (e.g., dicloxacillin 250 mg q.i.d.)
  - First-generation cephalosporin (e.g., cefalexin 250 mg q.i.d.)

Alternative
- Parenteral antibiotics

Course and Complications

Untreated lesions often rupture and drain spontaneously. After surgical or spontaneous drainage, healing usually occurs. Large lesions may leave scars.

In patients with recurrent furunculosis, an underlying predisposing systemic defect may be considered but is usually not found. Many such patients, however, harbor *S. aureus* in sequestered mucocutaneous sites, the most common of which is the nose. Other sites of colonization include the axillae and groin. Of US citizens, 1.5% are carriers of MRSA, harboring the bacteria in the anterior nares. In such patients, the regular use of antiseptic agents may decrease bacterial colonization and thereby prevent furuncles from recurring. The authors recommend a total body scrub every other day with an antiseptic cleansing agent such as chlorhexidine or benzoyl peroxide wash and daily nasal application of an antibiotic ointment such as prescription mupirocin ointment or over-the-counter bacitracin and polymyxin B ointment (Polysporin).

Patients with recurrent furuncles are often staphylococcal carriers.

Pathogenesis

For abscesses and furuncles, the bacteria usually gain entry into the dermis by an external route. For abscesses, this may be a traumatic inoculation such as a puncture wound, laceration, or surgical incision.

For furuncles, the bacteria enter through a hair follicle, in which they form deep folliculitis and extend into the surrounding dermis. In both instances, the presence of a large number of bacteria in the dermis elicits a vigorous inflammatory response and eventuates in a massive collection of inflammatory cells, primarily neutrophils.

In atopic dermatitis, low levels of the innate immune system's antimicrobial peptides, beta-defensins and cathelicidins, predispose patients to infections, such as abscesses from *S. aureus* (Fig. 15.6).

CELLULITIS

KEY POINTS

1. Frequently caused by *S. aureus* and group A streptococci
2. Fever is often present.
3. Resolves with antibiotics.

Definition

Cellulitis is a deep infection of the skin resulting in a localized area of erythema (Fig. 15.7). Group A streptococci (*Streptococcus pyogenes*) and *S. aureus* are the organisms most often responsible. MRSA is becoming a prevalent pathogen. Before the introduction of the *Haemophilus influenzae* vaccine, facial cellulitis in extremely young children was frequently caused by this bacterium. Streptococcal infection is now the most common cause, even in this age group. Rarely, other aerobic and anaerobic bacteria, as well as deep fungi such as *Cryptococcus neoformans*, cause cellulitis, particularly in patients who are immunosuppressed. In immunocompetent hosts, bacteria gain entry into the skin through a break in the skin's barrier, whereas in immunosuppressed hosts, bacteria or other organisms seed the skin from the blood.

Cellulitis is most frequently caused by infection with group A streptococci and *S. aureus*.

Erysipelas is sometimes considered separately from cellulitis, but the distinction between the two entities may be a matter

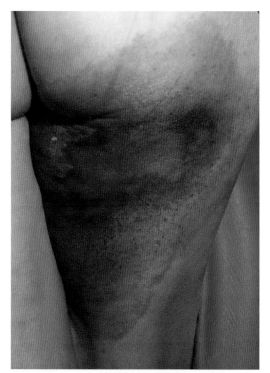

Fig. 15.7 **Cellulitis**—note erythema, edema, and bulla.

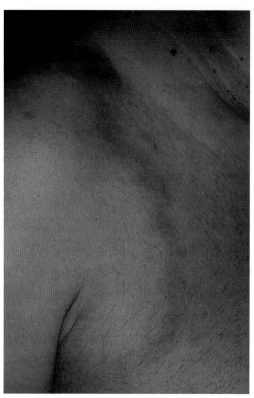

Fig. 15.9 **Cellulitis**—note the lymphangitic spread from an infected insect bite.

Incidence

Patients with this acute febrile disease are seen most often by their primary physician or an emergency physician. Only 0.1% of the present authors' new patients are seen for cellulitis.

History

Patients usually feel ill and febrile. The fever may precede the physical appearance of the skin involvement. A history of trauma or a preceding infected skin lesion is sometimes elicited (Fig. 15.9). Saphenous venectomy for coronary bypass surgery can predispose patients to recurrent cellulitis of the legs. Buccal cellulitis in children often accompanies otitis media, and symptoms of an ear infection may be present.

> Fever is almost always present.

Physical Examination

The involved skin shows all four cardinal signs of inflammation: redness (rubor), warmth (calor), swelling (tumor), and tenderness and pain (dolor). The epidermis is usually unaltered, although, rarely, blisters are present. The erythema in *H. influenzae* facial cellulitis is characteristically violaceous. Perianal fissures in children predisposed to perianal cellulitis are caused by group A streptococci (Fig. 15.10).

> The skin shows all four signs of inflammation:
> 1. Rubor
> 2. Calor
> 3. Tumor
> 4. Dolor

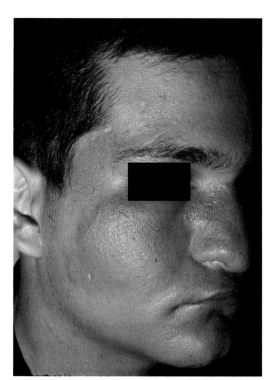

Fig. 15.8 **Erysipelas**—sharply demarcated, edematous, red plaque.

of semantics. The border of the involved area is more sharply demarcated in classic erysipelas than in cellulitis, and the surface looks more like an orange peel (Fig. 15.8). However, both disorders are caused by bacteria, most often group A streptococci; for diagnostic and therapeutic purposes, they can be considered the same.

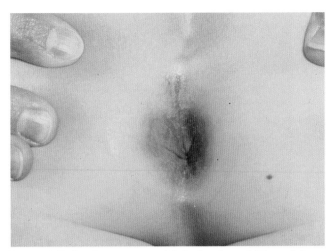

Fig. 15.10 Perianal streptococcal infection in a child—well-demarcated erythema with fissures.

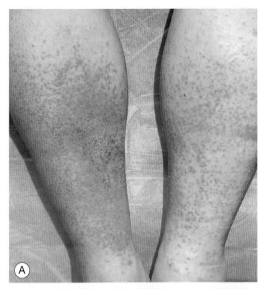

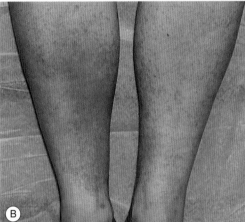

Fig. 15.11 Stasis dermatitis. (A) Bilateral lower leg involvement with significant epidermal change. (B) Near-complete resolution with topical corticosteroids and compression therapy.

In adults, cellulitis most often affects the lower legs, especially when lymphatic obstruction is present. In these patients, fissures between the toes owing to tinea pedis often serve as the initial portal of entry for bacteria.

Differential Diagnosis

Contact dermatitis, when severe, can mimic the erythema and swelling of cellulitis, but important distinguishing characteristics of contact dermatitis are the more marked epidermal involvement with vesicles, the symptom of itch rather than tenderness, and the absence of fever. A deep vein thrombosis may mimic cellulitis, and ultrasound evaluation will distinguish between the two conditions.

Stasis dermatitis is often confused with cellulitis, leading to inappropriate inpatient admissions for parenteral antibiotics. Distinguishing features include chronicity, bilateral involvement, epidermal involvement with crust and scale, and the absence of fever (Fig. 15.11).

Superficial thrombophlebitis of the lower legs can cause redness and tenderness and is sometimes difficult to distinguish from cellulitis. Fever is not present in superficial thrombophlebitis, however, and the involved vein can often be palpated as a hard cord.

Facial cellulitis in children can be confused with the "slapped cheek" appearance seen in *erythema infectiosum*. In erythema infectiosum, however, the erythema is bilateral and usually nontender, and the patient's condition does not appear toxic.

DIFFERENTIAL DIAGNOSIS FOR CELLULITIS

- Contact dermatitis
- Deep vein thrombosis
- Stasis dermatitis
- Superficial thrombophlebitis
- Erythema infectiosum (distinguish from facial cellulitis)

Laboratory and Biopsy

Skin and blood cultures may be obtained, but the bacterial pathogen responsible is not always recovered. A skin culture may be taken from the leading edge of the lesion by injecting and then aspirating 0.5 mL of nonbacteriostatic saline. The aspirate is Gram-stained and cultured. Unfortunately, the highest reported yield from this procedure is only 50%, and in most series, it is much less than this. Culture of a skin biopsy increases the yield but not to 100%.

Skin cultures are often negative.

A skin biopsy is usually not needed in ambulatory, immunocompetent patients. However, a biopsy is often done to identify a responsible organism in an immunocompromised patient whose cellulitis has not responded to antibiotic therapy. If a biopsy is performed, the examiner will see an inflammatory

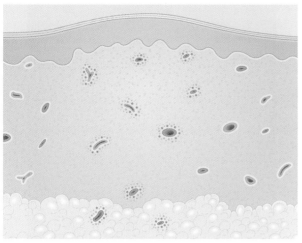

Fig. 15.12 Cellulitis. Epidermis—normal. Dermis—inflammation diffuses through the dermis, extending into the subcutaneous fat.

infiltrate composed primarily of neutrophils throughout the dermis, occasionally extending into the subcutaneous fat. Edema and dilation of lymphatics and small blood vessels are also present (Fig. 15.12). Special stains for bacteria may be positive. Fungal stains to search for cryptococcal organisms should also be done, particularly on tissue from immunocompromised patients.

Complete blood count reveals leukocytosis in immunocompetent patients.

Therapy

Systemic antibiotics are the mainstay of therapy. It is important to identify the organism and then tailor the antibiotic therapy. In most cases of cellulitis in immunocompetent hosts, empiric antibiotics are started along with warm wet compresses, bed rest, and close outpatient follow-up. Cefalexin (Keflex) or dicloxacillin, in doses of 500 mg four times daily, is prescribed for a 10-day course. Remember to account for MRSA if the patient is not responding to the antibiotics, and it is appropriate to use doxycycline or trimethoprim–sulfamethoxazole as first-line treatment. Patients who are more seriously ill, particularly those with facial cellulitis, should be hospitalized and administered appropriate parenteral antibiotics. Examples of parenteral antibiotics include cefazolin, nafcillin, and vancomycin plus cefepime, and their choice depends on history, the presence of risk factors for MRSA, and lack of response to antibiotics that do not include activity against MRSA. In immunocompromised patients, coverage may be needed for gram-negative bacteria or fungal organisms. In young children with facial cellulitis, antibiotic therapy must include coverage for *H. influenzae*, with amoxicillin combined with trimethoprim–sulfamethoxazole (Bactrim) or amoxicillin–clavulanate (Augmentin) combined with a third-generation cephalosporins such as ceftriaxone.

THERAPY FOR CELLULITIS

Initial
- Oral antibiotics
  - Doxycycline 100 mg b.i.d. or trimethoprim–sulfamethoxazole for methicillin-resistant Staphylococcus aureus (MRSA)
  - Cefalexin 500 mg q.i.d.
  - Dicloxacillin 500 mg q.i.d.

Alternative
- Intravenous antibiotics (if severe)
  - Nafcillin methicillin-sensitive Staphylococcus aureus (MSSA) or vancomycin plus cefepime MRSA
  - Or appropriate antimicrobial agent in an immunocompromised host

Course and Complications

With antibiotic therapy, the fever usually resolves within 24 hours. If it persists beyond 48 hours, a change in antimicrobial therapy should be considered, optimally guided by the initial culture results. The skin inflammation resolves more slowly than the fever, sometimes taking 1 or 2 weeks to subside completely. For most patients, a complete recovery can be expected.

Cutaneous inflammation is slow to subside.

Mortality is rare but can occur in neglected cases or in cases due to a virulent organism, such as *Pseudomonas aeruginosa*. Illnesses such as congestive heart failure, renal insufficiency, morbid obesity, alcoholism, and diabetes predispose to more serious complications. Facial cellulitis caused by *H. influenzae* is often accompanied by otitis media and less often by meningitis. Osteomyelitis due to cellulitis is a rare sequela.

Cellulitis was once a serious and sometimes life-threatening disease, but the use of antibiotics has reduced the mortality rate to near zero in immunocompetent hosts. In immunosuppressed patients, cellulitis from usual as well as unusual pathogens may still be a serious, sometimes life-threatening, infection (Fig. 15.13).

Pathogenesis

In cellulitis, the bacteria may enter the dermis by an external or a hematogenous route. In immunocompetent hosts, the source is usually external. In immunosuppressed hosts, the source is usually internal. Tissue edema predisposes to bacterial proliferation. Proteolytic enzymes elaborated by bacteria such as group A streptococci contribute to the spread of inflammation. Host defense mechanisms involve cellular infiltrates and the elaboration of cytokines, which rapidly kill the bacteria and thereby contribute to the inflammation. Damage to local lymphatics during an acute episode can result in residual lymphedema and may predispose the patient to recurrent episodes.

ERYTHEMA NODOSUM

KEY POINTS
1. Inflammatory reaction in subcutaneous fat
2. Tender nodules on lower legs
3. Treat underlying disease

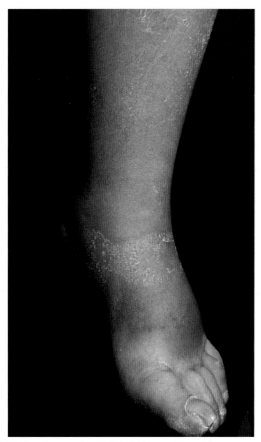

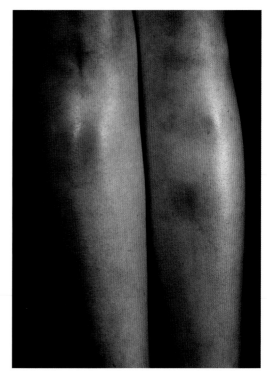

Fig. 15.14 Erythema nodosum—multiple, deep, tender nodules.

Fig. 15.13 Cryptococcal cellulitis in the setting of immunosuppression patient. An organism was diagnosed through biopsy after the patient failed to respond to standard antibiotics.

Definition

Erythema nodosum is an inflammatory reaction in the subcutaneous fat that, in most cases, represents a hypersensitivity response to a variety of infectious and inflammatory disorders. Clinically, erythema nodosum appears as deep, tender, red or purple nodules that are usually located on the lower legs and may be accompanied by fever and malaise (Fig. 15.14).

Incidence

Erythema nodosum is an uncommon disorder, representing 0.3% of the authors' new dermatology patients. It occurs most often in young adults, with females outnumbering males by a ratio of 3:1.

History

History is guided by consideration of etiologic possibilities. In erythema nodosum precipitated by streptococcal infection, the nodules occur within 3 weeks of pharyngitis. Fever and lower respiratory symptoms may be elicited in patients with pulmonary infections caused by deep fungi or tuberculosis. A history of abdominal pain and diarrhea suggests an inflammatory bowel disorder. Ulcerative colitis is the most common inflammatory bowel disease associated with erythema nodosum. Regional enteritis and *Yersinia* enterocolitis are encountered less frequently. An inquiry should be made regarding pregnancy. A complete drug history should be elicited, although, with the exception of

oral contraceptive pills, drugs are uncommon causes. Most cases are of unknown cause and labeled "idiopathic."

Causes:
1. Poststreptococcal infection
2. Sarcoidosis
3. Deep fungal infection: coccidioidomycosis, histoplasmosis
4. Tuberculosis
5. Inflammatory bowel disease
6. *Yersinia* enterocolitis
7. Pregnancy
8. Drugs
9. Idiopathic

Pain and tenderness are usually associated with the skin nodules. Fever and arthralgias may also be present, regardless of the cause. Joint symptoms most often affect the ankles and sometimes the knees and may precede the rash.

Physical Examination

Lesions of erythema nodosum appear as erythematous to violaceous, well-localized, extremely tender, deep nodules that are 1–5 cm in diameter and have indistinct borders. As lesions evolve, they become yellowish-purple and look like bruises. Multiple lesions are usually present, with the typical location being the pretibial areas. Much less often, lesions occur on the thighs and arms. Ulceration rarely occurs.

Typical nodules are:
1. On lower legs
2. Tender
3. Deep

Differential Diagnosis

The diagnosis is usually evident clinically. Lesions of later-stage erythema nodosum may appear as *traumatic bruises*, but history should discriminate between the two. *Superficial thrombophlebitis* also produces tender lesions on the lower legs, but these lesions are usually more linear and not multiple. *Pancreatic panniculitis* is a rare condition that produces tender nodules on the lower legs and occurs in the setting of pancreatitis or pancreatic carcinoma. Patients with this disorder usually have raised serum amylase and lipase levels and a diagnostic skin biopsy.

DIFFERENTIAL DIAGNOSIS FOR ERYTHEMA NODOSUM

- Traumatic bruise
- Superficial thrombophlebitis
- Pancreatic panniculitis

Laboratory and Biopsy

Laboratory testing takes into consideration the possible causes, and a few simple tests can screen for most of these conditions. Appropriate tests include a throat culture, antistreptolysin-O titer, tuberculosis skin test, and chest radiography. The chest radiograph is used to screen for both pulmonary infection and sarcoidosis. In patients with bowel symptoms, further gastrointestinal tract evaluation should be pursued.

Laboratory tests:
1. Throat culture
2. Antistreptolysin-O titer
3. Chest radiography
4. Tuberculosis skin test

A skin biopsy is usually not required. If a biopsy is performed, the changes will be found primarily in the subcutaneous fat, where vascular and perivascular inflammation are present in the fibrous septa separating the fat lobules. The septa become widened by edema and, subsequently, by fibrosis (Fig. 15.15).

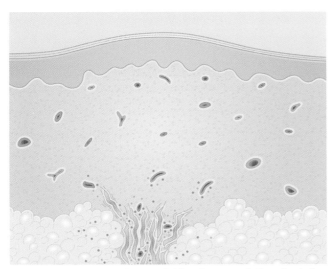

Fig. 15.15 Erythema nodosum. Epidermis—normal. Dermis—inflammation in the lower dermis and in widened septa in the subcutaneous fat.

Acutely, the inflammation shows numerous neutrophils and also involves the lower dermis. Hemorrhage may be present. In older lesions, a granulomatous infiltrate may be found.

Therapy

Therapy is aimed at removing or treating the underlying cause, if one is identified. Bed rest, leg elevation, and compression socks are general measures that may help with the associated pain. Symptomatic therapy may be achieved with nonsteroidal antiinflammatory drugs (NSAIDs) (e.g., 250–500 mg naproxen twice daily). In patients with extensive involvement and marked discomfort, a short course of systemic steroids (e.g., prednisone, starting with 40 mg daily and tapered over 2–3 weeks) often provides dramatic relief, provided the cause is not infectious. Some patients with chronic idiopathic erythema nodosum have been treated successfully with potassium iodide, given in granules, tablets, or as an oral solution. Other alternative medications include colchicine and dapsone. The mechanisms of action for these drugs are not known. Compression stockings may be helpful in patients with chronic or recurrent disease.

THERAPY FOR ERYTHEMA NODOSUM

Initial
- Identification of the precipitating disease, if any
- Bed rest, leg elevation, and/or compression stockings
- NSAIDs:
  - Naproxen—250 mg b.i.d.

Alternative
- Prednisone (if severe)
- Immunosuppressants if recurrent (mycophenolate mofetil or cyclosporine)
- Potassium iodide drops
- Colchicine

Course and Complications

The course is usually self-limiting, typically lasting 3–6 weeks. Erythema nodosum associated with inflammatory bowel disease may parallel the course of the underlying disorder, relapsing with the bowel disease. Erythema nodosum in most other settings does not often recur.

Cutaneous complications are infrequent and inconsequential. Although ulceration does not occur, slightly depressed scars may result.

Pathogenesis

Evidence suggests that erythema nodosum is mediated by immune complexes. Deposition of immunoglobulins and complement has been demonstrated in the blood vessels in early lesions of erythema nodosum. In addition, many patients have circulating immune complexes, presumably related to the underlying disorder. The usual localization of the disease to the skin of the lower legs may be related to hemodynamic factors. The relatively sluggish circulation in the dependent lower extremities predisposes patients to the deposition of immune complexes in those blood vessels.

UNCOMMON CAUSES OF LOCALIZED ERYTHEMA

Carcinoid Syndrome

Carcinoid syndrome is associated with cutaneous flushing and erythema, commonly located on the face (Fig. 15.16). This clinical feature becomes apparent only after hepatic metastases have occurred or when the primary tumor is in the lung (the venous drainage bypasses the liver). The diagnosis is established by high levels of 5-hydroxyindoleacetic acid in the urine. Treatment involves resection of the primary tumor, liver metastases or chemotherapy.

Carcinoma Erysipeloids

Cutaneous metastases can resemble erysipelas and cellulitis. Tumor cells infiltrate the superficial lymphatics and cause the appearance of a warm, red patch or plaque (Fig. 15.17). This occurs most commonly on the anterior chest wall in association with breast carcinoma. Patients fail to respond to antibiotics for a presumptive infection. Biopsy confirms the diagnosis.

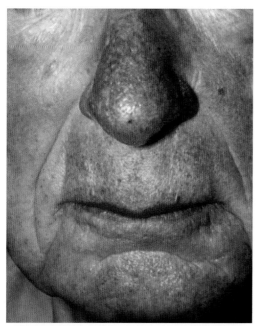

Fig. 15.16 **Carcinoid**—persistent erythema and flushing of face in a patient with liver metastases.

Fixed Drug Eruption

Fixed drug eruptions appear as sharply demarcated red to dark brown plaques (Fig. 15.18) that later take on a dusky hue. With the first exposure to the drug, the lesion appears in 1–2 weeks. On subsequent reexposures, the lesion appears within 24 hours at exactly the same location. The lesions can affect any part of the body but are most common on the distal extremities, face, lips, and genitalia. A biopsy confirms the diagnosis. The most common offenders are NSAIDs (e.g., ibuprofen, naproxen), sulfonamides, tetracyclines, and carbamazepine.

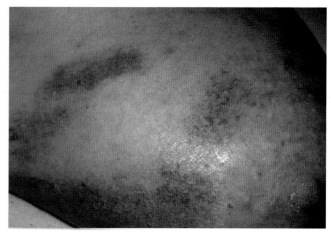

Fig. 15.17 **Carcinoma erysipeloids**—initially treated as cellulitis, biopsy of these red, slightly purpuric, patches confirmed the diagnosis.

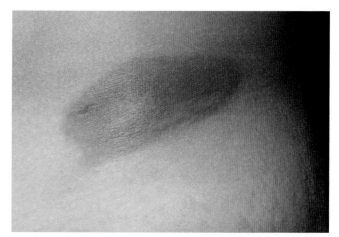

Fig. 15.18 **Fixed drug eruption**—well-demarcated red plaque that recurred after each exposure to trimethoprim–sulfamethoxazole.

Specialized Erythema

CHAPTER CONTENTS

Algorithm for specialized erythema

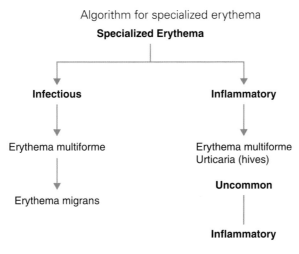

Specialized Erythema

Infectious

Erythema multiforme

Erythema migrans

Inflammatory

Erythema multiforme
Urticaria (hives)

Uncommon

Inflammatory

Erythema ab igne
Erythema annulare centrifugum
Erythema gyratum repens

ABSTRACT

Urticaria and erythema multiforme are characterized by lesions that are so distinctive that they are assigned special names. In urticaria, the lesion is a *hive* (or wheal), which is defined, in Chapter 3, as a papule or plaque of dermal edema, often with central pallor and an irregular, erythematous border. The *target lesion*, when present, is diagnostic of erythema multiforme and is characterized by three concentric zones of color. The third disease described in this chapter is erythema migrans, an expanding annular erythematous skin lesion found in Lyme disease. As demonstrated in these specialized erythema conditions, astute diagnosticians will recognize that "morphology is first in dermatology and everything else is a distant second." Additional features of these disorders are outlined in Table 16.1 and in the discussion that follows.

KEY POINTS

1. The distinctive morphology of the specialized erythemas is key to the diagnosis (e.g., erythema multiforme)
2. Specialized erythemas represent a reactive pattern to an underlying cause (e.g., erythema multiforme caused by herpes simplex infection)

ERYTHEMA MIGRANS

KEY POINTS

1. Hallmark sign of Lyme disease, the most common tick-borne disease in the United States
2. Caused by *Borrelia burgdorferi*, which is transmitted by a tick, *Ixodes* spp.
3. Treatment with antibiotics avoids late complications, notably arthritis

Definition

Erythema migrans represents the skin lesion associated with Lyme disease, a tick-borne illness caused by the spirochete *B. burgdorferi*, which is the primary cause in the United States. Erythema migrans begins as a small, erythematous macule or papule that expands slowly over days to weeks. It must achieve a diameter of at least 5 cm to qualify as erythema migrans (Fig. 16.1). Erythema migrans occurs in 60%–80% of patients with Lyme disease. The late manifestations include the involvement of the musculoskeletal, nervous, or cardiovascular system.

The size criterion for erythema migrans is a diameter of 5 cm.

TABLE 16.1	**Specialized Erythema**					
	Frequency (%)[a]	**Etiology**	**History**	**Physical Examination**	**Differential Diagnosis**	**Laboratory Test**
Erythema migrans	<0.1	Tick-borne spirochete (*Borrelia burgdorferi*)	Constitutional symptoms accompany rash Prior tick bite	One or more *expanding* red, annular macules at least 5 cm in diameter	Cellulitis Tinea corporis Granuloma annulare Fixed drug reaction Other insect bite reaction	Serology Skin biopsy
Erythema multiforme	0.3	Drugs Infection Idiopathic	Constitutional prodrome Prior herpes simplex infection	Erythematous plaques Bullae Target lesions Mucous membrane involvement	Urticaria Viral exanthem Drug reaction Blistering disease	May be indicated:Chest radiography Skin biopsy
Urticaria	2	Ingestants Drugs Foods Infection Physical agents Idiopathic	Lesions last <24 h	Wheals Generalized distribution	Erythema multiforme Drug reaction Urticarial vasculitis Erythema marginatum	–

[a]Percentage of new dermatology patients with this diagnosis seen in the Hershey Medical Center Dermatology Clinic, Hershey, Pennsylvania.

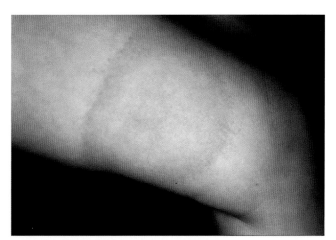

Fig. 16.1 **Erythema migrans**—expanding red patch with central clearing.

> Erythema migrans occurs in 60%–80% of patients with Lyme disease.

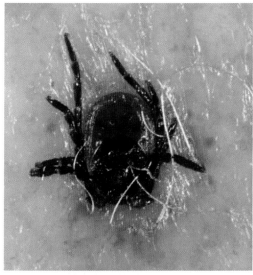

Fig. 16.2 **Ixodes scapularis**—tick that transmits Lyme disease.

Incidence

Lyme disease was first described in 1977, when it was diagnosed in a cluster of children living near Lyme, Connecticut, who were initially thought to have juvenile rheumatoid arthritis. Since then, the number of reported cases and their geographic distribution have increased steadily. Although cases have been reported from nearly every state in the United States, most cases occur in the northeast, midwest, and west coast. Cases are also seen in Central Europe and Scandinavia, where other species of *Borreliella* are pathogenic. Lyme disease is the most frequently reported arthropod-borne disease in the United States. Most cases occur between May and September.

> Lyme disease is the most frequent arthropod-borne disease in the United States.

History

Erythema migrans begins 3–30 days after a tick bite (Fig. 16.2). Because the tick is so small, many patients (75%) do not recall having received a bite. Most patients, however, do have a history of recent exposure to potential tick habitats such as woodlands or grassy areas. Many patients with erythema migrans have accompanying systemic symptoms such as fever, myalgia, arthralgia, headache, malaise, or fatigue. The skin lesion itself is usually asymptomatic but is noted by the patient to expand slowly over time.

> A history of tick bites is often lacking.

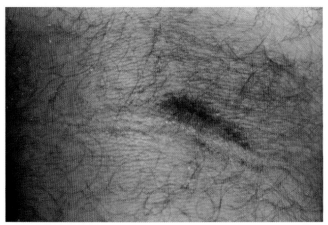

Fig. 16.3 Lyme disease—tick bite occurred in popliteal fossa, resulting in central purpura and red patch >5 cm. Patient developed stage 2 Lyme disease.

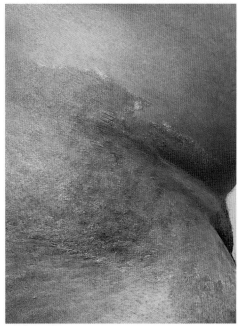

Fig. 16.5 Tinea corporis.

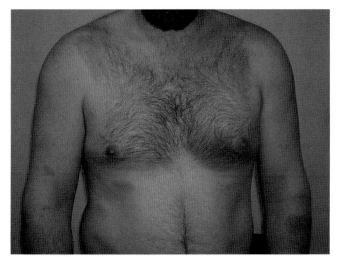

Fig. 16.4 Disseminated erythema migrans.

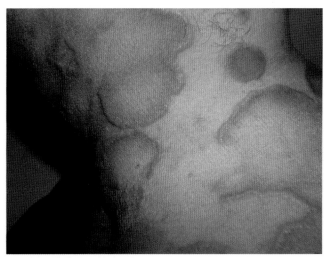

Fig. 16.6 Granuloma annulare.

Physical Findings

The erythema migrans lesion is located at a body site favored by a feeding tick, such as the waistband and intertriginous areas, as well as the extremities (Fig. 16.3). The diameter of the lesion must be at least 5 cm to qualify as erythema migrans and often reach a diameter of more than 20 cm.

A central punctum from the tick bite may be evident but is often not. Typical erythema migrans has a macular border and a clearing center, but less classic features are common and include a papular border, alternating rings of erythema and clearing, and a center that is intensely erythematous, vesicular, purpuric, necrotic, or even ulcerated. However, all erythema migrans lesions have an expanding border in common. Multiple skin lesions occur in 15% of patients, which is a sign of disseminated disease (Fig. 16.4). The erythema migrans rash may be more subtle in patients of darker skin tones, requiring clinicians to examine the skin more closely and with good lighting to ensure diagnosis.

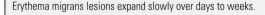

Erythema migrans lesions expand slowly over days to weeks.

Differential Diagnosis

The differential diagnosis includes cellulitis, tinea corporis, granuloma annulare, fixed drug reaction, and other insect bite reactions. Except for cellulitis, these conditions are not accompanied by systemic symptoms. In addition, compared with erythema migrans, cellulitis is more tender and usually more acute, warmer, and redder; *tinea corporis* has a scaling border that is potassium hydroxide-positive for fungal elements and is more chronic (Fig. 16.5); granuloma annulare, an idiopathic dermal granulomatous process, has a firm, elevated border, and persists for months to years (Fig. 16.6); *fixed drug eruption* has no central clearing, is violaceous, and characteristically recurs in the same spot within hours of ingestion of the offending agent (Fig. 16.7); other insect bite reactions often have more prominent

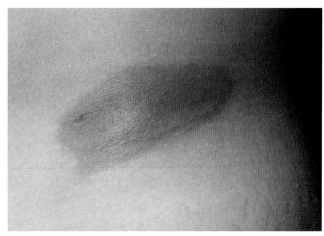

Fig. 16.7 Fixed drug eruption.

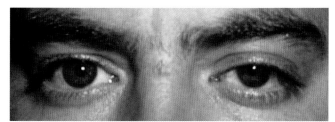

Fig. 16.8 Lyme disease—stage 2 Bell palsy. Note that patient cannot lift left upper eyelid.

central puncta, are smaller, and are usually more transient than erythema migrans.

DIFFERENTIAL DIAGNOSIS FOR ERYTHEMA MIGRANS

- Cellulitis
- Tinea corporis
- Granuloma annulare
- Fixed drug reaction
- Other insect bite reactions

Laboratory and Biopsy

Lyme disease is diagnosed clinically, especially in endemic areas. Therefore it is acceptable to prescribe antibiotic therapy without confirmatory testing because the skin lesions often appear before the patient develops antibodies for the serologic tests. Serologic tests (e.g., enzyme-linked immunosorbent assay) for immunoglobulin M (IgM) and IgG anti-*Borrelia burgdorferi* antibodies are commonly used, but this test is neither sensitive (antibodies do not appear until after the first 2–4 weeks of illness) nor specific (false-negative results in infected individuals and false-positive results in persons with other diseases, including systemic lupus erythematosus and rheumatoid arthritis). Positive or equivocal tests should be followed up with a standardized western blot.

Serologic tests have limited usefulness.

Therapy

The ideal treatment is prevention, including tick avoidance, protective clothing, DEET (*N,N*-diethyl-meta-toluamide) repellent, and prompt removal of ticks within 24 hours. All patients with erythema migrans are defined as having Lyme disease and thus require antibiotic therapy. The preferred agent for early localized disease is doxycycline, 100 mg twice daily for 10 days; however, doses can range up to 21 days. Alternatively, amoxicillin 500 mg three times daily for 10–21 days can be used. Cefuroxime axetil

500 mg twice daily for 14 days is a third but less preferable alternative. Manifestations and therapy of early disseminated infection and late persistent infection are discussed below.

THERAPY FOR ERYTHEMA MIGRANS (EARLY LOCALIZED LYME)

Initial
- Antibiotics for 10–21 days:
  - Doxycycline 100 mg b.i.d. or
  - Amoxicillin 500 mg t.i.d.
- For children aged <12 years:
  - Amoxicillin 50 mg/kg daily divided t.i.d.

Course and Complications

The course and manifestations of Lyme disease share many similarities with syphilis. In Lyme disease, even without therapy, the erythema migrans lesion usually resolves spontaneously within a month. However, without treatment of early localized infection (stage 1), the disease may progress to stage 2 or 3.

Stages:
1. Localized
2. Early disseminated
3. Late persistent

In stage 2 (early disseminated infection), the *B. burgdorferi* spirochete is spread hematogenously to distant sites. The skin is affected in approximately 50% of patients with annular lesions, which are usually smaller than the primary one. Patients are systemically ill with fever, chills, headache, arthralgia, and fatigue. Infection of other organ systems can result in a variety of symptoms, including arthritis, meningitis, cranial neuritis (particularly Bell palsy) (Fig. 16.8), lymphadenopathy, carditis, and atrioventricular conduction defects. After inoculation, neurologic involvement occurs weeks to months later and affects approximately 15%–20% of patients; cardiac involvement occurs within weeks and affects 4%–8%. Arthritis, the most common manifestation, occurs at a mean of 6 months, with a range of 2 weeks to 2 years. It affects 60% of patients with intermittent asymmetric arthritis that affects primarily large joints, especially the knee.

Arthritis is the most common manifestation of disseminated disease.

Without treatment, the disease may enter stage 3 (late disease), with a late persistent infection. The major manifestation of this stage is *continual* arthritis, lasting more than 1 year. Chronic central nervous system involvement also may occur with manifestations that include ataxia and mental disorder.

Treatment of more serious cardiac and neurologic manifestations requires parenteral therapy with 2 g ceftriaxone intravenously daily for 14–28 days. Lyme arthritis can be treated orally with 100 mg doxycycline twice daily for 30 days or amoxicillin 500 mg orally four times daily for 30 days.

> Cardiac and neurologic manifestations require parenteral antibiotic therapy.

Pathogenesis

The disease is caused by *B. burgdorferi*, a spirochete carried by *Ixodes* ticks. In the northeastern and midwestern United States, the tick species is *Ixodes dammini* (deer tick). In the western United States, the species is *Ixodes pacificus*, and in Europe, it is *Ixodes ricinus*. These ticks have a 2-year life cycle, and their preferred host in North America is the white-footed mouse, which asymptomatically carries the *Borrelia* infection and transmits it to a feeding larval tick. The white-tailed deer is the preferred host for the infected adult tick, hence the name deer tick. Deer, however, are not involved in the life cycle of the spirochete. The

Borrelia infection is transmitted to humans when an infected tick feeds, thereby injecting the spirochete from its salivary glands into the skin. Once injected, the spirochete produces a local infection with an inflammatory reaction that produces a visible skin lesion—erythema migrans. Untreated, the infection often disseminates, spreading hematogenously to internal organs.

ERYTHEMA MULTIFORME

KEY POINTS

1. Target lesions have concentric rings that are diagnostic.
2. Recurrent disease is most often precipitated by herpes simplex virus infection.
3. Involvement of two or more mucosal surfaces signifies a poorer prognosis.

Definition

Erythema multiforme (EM) is an immunologic reaction in the skin possibly triggered by circulating immune complexes. As its name suggests, the eruption is characterized clinically by a variety of lesions, including erythematous plaques, blisters, and "target" lesions (Fig. 16.9). Recurrent disease is caused most often by herpes simplex infection and is termed *erythema*

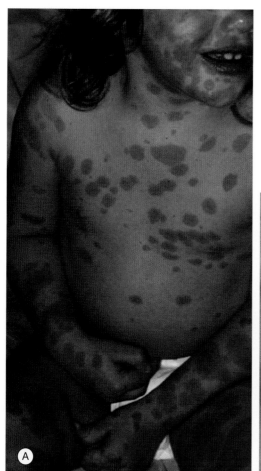
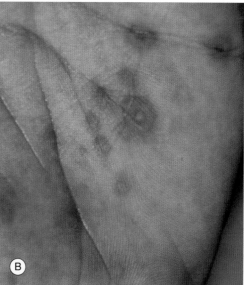

Fig. 16.9 Erythema multiforme. (A) Generalized, circular plaques with dusky centers secondary to upper respiratory infection. (B) Classic target lesions with *three zones* of color.

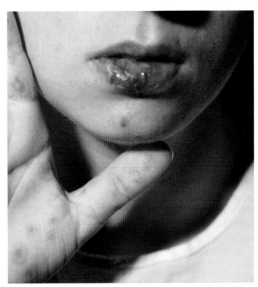

Fig. 16.10 Recurrent erythema multiforme secondary to herpes simplex virus.

multiforme minor. Mucous membrane involvement also occurs in the severe form of the disease—*erythema multiforme major*—and is usually caused by drugs or infection.

The most common causes of erythema multiforme:
1. Infection
2. Drugs

Incidence

Erythema multiforme, although not rare, is uncommon. Fewer than 1% of the authors' new dermatology patients are seen for this condition. The disorder most often affects older children and young adults.

History

The lesions usually appear abruptly within a 24-hour period. Some 50% of patients give a history of a coincident herpes infection. The lesions are pruritic and may have a burning sensation.

Recurrent herpes simplex infection is often the precipitating event in the majority of patients with *recurrent* erythema multiforme (Fig. 16.10). Other causes of recurrent erythema multiforme include repeated *Mycoplasma pneumoniae* infection, hepatitis, vaginal candidiasis, and menses; a thorough history is necessary to find a cause. The herpetic lesion usually precedes the erythema multiforme by a few days to 1 week or more. For the most extended intervals, the herpetic lesions may have healed by the time the patient presents for treatment, so the history is important.

Recurrent herpes simplex is the most common cause of recurrent disease.

M. pneumoniae infection is the precipitating event in some patients, particularly in children; a history of fever and cough is usually found. *Mycoplasma*-related and drug-induced erythema multiforme reactions are often severe, but they do not usually recur.

A cause is not always identifiable, particularly in patients with a single episode of erythema multiforme. In some patients, a febrile prodrome with upper respiratory symptoms precedes the cutaneous eruption by 1–14 days. Treatment of the prodrome with antibiotics probably led in the past to a falsely high rate of incrimination of these drugs as etiologic agents.

Physical Findings

The disorder ranges in severity from mild to severe. In the mild form of the disease (*erythema multiforme minor*), erythematous papules and plaques predominate. Characteristically, the distribution of the lesions favors the extremities and is strikingly symmetric when erythema multiforme is caused by an infection (e.g., herpes simplex); the distribution of lesions favors the trunk when caused by a drug (Fig. 16.11A and B) Target lesions are often present and are diagnostic. To meet the criteria for a target lesion, *three* zones of color must be present: (1) a central dark area or a blister surrounded by (2) a pale edematous zone surrounded by (3) a peripheral rim of erythema. Target lesions are seen most often on the palms and soles but may occur anywhere. Patients with erythema multiforme minor are not usually systemically ill. In the severe form of erythema multiforme (*erythema multiforme major*), the skin disease is more widespread, blisters develop frequently, and mucous membrane involvement is characteristic. The oral mucosa, lips, and conjunctivae are usually the most severely affected (Fig. 16.12). Blisters inside the mouth cause painful erosions that make eating difficult or even impossible when involvement is extensive. Purulent conjunctivitis may become so severe that the eyes swell shut. Patients with EM major may look and feel systemically ill with fever.

Target lesions have three zones of color and are diagnostic for erythema multiforme.

Differential Diagnosis

For the minor form of erythema multiforme, the usual differential diagnosis includes urticaria and viral exanthems. *Hives* may be confused with target lesions, but hives have only two zones of color (a central pale area surrounded by erythema), and individual lesions last fewer than 24 hours. *Viral exanthems* are usually monomorphous, less red, more confluent, and more centrally distributed than erythema multiforme. *Drug hypersensitivity reactions* can present as erythema multiforme with the involvement of the trunk and proximal extremities, but most reactions have a symmetric morbilliform appearance, which is distinguishable from erythema multiforme. The primary differential diagnosis for erythema multiforme major is Stevens-Johnson Syndrome (SJS). In the past, these were considered the same entity but now are known to be separate. Erythema multiforme major has the classic target papules with three distinct zones, typically on the extremities. In contrast, SJS lesions are more often irregular, dusky *macules* with two zones and lesion distribution favors the trunk. Body surface area should also be used to distinguish the two conditions— SJS covers more than 10% of the body while erythema multiforme major does not. Finally, a medication is often implicated

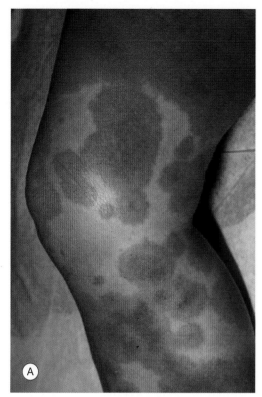

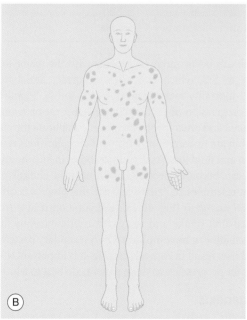

Fig. 16.11 **Distribution of erythema multiforme**. (A) Favors the extremities for infectious causes. (B) Favors the trunk for drug-related causes.

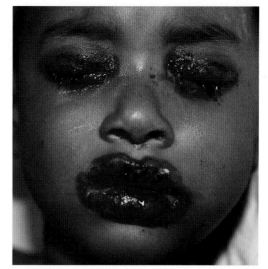

Fig. 16.12 **Erythema multiforme major** secondary to *Mycoplasma* pneumoniae.

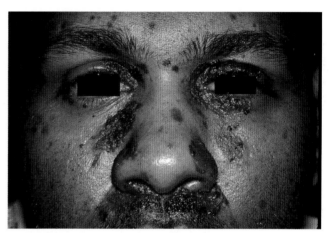

Fig. 16.13 **Pemphigus vulgaris**. Note erosions on the face.

in SJS, while in erythema multiforme major, infection is usually the cause. Other conditions to be considered in the differential diagnosis of the major form of erythema multiforme are the other blistering disorders, including *staphylococcal scalded skin syndrome*, in which the skin is diffusely red and the superficial epidermis strips off easily; *pemphigus*, in which histologic examination shows an intraepidermal blister (Fig. 16.13); and *bullous pemphigoid*, in which blisters often arise on clinically uninflamed skin and mucous membrane involvement is uncommon. As in erythema multiforme, the blister in

bullous pemphigoid is subepidermal, but immunofluorescent studies of a skin biopsy specimen enable distinction between the two. IgG is present at the dermal–epidermal interface in pemphigoid but not in erythema multiforme.

DIFFERENTIAL DIAGNOSIS FOR ERYTHEMA MULTIFORME
• Urticaria
• Viral exanthems
• Drug hypersensitivity reactions
• Blistering diseases for erythema multiforme major
• Staphylococcal scalded skin syndrome
• Bullous pemphigoid/pemphigus vulgaris
• Stevens-Johnson Syndrome

Laboratory and Biopsy

For herpes simplex–precipitated disease, if the responsible vesicular lesion is still present, a Tzanck preparation or viral culture can be obtained. Chest radiography is appropriate to screen for a pulmonary infection. *Mycoplasma* infection can be further confirmed with acute and convalescent cold agglutinin titers. For drug-induced cases, the laboratory is not helpful.

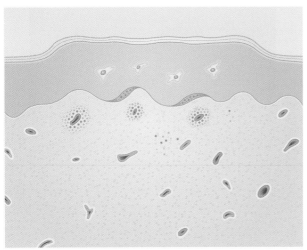

Fig. 16.14 Erythema multiforme. Epidermis—normal or may have individual cell necrosis or exocytosis of mononuclear cells. Dermis—subepidermal separation (center of target lesion); inflammation in the papillary dermis.

The disease is so clinically distinctive, particularly when target lesions are present, that a skin biopsy is usually not required for diagnosis. Biopsy of an erythematous plaque shows dermal changes with a lymphohistiocytic perivascular infiltrate and edema in the papillary dermis. Histologically, the epidermis may also be involved, with changes ranging from spongiosis and individual cell necrosis to full-thickness epidermal necrosis. Subepidermal separation is found in blisters and in the center of target lesions (Fig. 16.14).

Therapy

No convincing evidence indicates that medical therapy favorably alters the course of this disease once the disease is established. Treatment of a precipitating infection is appropriate; erythromycin, azithromycin, or clarithromycin is recommended for *M. pneumoniae*, and a 5-day course of oral valacyclovir (Valtrex) 500 mg twice daily or famciclovir (Famvir) 125 mg twice daily for herpes simplex infection. Recurrent herpes-associated erythema multiforme can be prevented with maintenance antiviral therapy. A medium-potency topical corticosteroid can alleviate pruritus and skin discomfort, mainly burning.

> Initial therapy: treat infection, if present.

For oral mucosal involvement, systemic steroids have often been used, but their value remains controversial. Systemic prednisone in doses starting at 1 mg/kg/day and then tapered over 2–3 weeks is still used frequently in patients with severe erythema multiforme. A prospective study is needed to evaluate the wisdom of this approach more thoroughly. Supportive measures are directed toward restoring and maintaining hydration, preventing secondary infection, and providing pain relief. Intravenous fluids are required in patients with severe oral involvement. Local therapy with antiseptics and dressings may help to prevent secondary infections, and systemic

analgesics are used for pain. The intraoral use of topical anesthetics helps to provide temporary relief for patients with painful mouth lesions; viscous lidocaine or dyclonine liquid can be used. It is always important to monitor these patients so as not to miss SJS.

> Systemic steroids are controversial but used frequently.

THERAPY FOR ERYTHEMA MULTIFORME

Initial
- Treat infection, if present
- For *M. pneumoniae*: erythromycin, azithromycin, or clarithromycin
- For recurrent herpes simplex: valacyclovir 500 mg b.i.d. or famciclovir 125 mg b.i.d.
- Discontinue responsible drug, if any
- For severe mucosal involvement:
  - Supportive care
  - Systemic steroids

Course and Complications

The mild form of erythema multiforme usually resolves spontaneously within 2–3 weeks. The time course is longer in patients with more severe involvement, lasting up to 6 weeks.

> Spontaneous resolution occurs in 2–6 weeks.

Death can occur rarely in patients with the major form who progress to SJS, which is likely the correct initial diagnosis; reported mortality rates range from 0% to 5%. Monitoring for disease progression of erythema multiform major is important. Pneumonia and renal involvement can complicate the cutaneous picture but are uncommon. The major complications result from infection and fluid loss. As discussed above, in SJS, the entire skin surface can become involved, resulting in a clinical presentation that resembles an extensive burn; this process is called *toxic epidermal necrolysis* (Fig. 16.15). Dehydration results from both decreased oral intake and increased transcutaneous fluid loss. Conjunctivitis can be complicated by a secondary bacterial infection and may result in corneal scarring. It is important to monitor patients for progression as these patients do best in a burn unit.

Pathogenesis

Circulating immune complexes have been found in patients with erythema multiforme. The antigen is presumed to be derived from the implicated drug or infectious agent. Evidence supporting a pathogenic role for immune complexes includes the localization of IgM deposits around dermal blood vessels in affected skin and the finding of immune complexes containing herpes antigen in the serum in patients with herpes-associated recurrent erythema multiforme but not in patients with recurrent herpes simplex alone or in those with drug-induced erythema multiforme.

Some investigators favor a cellular immune mechanism. The predominance of mononuclear cells and the absence of leukocytoclastic vasculitis in the skin biopsy favor this mechanism.

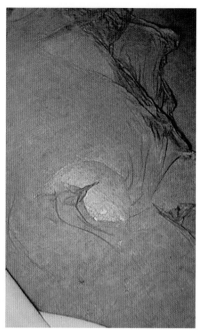

Fig. 16.15 Toxic epidermal necrolysis, a severe form of SJS. Note confluent erythema on the trunk and full-thickness skin separation. Transfer to a burn unit is critical.

URTICARIA (HIVES)

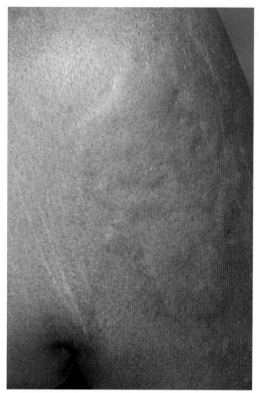

Fig. 16.16 Urticaria (hives)—edematous plaques with scratch marks on the shoulder.

> ## KEY POINTS
> 1. Characterized by evanescent, edematous papules and plaques.
> 2. Acute urticaria is often caused by upper respiratory infection in children.
> 3. A cause is rarely found in chronic urticaria (>6 weeks).
> 4. Treat with antihistamines.

Definition

Urticaria is a condition characterized by pruritic, transient wheals in the skin resulting from acute dermal edema (Fig. 16.16). Acute urticaria is often caused by upper respiratory infections, viral infections in children, and drugs (e.g., antibiotics) and foods (e.g., shellfish) in children and adults. For chronic (lasting >6 weeks) urticaria, a cause is usually not found and physical causes of urticaria must be ruled out.

Incidence

Urticaria is common, with the highest incidence in young adults. Some 20% of the general population will have hives at some point. Patients with acute urticaria often present to the emergency department.

History

Acute urticaria presents with a new onset of pruritus and urticaria. In addition to pruritus and urticaria, patients with chronic urticaria are distressed owing to the longevity of signs and symptoms. Itching is nearly always present. Diagnosis is based mainly on history. For example, in acute urticaria the most common cause is upper respiratory infection from viral or bacterial causes (e.g., strep throat) in children, and hence

associated symptoms such as cough and fever may be present. The drug history is most important, including over-the-counter medications, which the patients may perceive as being unimportant. Inquiry regarding specific medications (e.g., vitamins, analgesics, and laxatives) may help to jog the patient's memory. Virtually all classes of antibiotics have been associated with urticaria, not just beta-lactams, like penicillin and cephalosporins. A history of aspirin and other nonsteroidal antiinflammatory drug (NSAID) ingestion, for example, is particularly important because salicylates cause hives in some patients and aggravate them in as many as one-third of all patients with urticaria, regardless of the cause. A detailed food history (e.g., milk and peanuts in children and fish and shellfish in adults) may also uncover the cause of the urticaria. Stinging insects can cause urticarial lesions.

> Itching is a prominent symptom.

> Ask about over-the-counter medications as well as prescription drugs.

For chronic urticaria, occult infections (e.g., dental and sinus) and physical modalities of urticaria (e.g., cold, pressure, sunlight, physical exercise, heat, and stress) should be evaluated. Foods are a rare cause of acute and chronic urticaria. A history of obstructive airway or other anaphylactic symptoms imparts greater seriousness to the problem. Urticaria accompanied by fever and arthralgia occurs in serum sickness reactions and in prodromal viral hepatitis.

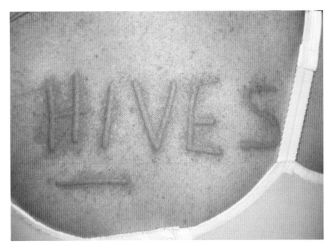

Fig. 16.17 **Dermographism**.

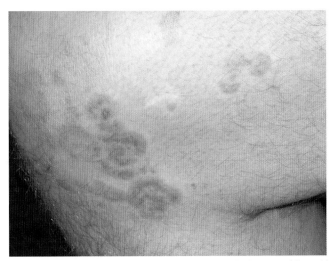

Fig. 16.18 **Urticarial vasculitis**—annular urticarial plaques with residual purpura.

Although allergy to an external allergen is most often manifested by contact dermatitis, in some patients contact of the skin with certain chemicals can cause an urticarial response, such as contact urticaria. For example, the latex in rubber gloves and other rubber objects is a relatively common cause of contact urticaria in medical and dental personnel.

Physical Findings

Hives are skin lesions that are easily recognized. They appear as edematous plaques, often with pale centers and red borders. They frequently assume geographic shapes and are sometimes confluent. The lesions may be scattered but are usually generalized. By definition, an individual hive is transient, lasting less than 24 hours, although new hives may develop continuously. Serum sickness reactions include lymphadenopathy, fever, and arthralgias.

> An individual hive lasts less than 24 hours.

Dermographism can be elicited in many patients with urticaria, including patients who have no visible hives at the time. This "writing with wheals" reaction represents a wheal and flare response to scratching the skin (Fig. 16.17). It indicates that the cutaneous mast cells are unstable and are easily provoked to release their histamine content. Many healthy patients develop erythema after stroking the skin, but wheal formation is limited mainly to patients with urticaria. In eliciting this reaction, one should realize that it takes several minutes for the wheal to develop after the skin has been scratched.

Differential Diagnosis

Lesions sometimes mistaken for urticaria include those seen in erythema multiforme, acute febrile neutrophilic dermatosis (Sweet syndrome), insect bite reactions, urticarial drug reactions, erythema marginatum, and urticarial vasculitis. In *erythema multiforme*, erythematous plaques are often seen, but they last much longer than 24 hours. In *Sweet syndrome*, urticarial plaques favor the head, neck, and upper extremities and are associated with fever and malaise. *Insect bite reactions* can

present as papular urticaria, and the determination of the vector confirms the diagnosis. *Urticarial drug reactions* have a temporal association with a culprit drug, and the lesions are not transient but rather fade when the culprit drug is stopped. *Erythema marginatum* is associated with acute rheumatic fever. The skin lesions are erythematous, annular, and either macular or papular. They are also often transient but rarely itch. *Urticarial vasculitis* is associated with hives that last longer than 24 hours, typically have a burning sensation, and resolve with residual hyperpigmentation (Fig. 16.18).

DIFFERENTIAL DIAGNOSIS FOR URTICARIA

1. Erythema multiforme
2. Acute febrile neutrophilic dermatosis (Sweet syndrome)
3. Insect bite reaction
4. Urticarial drug reaction
5. Erythema marginatum
6. Urticarial vasculitis

> A biopsy shows the evidence of vasculitis, and workup for systemic involvement is important.

Laboratory and Biopsy

History confirms the diagnosis and is supported by appropriate investigations. In acute urticaria, 40% of cases are caused by upper respiratory infections, 9% by drugs, 1% by foods, and 50% by unknown causes. In chronic urticaria, 60% are idiopathic (most of these cases are likely owing to autoimmune factors), 35% are physical, and 5% are vasculitic. For chronic urticarias, it is always important to rule out physical causes of urticaria (e.g., cold, solar, cholinergic, heat, stress, and pressure) (Fig. 16.19). Rarely, chronic urticaria can be associated with malignancy, so a complete history and physical examination are recommended. Liver function tests are appropriate in patients with urticaria and fever to rule out hepatitis. However, for most patients, the laboratory is rarely helpful in eliciting a cause. A biopsy is rarely

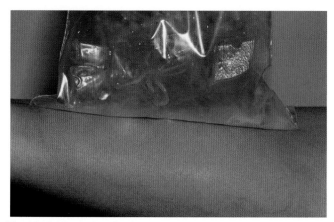

Fig. 16.19 **Physical urticaria**—cold induced.

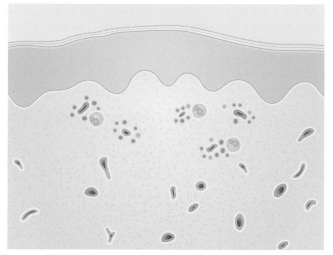

Fig. 16.20 **Urticaria**. Epidermis—normal. Dermis—papillary dermal edema; sparse inflammatory cell infiltrate around dilated vessels; eosinophils sometimes present.

required. If a biopsy is performed, the pathologic findings are minimal, with vasodilation, dermal edema, and a sparse perivascular inflammatory infiltrate composed mainly of lymphocytes, sometimes admixed with eosinophils (Fig. 16.20).

Therapy

Any suspected medication, including aspirin, should be discontinued. Avoidance may be helpful for some of the physical urticarias, such as solar and cold urticaria. Symptomatic therapy is usually achieved with H1 antihistamines given on a regular, rather than an intermittent as needed, basis. Taking an antihistamine after the hives break out, as in the as needed schedule, is analogous to closing the barn door after the horses have escaped. Hydroxyzine (Atarax) is often used in doses of 10–25 mg four times daily for 1–2 weeks in acute urticaria. For chronic diseases, long-term therapy (months to years) may be required, with frequent attempts to taper the dose. Patients who are bothered by sedation from hydroxyzine can be treated with the nonsedating (but more expensive) antihistamines: loratadine (Claritin) or cetirizine (Zyrtec) 10 mg daily, or fexofenadine (Allegra) 180 mg daily.

Initial therapy: antihistamines.

A second-line therapy, in combination with the antihistamines mentioned, includes omalizumab (Xolair) at 300 mg every 4 weeks, which is US Food and Drug Administration approved for the treatment of chronic urticaria in those older than 12 years of age. This medication is administered in an office or an infusion center due to the risk of postinjection anaphylaxis. The tricyclic antidepressant doxepin (Sinequan), in a dose of 25 mg once or twice daily, is also effective and has been shown to have both H1 and H2 antihistamine activity. Prednisone is effective but not usually needed and is to be avoided in long-term therapy given its side-effect profile. Other therapies with less evidence for efficacy include dapsone, hydroxychloroquine, and several immunosuppressants, such as azathioprine or mycophenolate mofetil, which may be necessary for the treatment of uncontrolled, chronic urticaria which is driven by an autoimmune response.

THERAPY FOR URTICARIA

Initial
- Discontinue drugs suspected to be responsible
- Avoid aspirin and other NSAIDs
- Antihistamines:
  - Hydroxyzine 10–25 mg q.i.d.
  - Cetirizine 10 mg daily
  - Fexofenadine 180 mg q.i.d.

Alternative
- Omalizumab 300 mg every 4 weeks
- Tricyclic drugs:
  - Doxepin 25 mg b.i.d.
- Less frequently used agents:
  - Prednisone 0.5 mg/kg daily
  - Dapsone
  - Hydroxychloroquine
  - Immunosuppressants

Course and Complications

Acute urticaria usually resolves within 2 weeks, whereas chronic urticaria can last several years. Drug-induced urticaria usually clears within several days of discontinuation of the responsible medication. Physical urticarias often have a prolonged course. Hives have no complications other than discomfort from intense itching. Hives, however, may precede or accompany a potentially life-threatening anaphylactic response in patients with a severe reaction.

Chronic urticaria may last for years.

Pathogenesis

As summarized below, hives can be mediated immunologically or nonimmunologically. IgE mediation is the most common immunologic mechanism. In this pathway, a sensitized individual possesses IgE antibodies against a specific antigen, such as penicillin. These IgE antibodies are attached to the surface of mast cells and, when rechallenged, are bridged by the antigen. This results in a sequence of reactions leading ultimately to the release of numerous biologically active products from the mast cells, the most important of which appears to be histamine. It would make sense then, why omalizumab, an IgG monoclonal antibody, is an effective treatment for chronic urticaria, as its mechanism of action involves inhibition of IgE from binding to the high-affinity IgE receptors on mast cells and basophils.

Mechanisms for the Production of Hives
- Immunologic
- IgE mediated
  - Complement mediated
- Nonimmunologic
  - Agents that directly cause mast cell degranulation (e.g., opiates and radiocontrast media)
  - Agents that cause alteration in arachidonic acid metabolism (e.g., aspirin and other NSAIDs)
- Idiopathic

Autoantibodies to the high-affinity IgE receptor or to IgE itself have been identified in some patients with chronic idiopathic urticaria. These autoantibodies possess histamine-releasing activity, and this activity may play a role in this disorder.

Complement-mediated urticaria occurs in several settings, the most spectacular of which is the syndrome of hereditary or acquired *angioedema*, in which patients have a deficiency of the inhibitor of the activated first component of the complement system (C1 esterase). Trauma often precipitates attacks that result clinically in massive local swelling and, occasionally, fatal laryngeal edema (Fig. 16.21). The complement system also participates in the hives that occur in *serum sickness*. The postulated mechanism is the deposition of immune complexes in blood vessel walls, followed by fixation of complement and ensuing inflammation. Several drugs can cause direct release of histamine from mast cells. The most commonly encountered are opiates and radiocontrast media.

The mechanism by which aspirin and other NSAIDs causes hives is thought to be their effect on arachidonic acid metabolism. By blocking the production of prostaglandins from arachidonic acid, the pathway is shifted to the production of other metabolites, including leukotrienes, a family of compounds that

includes the previously designated slow-reacting substance of anaphylaxis. As that name suggests, this chemical has the ability to induce urticarial reactions. All these pathways ultimately result in the release of vasoactive substances (e.g., histamine) that alter vascular permeability and produce dermal edema, which appears clinically as a hive.

UNCOMMON CAUSES OF SPECIALIZED ERYTHEMA

Erythema Ab Igne

Erythema ab igne results from chronic exposure to a heating source, most commonly a space heater (affects lower anterior legs) and a heating pad (affects lower back). The pathophysiology is unknown. The skin lesions have a net-like (reticulated) erythema and hyperpigmentation (Fig. 16.22). There is a low risk of developing squamous cell carcinoma within the lesion. Treatment involves the removal of the heating source.

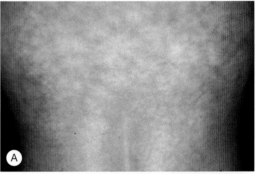

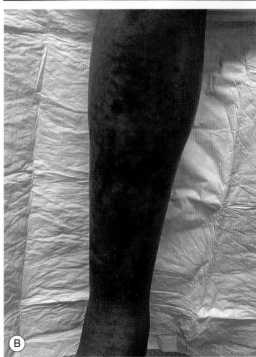

Fig. 16.22 Erythema ab igne. (A) reticulated brownish erythema on back secondary to heating pad. (B) Reticulated brownish hyperpigmentation in a Black patient due to a space heater.

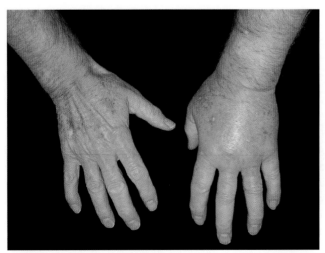

Fig. 16.21 Hereditary angioedema—soft-tissue swelling results in the loss of vein markings of affected hand.

Erythema Annulare Centrifugum

Erythema annulare centrifugum is characterized by annular red plaques that expand centrifugally (Fig. 16.23). There are two forms of the disease: (1) a superficial form with a trailing edge of white scale and (2) a deep form with infiltrated borders and no scale. The most common locations for involvement are the axillae, hips, and thighs. The lesions can be episodic and last for months. The cause remains unknown, and the treatment is often unsatisfactory. Some investigators believe the condition to be a cutaneous response to a distant infection, most often tinea pedis.

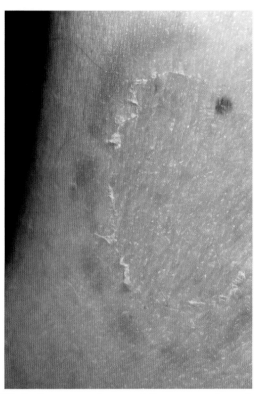

Fig. 16.23 Erythema annulare centrifugum—annular red plaques with characteristic trailing edge of scale.

Erythema Gyratum Repens

Erythema gyratum repens most often represents a paraneoplastic figurate erythema. The most common underlying neoplasms are from the lungs, breast, or esophagus. The rash can appear either before or after the detection of the malignancy. The rash is striking, characterized by gyrate red plaques (Fig. 16.24) that can advance their edges by up to 1 cm per day. The skin lesions resolve when the malignancy is treated.

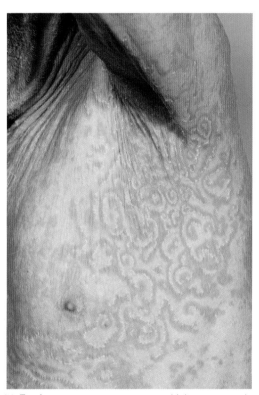

Fig. 16.24 Erythema gyratum repens—multiple gyrate erythematous plaques (wood grain appearance).

Purpura

CHAPTER CONTENTS

Algorithm for Purpura

Purpuric rash

- **Febrile, toxic**
  - Palpable
    - Meningococcemia
      - Disseminated gonococcal infection
  - Nonpalpable
    - DIC
      - TTP
- **Afebrile, nontoxic**
  - Palpable
    - Nonsystemic vasculitis (e.g., vasculitis)
  - Nonpalpable
    - Actinic purpura hypersensitivity
      - ITP

Rocky Mountain spotted fever

Systemic vasculitis (e.g., ANCA-associated vasculitis, polyarteritis nodosa)

ABSTRACT

The word *purpura* is derived from the Latin word for "purple," a clinical characteristic that helps to differentiate the lesion from erythema, which is red in color. Blanchability is the clinical sign that best distinguishes the two. Purpura is nonblanchable because the blood is extravasated outside the vessel walls.

KEY POINTS

1. Purpura (Latin for purple) is the extravasated blood outside the blood vessels and therefore does not blanch.
2. Distinguish palpable from nonpalpable purpura.
3. Palpable purpura represents vasculitis.
4. Always rule out infection first in a patient with purpura.

Purpura is purple and nonblanchable.

Purpura is categorized by size. Small purpura less than 3 mm are called petechiae. Larger purpura more than 3 mm are termed ecchymoses. The differential diagnosis for purpura is determined by two key clinical features: (1) whether or not the patient is febrile and toxic and (2) whether or not the purpura is palpable (stated otherwise, whether the purpura is macules or papules). Nonpalpable purpura results from bleeding into the skin without inflammation of the vessels and is caused by trauma bleeding disorder or blood vessel fragility. Nonpalpable petechiae (small purpura) typically derive from platelet dysfunction or thrombocytopenia (aspirin use, immune thrombocytopenia), forceful venous pressure increases (vomiting or coughing as examples), or other rarer conditions (scurvy). These patients will be afebrile and nontoxic. Nonpalpable ecchymoses develop from trauma or blood vessel fragility (Ehlers–Danlos disease, actinic purpura) in nonfebrile, nontoxic patients. More serious conditions such as disseminated intravascular coagulation (DIC), thrombotic thrombocytopenic purpura (TTP), serious infections (angioinvasive fungus), embolic phenomenon (cholesterol emboli following cardiac catheterization, endocarditis, sickle cell crisis) or rarer conditions like paroxysmal nocturnal hemoglobinemia present as nonpalpable ecchymoses in toxic and/or febrile patients. Necrosis is often observed in many of these nonlatter conditions, particularly DIC, owing to thrombi forming in dermal vessels.

> Nonpalpable purpura:
> 1. Petechiae are found in platelet disorders.
> 2. Ecchymoses result from trauma, fragile blood vessels, or more serious conditions in toxic or febrile patients.
> 3. Necrotic ecchymoses occur in DIC.

Palpable purpura results from inflammatory damage of blood vessels (vasculitis). The inflammation accounts for the elevation of the lesions and allows leakage of blood through the vessel wall. Features of these disorders are outlined in Table 17.1. Minor, often self-limited types of vasculitis (hypersensitivity vasculitis) occur in patients with palpable purpura without fever or toxic appearance. Palpable purpura in patients with a fever or toxic appearance often represents serious types of systemic vasculitis (antineutrophil cytoplasmic antibody [ANCA]–associated vasculitis, rheumatic disease–associated vasculitis) or serious infection (disseminated meningococcemia). Infection needs to be ruled out in patients with purpura and petechiae, especially in those with an accompanying fever. Most causes of purpura, except for actinic purpura, are uncommon. Other uncommon causes of purpura are highlighted in the differential diagnosis sections.

> Palpable purpura represents vasculitis in the skin.

ACTINIC PURPURA (AKA SENILE PURPURA)

> ### KEY POINTS
> 1. Incidental findings most often found in the elderly.
> 2. Appears as purpuric macules on forearms secondary to minor trauma.
> 3. Caused by dermal atrophy from sun exposure and aging.
> 4. There is no specific treatment.

Definition

Purpura resulting from blood vessel fragility appears clinically as ecchymoses, that is, purpuric macules of more than 3 mm in diameter (Fig. 17.1). Dermal tissue atrophy resulting from sun exposure and aging is the most common cause. Blood thinners such as low-dose aspirin or corticosteroid use also lead to additive susceptibility.

Incidence

Actinic purpura is extremely common in elderly people, in whom it is usually noted only as an incidental finding. Patients with darker skin types are rarely affected by this disorder because the melanin in their skin prevents dermal tissue from sun exposure.

TABLE 17.1	**Purpura**					
	Frequency (%)[a]	Etiology	History	Physical Examination	Differential Diagnosis	Laboratory Test
Thrombocytopenic purpura	Uncommon	Drugs Malignancy Autoimmune	Drugs Fever	Petechiae, often on the legs Mucosal bleeding	Identify cause Pigmented purpura disease Scurvy	Complete blood count with platelet count
Actinic purpura	Uncommon	Blood vessel fragility from sun and aging	Sun exposure Steroid use	Ecchymoses confined to hands and arms	Steroid purpura Amyloidosis	Skin biopsy if amyloid is suspected
Disseminated intravascular coagulation (DIC)	Rare	Sepsis Malignancy Obstetric complications Idiopathic Warfarin	Fever (sepsis) Antecedent viral or streptococcal infection	Necrotic ecchymoses and/or: Petechiae Acral cyanosis Palpable purpura Mucosal bleeding Bleeding from venipuncture site	Vasculitis	Coagulation studies Protein C levels
Vasculitis	0.3[b]	Sepsis Collagen vascular disease Cryoglobulinemia Drugs Malignancy	–	Purpuric papules, nodules, or bullae Legs are most commonly affected	DIC	Skin biopsy Screening tests for systemic involvement

[a]Percentage of new dermatology outpatients with this diagnosis seen in the Hershey Medical Center Dermatology Clinic, Hershey, Pennsylvania.
[b]Of inpatient dermatology consultations, 2% are for vasculitis.

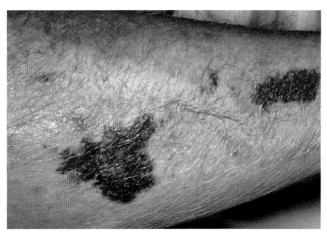

Fig. 17.1 **Actinic purpura**—macular purpura with a regular border (ecchymosis).

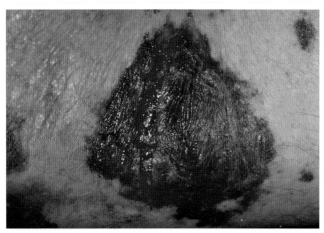

Fig. 17.2 **Actinic purpura** with tear in skin secondary to slight trauma.

History

The trauma that induces the purpura is often so minor that it is not remembered by the patient. The patient has no symptoms, and health is unaffected.

Physical Findings

In actinic purpura, ecchymoses are characteristically confined to the dorsa of the hands and forearms and are vaguely round or oval. The skin itself in these areas may also be more fragile and may tear easily (Fig. 17.2).

> Actinic purpura occurs only on the hands and forearms.

Another clinical finding is the development of stellate pseudoscars (Fig. 17.3). These thin-line scars result from the healing of the skin tears.

Differential Diagnosis

The diagnosis of actinic purpura is relatively straightforward, thereby making a differential diagnosis not necessary. It is important to recognize exacerbating factors for actinic purpura,

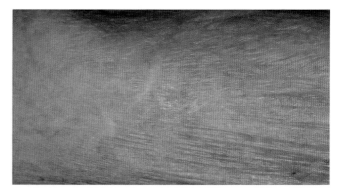

Fig. 17.3 **Stellate pseudoscars on forearm**—thin white scars resulting from the healing of skin tears, commonly seen with actinic purpura.

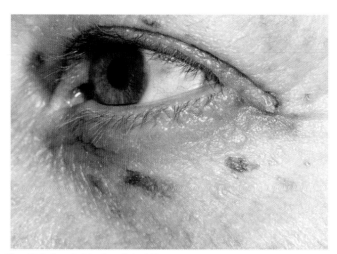

Fig. 17.4 **Amyloidosis**—"pinch" purpura.

mainly medications that increase the risk of bleeding with trauma. Other causes of blood vessel fragility, in declining order of frequency, are corticosteroid use, amyloidosis, and Ehlers–Danlos syndrome. Steroid purpura with skin atrophy can result from topically or systemically administered corticosteroids. Patients with excessive systemic steroids also have moon facies, a "buffalo hump" on the upper back, purple striae, and, in younger patients, steroid acne.

> Common Medications That Contribute to Blood Vessel Fragility
> 1. Nonsteroidal antiinflammatory drugs
> 2. Anticoagulants
> 3. Systemic and topical steroids
> 4. Supplements (*Ginkgo biloba*, vitamin E)

In patients with amyloidosis, the amyloid may infiltrate the skin and result in papules and nodules, which are most often present on the face, particularly the eyelids. These characteristically bleed easily. Purpura also occurs in the absence of papules and can be precipitated by minor trauma or the Valsalva maneuver, referred to as "pinch" purpura (Fig. 17.4). The tongue may also be enlarged.

Ehlers–Danlos syndrome is the least common cause of blood vessel fragility. Several variants of this syndrome are known, in which joint hyperextensibility, skin hyperelasticity, increased fragility of the skin, and an increased tendency to bruise occur in varying combinations. Ecchymoses resulting from blood vessel fragility are distinguished from vasculitis by being macular and from the ecchymoses in DIC by their usually smooth rather than ragged contour and by the absence of necrosis. Additionally, patients with DIC will be febrile and toxic appearing.

DIFFERENTIAL DIAGNOSIS FOR ACTINIC PURPURA

- Steroid purpura
- Amyloidosis (rare)
- Ehlers–Danlos syndrome (rare)

Ecchymoses resulting from fragile blood vessels have a smooth border and are not necrotic.

Laboratory and Biopsy

Because the diagnosis of actinic purpura is obvious clinically, a biopsy is not required. If a biopsy is done, hemorrhage without inflammation will be noted in the dermis, along with actinically damaged collagen, which appears disorganized, smudged, fragmented, and more basophilic than normal collagen on routine hematoxylin and eosin staining (Fig. 17.5).

Therapy

No therapy exists for actinic purpura. Protection against sun exposure with sunscreens is advisable to prevent further damage. Avoidance of prolonged topical steroid use is recommended. It is important to offer reassurance that the condition is benign.

Course and Complications

Ecchymoses slowly fade, leaving brown macules from residual hemosiderin. New ecchymoses, however, continue to develop.

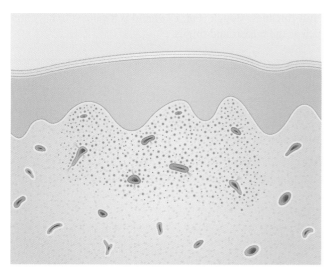

Fig. 17.5 Actinic purpura. Epidermis—normal. Dermis—confluent hemorrhage in the superficial dermis; damaged collagen.

Scars frequently occur after tearing of the skin and are referred to as stellate pseudoscars.

Pathogenesis

The diseases of blood vessel fragility have the problem of defective collagen in common, which weakens the vessels and makes them more susceptible to bleeding from minor trauma. In actinic purpura, blood vessel fragility results from both aging and the damaging effect of sunlight on the connective tissue that provides support to blood vessels in sun-exposed skin. Steroid purpura results from the inhibition of collagen metabolism by high-dose corticosteroids. In amyloidosis, amyloid material infiltrates and weakens the vessel walls. In Ehlers–Danlos syndrome, fragility of blood vessels results from an intrinsic abnormality in collagen biosynthesis.

DISSEMINATED INTRAVASCULAR COAGULATION

KEY POINTS

1. Life-threatening
2. Seen in bacterial sepsis (meningococcemia)
3. Stellate purpura with central necrosis is characteristic
4. Treat underlying condition

Definition

Disseminated intravascular coagulation (also called consumption coagulopathy and defibrination syndrome) is a condition in which uncontrolled clotting results in diffuse thrombus formation. The skin is frequently affected, with thrombosed vessels causing skin necrosis. Hemorrhage from these vessels appears as ecchymoses (Fig. 17.6). Petechiae also occur as a result of thrombocytopenia from platelet consumption. Purpura fulminans can be confused with the term DIC. Purpura fulminans is the cutaneous marker of DIC, characterized by the sudden appearance of very large ecchymosis, symmetrically distributed mainly on the extremities. Skin necrosis often develops in purpura fulminans in the setting of DIC and is most commonly associated with an infection (Fig. 17.7).

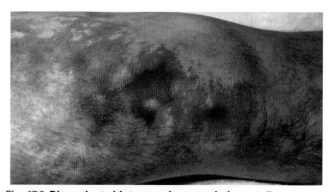

Fig. 17.6 Disseminated intravascular coagulation—stellate purpura. Dark gray areas are necrotic and eventually slough; petechiae are also present.

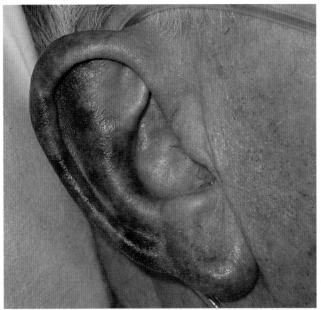

Fig. 17.7 Purpura fulminans. This patient had *Escherichia coli* sepsis and developed acral gangrene, including necrosis of the ear skin tissue.

Incidence

As an uncommon, life-threatening disease, DIC usually occurs in the setting of bacterial sepsis (particularly meningococcemia). DIC may be also associated with malignancy, particularly prostatic carcinoma and acute promyelocytic leukemia. It can also be precipitated by massive trauma. Occasionally, it may result from amniotic fluid embolism, or it may occur as an idiopathic or "postinfection" phenomenon. Localized intravascular coagulation occurs in patients with protein C deficiency who are given warfarin (warfarin-induced skin necrosis).

Causes of DIC:
1. Bacterial sepsis
2. Malignancy
3. Amniotic fluid embolism
4. Massive trauma
5. Idiopathic

History

Patients with DIC are usually systemically ill, often severely so. Fever and shock are frequently present. Symptoms of infection (e.g., headache and stiff neck with meningococcal meningitis) should be sought. A history of a malignancy may be important. Patients with purpura fulminans often have a prodrome of upper respiratory tract symptoms from viral or streptococcal infection. Patients with warfarin-induced skin necrosis are not affected systemically but rather develop localized areas of skin hemorrhage and necrosis approximately 1 week after starting warfarin.

Physical Findings

Patients are febrile or toxic appearing. Various hemorrhagic skin lesions may be present. The most distinctive is a purpuric, stellate or retiform (net-like) ecchymosis, which often appears

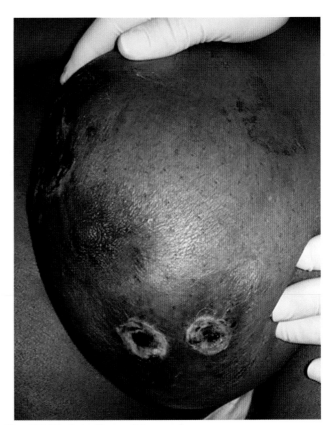

Fig. 17.8 Warfarin (Coumadin) **necrosis**.

to be necrotic in the center. The stellate shape is characteristic of blood vessel thrombosis with infarction. Dark gray central areas indicate necrosis and impending slough. Most lesions are flat, but palpable purpura occurs in approximately 20% of patients as a result of edema associated with skin infarction and necrosis, rather than inflammation. Petechiae may be present, but ecchymoses are more than two-thirds of lesions, and hemorrhagic bullae, acral cyanosis, mucosal bleeding, dissecting hematomas, and prolonged bleeding from wound sites can also occur. Warfarin-induced skin necrosis is usually limited to one or a few body sites, but the skin involvement is severe and results in a full-thickness slough (Fig. 17.8) and is localized to fatty areas such as the breasts and thighs.

Stellate purpura with dark gray central areas indicates thrombosis and infarction.

Differential Diagnosis

Ecchymoses from fragile blood vessels are round or oval, have smooth borders, and are not necrotic; DIC-related ecchymoses are irregular (stellate or retiform) in outline and often become necrotic. In addition, patients with DIC are usually severely systemically ill. In contrast to vasculitic lesions, the purpura in DIC is usually flat but may be occasionally palpable following necrosis. Elevated lesions in DIC can be distinguished from those of vasculitis by a skin biopsy. In bacterial sepsis, vasculitis and DIC can coexist. TTP can lead to purpura but from

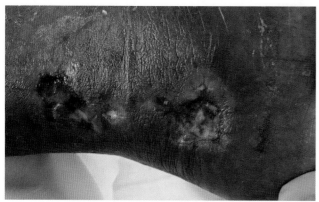

Fig. 17.9 Calciphylaxis. Note that purpura surrounding ulceration is more difficult to notice on the posterior thigh in this Black patient.

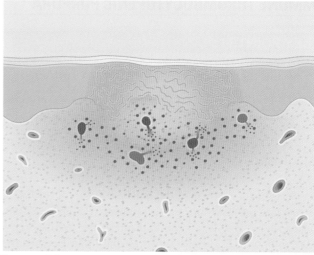

Fig. 17.10 Disseminated intravascular coagulation. Epidermis—central necrosis. Dermis—fibrin thrombi in the capillaries of the middle to upper dermis; hemorrhage from necrotic vessels; no inflammation.

a distinct mechanism; widespread endothelial damage causes platelet activation, leading to thrombosis. TTP does not occur in the setting of sepsis, as in DIC. Severe liver disease can cause a reduction in the production of coagulation factors, leading to blood vessel fragility. Calciphylaxis can appear clinically similar to DIC but is distinguished by its association with chronic renal failure and firmness to palpation secondary to underlying skin vessel calcification. Calciphylaxis is very painful, tends to localize the legs, and impends a poor prognosis (Fig. 17.9).

Laboratory and Biopsy

DIFFERENTIAL DIAGNOSIS FOR DISSEMINATED INTRAVASCULAR COAGULATION
• Ecchymoses
• Vasculitis
• TTP
• Coagulopathy secondary to liver disease
• Calciphylaxis

The laboratory findings characteristic for DIC are thrombocytopenia, prolonged prothrombin time, hypofibrinogenemia, and the presence of fibrin and fibrinogen degradation products. Of these tests, the platelet count and fibrinogen levels are the most useful for diagnosing and following patients with DIC.

A skin biopsy reveals the presence of intravascular thrombi, blood vessel necrosis, and extravasated red blood cells with little or no associated inflammation. Epidermal and dermal necrosis may result from infarction (Fig. 17.10).

Therapy

In DIC, the most important principle is to treat the underlying condition. Clotting factors should be repleted with infusions of platelets, cryoprecipitate (for fibrinogen and factor VIII), and fresh plasma (for factor V). Clinical thromboses, which occur particularly in patients with malignancy-associated DIC, are additionally treated with heparin to help control the clotting. Patients with warfarin necrosis are also treated with heparin. Full-thickness skin necrosis may occur, particularly in warfarin necrosis, and requires skin grafting for repair.

THERAPY FOR DISSEMINATED INTRAVASCULAR COAGULATION
Initial
• Treatment of underlying condition
• Repletion of clotting factors
• Heparin (in select patients with intravascular thromboses)

Course and Complications

A serious disorder, DIC has an overall mortality rate of about 50%. Early diagnosis and prompt therapy improve survival. Cutaneous complications result from infarction, causing necrosis of the skin and the tips of the digits.

Pathogenesis

The primary process appears to be widespread thrombus formation, in which coagulation factors are consumed. Fibrinogen, the target protein, is acted on by thrombin and plasmin, and fibrin clots are formed. In DIC associated with gram-negative bacterial sepsis, bacterial endotoxins are thought to induce this process. Cytokines such as tumor necrosis factor may also play a role. The clotting process also produces fibrinogen and fibrin degradation products that act as anticoagulants. These anticoagulants compound the bleeding diathesis produced by the consumption of clotting factors.

Patients with inherited or acquired protein C deficiency are also susceptible to intravascular coagulation. Protein C is a vitamin K-dependent anticoagulant. Patients with congenital absence of protein C die early in life from purpura fulminans with internal thromboses. Patients who have inherited or acquired protein C deficiency are susceptible to recurrent venous thromboses and to skin necrosis if warfarin is administered. Warfarin causes necrosis in these patients by depleting their marginal reserves of protein C before depleting the vitamin K-dependent clotting factors. The resultant imbalance in the anticoagulation-to-coagulation ratio allows the formation of clots with subsequent skin necrosis.

IMMUNE THROMBOCYTOPENIC PURPURA

KEY POINTS

1. Petechiae are a major clinical finding.
2. Drugs are a common cause.
3. Check platelet count.
4. Treatment depends on cause.

Definition

Immune thrombocytopenic purpura (ITP) is a blood disorder caused by a decrease in the number of blood platelets due to autoantibodies against platelet antigens. Petechiae are purpuric macules less than 3 mm in diameter that can be seen in this condition (Fig. 17.11). Larger purpura called ecchymoses can sometimes be seen. Examples of conditions leading to deficient platelet production include drugs (e.g., heparin), preceding viral infection, rheumatic disease (e.g., lupus), hematologic malignancy, and idiopathic (no clear association). TTP is a rare blood disorder associated with small-vessel thromboses, resulting in low platelets. Patients with TTP are severely ill and manifest ecchymoses, as opposed to patients with ITP.

Causes of thrombocytopenic purpura:
1. Drugs
2. Viral infections
3. Collagen vascular disease
4. Hematologic malignancy
5. Pregnancy (unique cause and not discussed)
6. Idiopathic
7. TTP (rare)

Incidence

Of the causes listed, drugs are often associated with thrombocytopenic purpura in adults. In children, especially younger than age 10 years, ITP is most often precipitated by a viral infection and has an annual incidence of 4 per 100,000 children; spontaneous remission often occurs. About 15,000 new cases of ITP are diagnosed in the United States each year. TTP is uncommon.

History

In patients with petechiae, a drug history is important. Systemic symptoms should also be sought. For example, children with ITP usually have a history of a viral infection within the preceding 1–3 weeks. TTP is accompanied by fever, hemolytic anemia, and neurologic symptoms. It can be associated with pregnancy and rheumatic disease. Ecchymoses dominate in TTP, though petechiae may be present, and the physical examination findings can be similar to DIC.

Physical Findings

Petechiae may be generalized but are usually most pronounced in areas of dependency. Easy bruising, described as ecchymoses or nonpalpable purpura, may be noted, and mucosal bleeding may also be present, so the conjunctivae and oral cavity should be examined carefully. Splenomegaly is frequent in patients with hematologic malignancies or chronic ITP.

Differential Diagnosis

It is most important to determine the etiology of the petechiae by extensive history and physical examination, with close attention to causes of increased platelet destruction. High-risk conditions associated with ITP include infections (e.g., hepatitis), autoimmune disorders, and malignancy. Certain medications (discussed below) and alcohol abuse can lead to low platelets and should be considered in the differential diagnosis. Petechiae can also result from increased intravascular pressure with forceful retching or coughing (Fig. 17.12). This Valsalva maneuver results in nonpalpable petechiae on the face, neck, and upper trunk. Leakage of blood from capillaries also occurs in pigmented purpura (a.k.a. Schamberg disease), an idiopathic capillaritis, in which inflammation (although not sufficient to cause elevation of the lesion) weakens the capillaries so they leak (Fig. 17.13). Pigmented purpura is one of the most commonly encountered petechial diseases in dermatology. This causes nonpalpable petechiae of the lower legs that have been likened in appearance to cayenne pepper. Petechiae in the lower extremities can also occur in the setting of venous stasis, particularly if the patient also has dermatitis. Scurvy results from a vitamin C deficiency and can present with perifollicular petechiae,

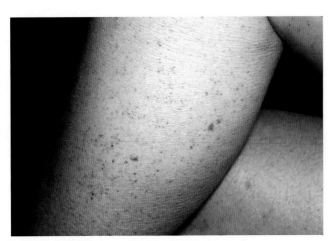

Fig. 17.11 **Petechiae**—small (<3 mm) purpuric macules.

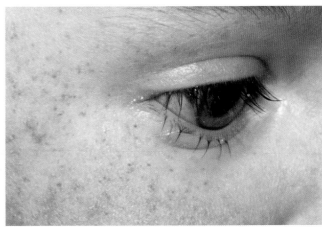

Fig. 17.12 **Petechiae on the cheek** in a 2-year-old child after forceful retching.

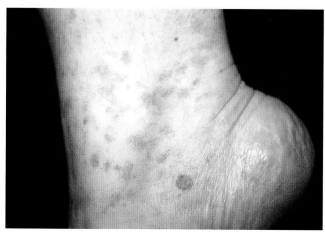

Fig. 17.13 Pigmented purpura—patches of petechiae (best seen under magnification) on lower leg.

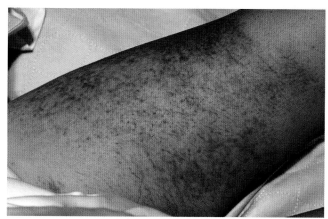

Fig. 17.14 Scurvy—petechiae, purpura, and corkscrew hairs on leg. (Photo courtesy Bryan E. Anderson, MD.)

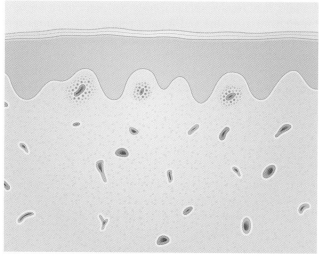

Fig. 17.15 Petechiae. Epidermis—normal. Dermis—hemorrhage around superficial vessels.

Screening tests:
1. Complete blood cell count
2. Platelet count
3. Urinalysis
4. Stool guaiac

Therapy

Therapy is aimed at the underlying disorder. If a drug is the cause, its discontinuation solves the problem, usually within several days. Therapy is not always needed in children with acute thrombocytopenic purpura, as spontaneous remission often occurs. Both prednisone and intravenous γ-globulin (IVIG) have been used with good effect in symptomatic children. Chronic ITP (defined by a platelet count of <100,000 cells/mm^3 for >6 months) is often treated with several therapies, including therapeutic plasma exchange (TPE), glucocorticoids, rituximab, and caplacizumab, a humanized monoclonal antibody that prevents von Willebrand factor from binding to platelets, which reduces the formation of microthrombi. A referral to a hematologist is in order!

THERAPY FOR ITP

Initial
- Discontinue drug (if drug induced)
- TPE
- Prednisone (for ITP)

Alternative
- Rituximab
- Caplacizumab

ecchymosis, most commonly on the lower extremities, and characteristic corkscrew hairs (Fig. 17.14). Scurvy is most commonly seen in alcoholics and patients on restrictive diets.

DIFFERENTIAL DIAGNOSIS FOR ITP
- DIC
- Identify high-risk conditions associated with ITP
- Medications
- Pigmented purpura
- Scurvy

Laboratory and Biopsy

In patients with nonpalpable petechiae, a complete blood cell count and platelet count should be taken. Bleeding from thrombocytopenia usually does not occur unless the platelet count is less than 50,000/mm^3. A platelet count of less than 20,000/mm^3 results in bleeding from even minor trauma, and a count of less than 10,000/mm^3 predisposes the patient to internal bleeding.

Urinalysis and guaiac testing of the stool help to screen for bleeding from the urinary and gastrointestinal tracts. Skin biopsy enables noninflammatory petechiae to be distinguished from vasculitis, although the clinical picture is usually so distinctive that a biopsy is not required (Fig. 17.15).

Course and Complications

The course and complications depend on the nature of the underlying disease. Drug-induced thrombocytopenia can produce bleeding at other sites, particularly the gastrointestinal tract. Virus-induced acute thrombocytopenia resolves without therapy and without complications in 90% of children. ITP in adults may resolve spontaneously but more often becomes chronic with a waxing and waning course that requires splenectomy in many patients. ITP is the presenting problem in some patients with underlying "autoimmune" diseases such as systemic lupus erythematosus. TTP, a distinct and much more severe disorder, was associated with a 75% mortality rate. With plasma exchange and infusion therapy, this rate has been reduced to 25%.

Pathogenesis

Platelets normally plug small defects in capillary walls and also help to initiate the clotting mechanism. Deficiency or dysfunction of platelets leads to "leaky" vessels.

Drugs can cause both thrombocytopenia and platelet dysfunction. Drug-induced thrombocytopenia results from either a toxic or an antibody-mediated mechanism. Drugs causing immunologic platelet destruction include quinidine, quinine, sulfonamides, heparin, digitoxin, phenytoin (Dilantin), and methyldopa. Aspirin causes platelet dysfunction through the inhibition of thromboxane production.

Drugs that can cause thrombocytopenia:
- Quinidine
- Quinine
- Sulfonamides
- Heparin
- Digitoxin
- Phenytoin
- Methyldopa

Cancer chemotherapy causes thrombocytopenia through the inhibition of marrow production. Decreased platelet production occurs in hematologic malignancies as a result of bone marrow replacement with malignant cells.

An autoimmune mechanism is operative in virus-induced acute childhood thrombocytopenia and chronic ITP. In these disorders, immunoglobulin G (IgG) antiplatelet antibodies bind to specific platelet membrane glycoproteins. The immunoglobulin-coated platelets are then recognized and removed by the reticuloendothelial system, especially the spleen.

VASCULITIS

KEY POINTS

1. Palpable purpura represents vasculitis.
2. Rule out systemic involvement.
3. Biopsy confirms the diagnosis.
4. Treatment depends on the cause.

Definition

Strictly speaking, any inflammation of blood vessels could be called "vasculitis," although the term is generally used to describe an autoimmune necrotizing reaction in blood vessels. Numerous vasculitides have been described and are best

---

TABLE 17.2 Types of Vasculitis (note that not all conditions will be discussed in this chapter)

1. Small-vessel vasculitis:
   a. Hypersensitivity vasculitis
   b. Rheumatic disease–associated vasculitis (lupus vasculitis, rheumatoid vasculitis)[a]
   c. Malignancy-associated vasculitis
   d. IgA vasculitis[a]
   e. ANCA-associated vasculitis[a]
   f. Hypocomplementemic urticarial vasculitis[a]
   g. Antiglomerular basement membrane disease (no skin findings)
   h. Cryoglobulinemic vasculitis[a]
   i. Other:
      i. Erythema elevatum diutinum
      ii. Golfers vasculitis (also called Disney vasculitis)
      iii. Hemorrhagic edema of infancy
2. Medium-vessel vasculitis[a]:
   a. Polyarteritis nodosa
   b. Kawasaki disease
3. Large-vessel vasculitis[a]:
   a. Takayasu arteritis
   b. Giant cell arteritis
   c. Thrombangiitis obliterans

ANCA, Antineutrophil cytoplasmic antibody; *IgA*, immunoglobulin A.
[a]Systemic vasculitis.

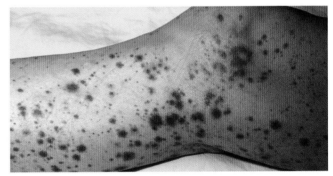

Fig. 17.16 Vasculitis—purpuric papules.

---

categorized by the size of the vessel affected, small, medium, or large—see Table 17.2 (such as the Chapel Hill Consensus Criteria). Vasculitis can affect multiple organ systems (systemic vasculitis) or just the skin (nonsystemic or isolated cutaneous small-vessel vasculitis). The small-vessel vasculitis category affects capillaries and postcapillary venules and represents the plurality of cases. Small-vessel vasculitis presents with palpable petechiae (often called palpable purpura, though this term is less accurate) (Fig. 17.16). The lesions are elevated (palpable) because of inflammation and edema, and purpuric because of the extravasation of blood from damaged blood vessels.

Palpable purpura indicates small-vessel vasculitis.

This process is mediated by immune complexes and neutrophils. The key histopathologic findings are termed *leukocytoclastic vasculitis*. Leukocytoclastic vasculitis is not a diagnosis and can occur in a variety of settings. Most small-vessel vasculitis is a secondary process, with causes including sepsis, viral infections, collagen vascular disease (particularly systemic lupus erythematosus and rheumatoid arthritis), cryoglobulinemia, drug reactions, and, occasionally, malignant lymphoma and myeloma. Small-vessel vasculitis confined to the skin following a viral infection, caused by a medication, or in which an underlying cause cannot be found is called *hypersensitivity vasculitis*. This is the most common type of vasculitis across all categories.

Systemic vasculitis results in the inflammation of blood vessel walls of any organ, including the skin, and is often a serious life-threatening condition. Systemic vasculitis incorporates a few types of small-vessel diseases and all cases of medium- and large-vessel vasculitis. Systemic vasculitis commonly involves the kidneys, peripheral nerves (often asymmetric mononeuropathy), the respiratory tract, and the gut. The most common *systemic vasculitis* is IgA vasculitis, formerly known as Henoch–Schönlein purpura. This small-vessel condition often follows a mild infection. Children manifest the tetrad of palpable purpura, arthritis, abdominal pain, and minor transient kidney disease (Fig. 17.17). Adults are at higher risk for serious kidney involvement.

ANCA-associated vasculitis (AAV) is a serious primary small-vessel systemic vasculitis. Devastating renal and sinopulmonary involvement are common.

ANCA-associated vasculitides:
1. Granulomatosis with polyangiitis
2. Eosinophilic granulomatosis with polyangiitis
3. Microscopic polyangiitis

Medium-vessel vasculitides, such as polyarteritis nodosa (PAN), do not feature petechiae, but rather feature tender subcuticular nodules, stellate or retiform purpura that may feature necrosis, and livedo reticularis. Patients with AAV or PAN are often febrile or toxic appearing. Large-vessel vasculitis rarely has skin findings, outside of rare cases of watershed necrosis.

Causes of cutaneous vasculitis:
1. Infections
   - Bacterial
   - Rickettsial sepsis
   - Viral (hepatitis C virus)
2. Collagen vascular diseases
   - Systemic lupus erythematosus
   - Rheumatoid arthritis
3. Cryoglobulinemia
4. Drugs
5. Lymphoma and myeloma
6. Idiopathic
   - Henoch–Schönlein purpura
   - Hypersensitivity

Incidence

Cutaneous vasculitis is uncommon. Among new patients seen in the authors' dermatology clinic, 0.3% had cutaneous vasculitis. It was more common in their hospital practice: 2% of the dermatology consultations were for vasculitis.

History

Systemic disease must be ruled out, and history is the first step in doing so. In febrile or toxic-appearing patients with cutaneous vasculitis, infection must be considered. Bacteria causing septic vasculitis include *Neisseria meningitidis*, *Neisseria gonorrhoeae*, *Staphylococcus aureus*, *Streptococcus pneumoniae*, Viridans streptococci, and *Pseudomonas aeruginosa*. Fever may also occur in patients with viral infection, collagen vascular disease, AAV, and even drug reactions, but the first responsibility is to rule out infection. Rickettsial sepsis (Rocky Mountain spotted fever [RMSF]), in which the abrupt onset of fever is accompanied by headache and myalgia, is followed several days later by an erythematous rash, which characteristically begins on the wrists and ankles and then involves the palms and soles as it becomes generalized and petechial (Fig. 17.18). The history and appearance of the rash permit an early clinical diagnosis of this disease, which is fatal if not treated promptly.

First, rule out infection as the cause of vasculitis in the febrile or toxic-appearing patient.

The rash in RMSF starts on the wrists and ankles.

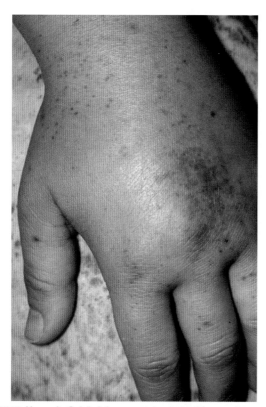

Fig. 17.17 **Henoch–Schönlein purpura**—petechiae and purpura in association with joint swelling from arthritis.

Symptoms of multisystem involvement in systemic vasculitis may include arthritis, hematuria, abdominal pain and melena, cough and hemoptysis, and neurologic involvement with headaches and peripheral neuropathy. The presence of these features

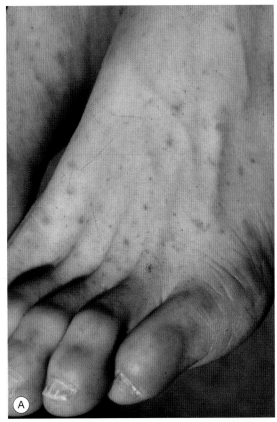

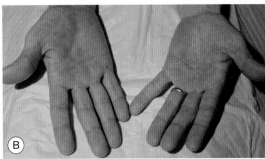

Fig. 17.18 Rocky Mountain spotted fever. (A) Petechiae on dorsal feet. (B) Palmar involvement with dusky papules, which evolved into purpura.

should prompt serological evaluation for systemic vasculitis, described below. Although drug-induced vasculitis is uncommon, drug history is important. The drugs most frequently implicated include aspirin, phenothiazines, penicillin, sulfonamides, and thiazides.

Workup for patients with systemic vasculitis:
- Complete blood count (CBC)
- Comprehensive Metabolic Panel (CMP)
- Hepatitis B/C/HIV
- Erythrocyte sedimentation rate (ESR)/ C-reactive protein (CRP)
- ANCA
- Rheumatoid factor (RF)/ Cyclic citrullinated peptide (CCP)
- Antinuclear antibodies (ANA)
- Compliment component 3 (C3)
- Compliment component 4 (C4)
- Cryoglobulins
- Serum protein electrophoresis (SPEP) with immunofixation

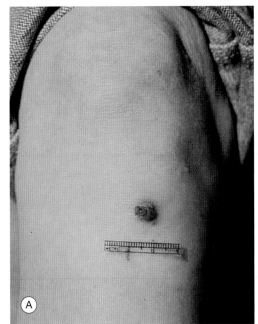

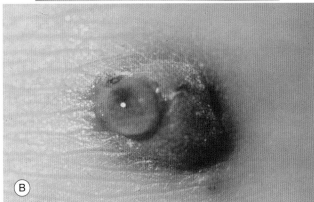

Fig. 17.19 Gonococcemia. (A) Hemorrhagic (purpuric) pustules sparsely distributed on distal extremities. (B) Close-up of hemorrhagic pustule.

Physical Examination

The primary lesion in cutaneous vasculitis is a purpuric papule (palpable petechiae, or less accurately, palpable purpura). Necrosis sometimes follows; it is heralded by the appearance of a dark gray color in the center of a lesion, followed by slough. In the absence of necrosis, lesions evolve by flattening and fading. The flattening may occur surprisingly quickly, so a lesion that is palpable on the first day may be flat by the second. As lesions fade, hemosiderin remains, leaving the affected skin brown. In gonococcemia, lesions are distinctive in that they are pustular as well as purpuric, sparse, and distributed distally on the extremities (Fig. 17.19). Lesions of vasculitis are most often located on the lower extremities, but they may be generalized in patients with extensive disease.

Gonococcemia is characterized by purpuric pustules in acral distribution.

Differential Diagnosis

Most cases of cutaneous vasculitis are secondary, following any of the long list of causes discussed above. Hypersensitivity

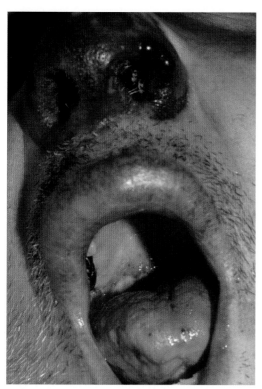

Fig. 17.20 Granulomatosis with polyangiitis—a type of antineutrophil cytoplasmic antibody–associated vasculitis—necrotic lesions of the nose and ulcerations in the mouth are due to the vasculitis of larger vessels.

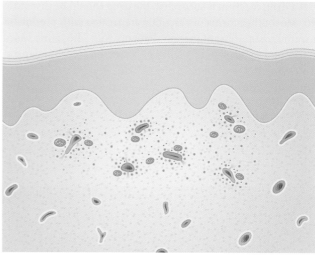

Fig. 17.21 Vasculitis. Epidermis—normal. Dermis—neutrophils and nuclear debris in and around the blood vessels; endothelial swelling and necrosis of blood vessel walls; hemorrhage.

Laboratory and Biopsy

The diagnosis of vasculitis is confirmed by a skin biopsy. The histologic features are as follows: (1) the presence in and around the blood vessel walls of neutrophils with leukocytoclasis (i.e., destruction of neutrophils leaving nuclear debris), (2) hemorrhage, (3) endothelial cell swelling, and (4) fibrinoid necrosis of the vessel wall (Fig. 17.21). Immunofluorescent evaluation is mandatory in small-vessel vasculitis to evaluate for the presence of IgA, which confirms the diagnosis of IgA vasculitis.

All patients with small-vessel vasculitis require a baseline urine analysis (UA) to assess for protein or red cell casts. Laboratory tests are used to rule out systemic involvement or specific systemic diseases, but only in patients with a positive review of systems (fever, arthritis, neuropathy, hemoptysis, epistaxis, etc.) or a UA demonstrating protein or red cell casts. Blood cultures should be obtained in all patients with vasculitis and fever. Acute and convalescent serologic titers confirm (posthumously, if treatment is not instituted early in the disease) a diagnosis of RMSF. Other laboratory work includes a complete UA, guaiac test of stool, CBC with differential and platelet count, sedimentation rate, serum creatinine, serum protein electrophoresis, cryoglobulins, antinuclear antibody test, RF, viral hepatitis serology, and chest radiography.

> Obtain blood cultures in patients with vasculitis and fever.

Therapy

The treatment is for the underlying disease, if one is found. In patients with suspected bacterial sepsis, treatment should be instituted immediately, not after culture results are returned. Meningococcemia is a dramatic example in which a treatment delay of a few hours can mean the difference between a favorable and a fatal outcome. The same is true for RMSF, in which early treatment (with tetracycline) is life-saving and must be instituted on the basis of clinical suspicion.

vasculitis is overwhelmingly the most common type of vasculitis, following URI, medication, or may be idiopathic. Ruling out infectious causes of vasculitis in febrile toxic-appearing patients is most important because of the threat of mortality (e.g., RMSF). Other broad categories for the causes of vasculitis include inflammatory (e.g., collagen vascular), drug, and underlying malignancy. Distinguishing vasculitis from causes of nonpalpable purpura can usually be accomplished by an examination alone. The causes of nonpalpable purpura were listed above. Lesions in DIC may be flat or elevated. Those that are elevated are so because of the edema that acutely accompanies necrosis. Vasculitis may coexist with DIC in some patients who have bacterial sepsis (e.g., meningococcemia)—bacterial emboli cause the vasculitis, and endotoxin initiates the DIC. Patients with medium-vessel vasculitis (e.g., PAN) frequently experience necrosis and ulcerations of the skin as a manifestation of the destruction of vessels that are larger than those involved in the vasculitis lesions discussed above (Fig. 17.20).

DIFFERENTIAL DIAGNOSIS FOR VASCULITIS

- Identify the category of the cause
  - Rule out infection first
  - Inflammatory
  - Drug
  - Malignancy
- DIC

If a drug reaction is suspected, the drug should be discontinued. Most other forms of vasculitis are treated with prednisone or immunosuppressant therapy. Patients with idiopathic vasculitis limited to the skin respond well to prednisone, but dapsone also frequently controls the process and is safer for long-term administration. Colchicine has also been used with success in some patients. One should not be overzealous in the treatment of cutaneous vasculitis because this condition is chronic and often does not affect the viscera. Systemic vasculitis like AAV or PAN often requires advanced specialist care in an inpatient setting, utilizing medications like rituximab or cyclophosphamide.

THERAPY FOR VASCULITIS

Initial
- Treat infection if suspected
- Treat underlying disease
- Discontinue implicated drugs, if any
- For acute noninfectious vasculitis: prednisone

Alternative
- For chronic cutaneous vasculitis:
  - Dapsone
  - Colchicine
  - Immunosuppressants

Course and Complications

The course and complications depend on the underlying disease and extent of organ involvement by the vasculitis. Vasculitis associated with bacterial or rickettsial sepsis responds promptly to antibiotic therapy. If a drug is responsible, its withdrawal solves the problem. Purpuric lesions associated with viral diseases (e.g., enterovirus infections and atypical measles) resolve spontaneously. Idiopathic cutaneous vasculitis has a tendency to wax and wane, frequently over a period of years, and is not usually a harbinger of serious internal involvement. The skin disease in IgA vasculitis is usually self-limited, but renal impairment persists in nearly 30% of adult patients (persistent renal disease is rare in children). Cutaneous vasculitis associated with rheumatic diseases may be severe but often improves with control of the underlying disease. AAV and PAN are often life-threatening and may cause lasting damage or necrosis in the kidneys, lungs, or gut.

Serious complications are related less to the skin than to internal organ involvement, with the kidney most often and usually most seriously affected.

Kidney is the most frequently involved internal organ.

Pathogenesis

Most small-vessel vasculitis is an immune complex-mediated disease. The antigen in the immune complex may be exogenous (e.g., bacterial, drug) or endogenous (e.g., another antibody, as in RF, or nuclear antigens, as in lupus). These circulating immune complexes lodge in the walls of blood vessels; in the skin, small venules are most often involved. The propensity for involvement in the lower legs may relate to hydrostatic forces that predispose to sluggish blood flow and immune complex deposition. The complement cascade is then activated, producing chemotactic factors that attract polymorphonuclear leukocytes into the vessel wall. Lysosomes are released from the leukocytes and cause sufficient damage to the vessel wall to permit the extravasation of red blood cells.

Most small-vessel vasculitis is a type III immune complex reaction.

The antibodies in the immune complexes are usually of the IgG or IgM class, with the exception of Henoch–Schönlein purpura, in which they are characteristically IgA. AAV is caused by autoimmune intravascular neutrophil degranulation caused by ANCA binding.

Dermal Induration

CHAPTER CONTENTS

Algorithm for dermal induration

Dermal induration

↓

Inflammatory

Granuloma annulare

↓

Uncommon

Lichen sclerosus
Necrobiosis lipoidica
Scleroderma/morphea
En coup de sabre
Sarcoidosis

ABSTRACT

Induration represents dermal thickening, resulting in skin that feels thicker or firmer than normal. Scleroderma is the disease that best exemplifies this process. All the diseases included in this chapter are uncommon conditions, except for granuloma annulare. Stasis dermatitis, a cause of dermal induration of the lower extremities, has a significant epidermal component and is discussed in Chapter 8. For all causes of dermal induration, a skin biopsy is often necessary to confirm the diagnosis, where the degree of dermal inflammation varies depending on whether the biopsy is performed at an early or late (burned out) stage of the disease process. Treatment options are limited and usually have minimal impact on the disease course.

KEY POINTS
1. Dermal induration presents with firm and thickened skin.
2. A skin biopsy is often necessary for the diagnosis.
3. Diseases tend to run a natural course despite treatment intervention.

GRANULOMA ANNULARE

KEY POINTS
1. Self-limiting, asymptomatic condition with papules arranged in an annular configuration
2. Commonly affects children and young adults
3. Occurs mostly on dorsal hands and feet

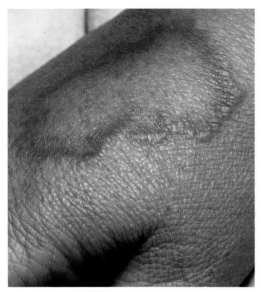

Fig. 18.1 **Granuloma annulare**—annular dermal plaque.

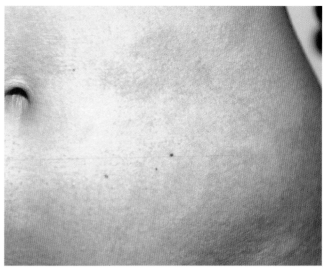

Fig. 18.2 **Generalized granuloma annulare**—brownish plaques with serpiginous borders.

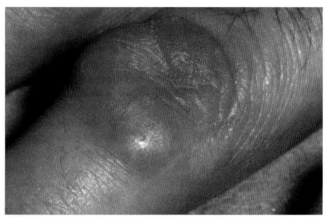

Fig. 18.3 Subcutaneous granuloma annulare.

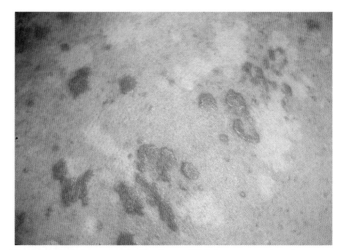

Fig. 18.4 **Cutaneous sarcoidosis**—reddish brown, annular plaques.

Definition

Granuloma annulare (GA) is an asymptomatic skin condition characterized by dermal papules (no overlying epidermal change), forming annular plaques and commonly arising on the dorsal hands and feet (Fig. 18.1). Although the center of the plaques becomes depressed, the leading edge of the papules represents dermal induration. GA is most often localized but can be generalized.

Incidence

GA appears most commonly in children and young adults and affects females more commonly than males. The localized form of GA is much more common than the generalized form of GA.

History

The lesions are usually asymptomatic and come to the attention of the physician because of cosmetic concerns. Some patients mistakenly treat the condition for tinea corporis because of the annular configuration.

Physical Examination

The localized variant appears as shiny dermal papules and annular plaques that are centrally depressed. GA can be skin colored, violaceous, or erythematous. Generalized GA can affect the entire body (Fig. 18.2). Other, less common, variants are subcutaneous (deep dermal solitary nodules) (Fig. 18.3) and perforating (papules with central umbilication that is crusted and ulcerated). Both the subcutaneous and perforating variants of GA appear on the distal extremities.

Clinical variants of GA:
1. Localized
2. Generalized
3. Subcutaneous
4. Perforating

Differential Diagnosis

GA can be confused with other, often more serious, conditions. Papular GA can appear similar to papular *sarcoidosis* (Fig. 18.4) and *lichen planus*. A skin biopsy easily distinguishes between these conditions. Necrobiosis lipoidica (NL), also called necro-biosis lipoidica diabeticorum (NLD), can appear clinically and histologically similar to GA. NLD often has a yellowish hue, and telangiectasias are present centrally within the depressed plaques on the lower legs. NL has a stronger association with diabetes mellitus than GA, hence its alternative name NLD. Subcutaneous GA can appear similar to a rheumatoid nodule, both clinically and histologically. Arthritis is not present with GA. Annular GA is most often confused with tinea corporis, but a lack of scale in GA should enable the clinician to distinguish between the two.

DIFFERENTIAL DIAGNOSIS FOR GRANULOMA ANNULARE
• Sarcoidosis • Lichen planus • NL • Rheumatoid nodule • Tinea corporis

Annular plaques of GA have no scale; tinea corporis has scale.

Laboratory and Biopsy

Laboratory workup with GA is not usually necessary. Diabetes mellitus has been reported to be associated with generalized GA. A skin biopsy shows necrobiosis (degenerative collagen) in the dermis with a predominantly histiocytic (i.e., macrophages) and multinucleated giant cell infiltrate on the periphery (Fig. 18.5).

Therapy

Treatment of GA is unsatisfactory. For young children, spon-taneous resolution occurs. Therefore no treatment is the best

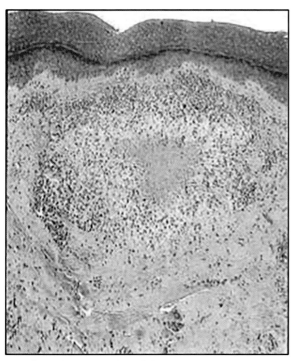

Fig. 18.5 Granuloma annulare. Epidermis—normal. Dermis—note a central area of collagen degeneration surrounded by an inflammatory infiltrate necrobiosis (degenerative collagen).

treatment (i.e., benign neglect). For cosmetically disfiguring lesions, treatment with potent topical corticosteroids, such as fluocinonide 0.05% cream, or intralesional triamcinolone 5–10 mg/mL may be effective. Skin atrophy is always a con-cern with prolonged topical or intralesional corticosteroid use. Topical calcineurin inhibitors (topical tacrolimus 0.1% and topical pimecrolimus 0.1%) can be helpful for long-term treatment of GA in skin areas at high risk for steroid-induced skin atrophy or patients who do not respond to topical cor-ticosteroids. Narrow-band ultraviolet B (UVB) light therapy and the antimalarial hydroxychloroquine (200 mg b.i.d.) are reserved for patients with generalized GA. In refractory cases, biologic agents have been utilized (e.g., adalimumab). No well-designed studies favor any systemic therapy.

Localized GA often resolves spontaneously.

THERAPY FOR GRANULOMA ANNULARE
Initial • Observation • Topical steroids (fluocinonide 0.05% cream) • Intralesional steroids (triamcinolone 5–10 mg/mL) • Topical calcineurin inhibitors (tacrolimus 0.1% ointment or pimecrolimus 1% cream) **Alternative (for Generalized Variant)** • Narrow-band UVB • Antimalarial (hydroxychloroquine 200 mg b.i.d.)

Course and Complications

After 2 years, approximately 75% of GA lesions will disap-pear. Recurrences are not uncommon. This is a self-limiting disease.

Pathogenesis

The cause remains unknown.

LICHEN SCLEROSUS

KEY POINTS
1. Sclerotic white plaques 2. Often affects genital skin 3. Pruritic

Definition

Lichen sclerosus is a chronic inflammatory condition that results in sclerotic white plaques due to thickening of the super-ficial dermis with an overlying, thinned, finely wrinkled epider-mis (Fig. 18.6). Genital involvement of lichen sclerosus is more common than nongenital involvement, and it can coexist with morphea, suggesting that the two diseases are related. Pruritus is often a major complaint.

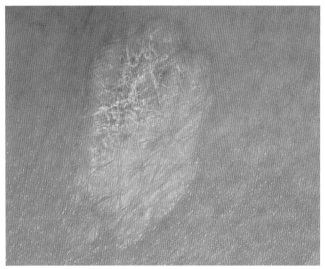

Fig. 18.6 Lichen sclerosus et atrophicus—sclerotic white plaque with wrinkled, atrophic epidermis.

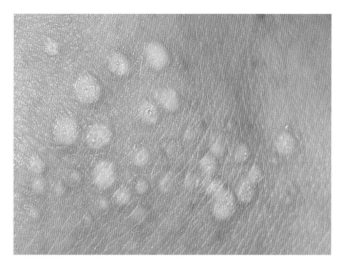

Fig. 18.7 Lichen sclerosus et atrophicus—guttate papules.

Incidence

Lichen sclerosus is an uncommon disease that typically occurs in middle-aged adults, although uncommon cases in children have been reported. There does not seem to be a sex predilection.

History

Lichen sclerosus involving nongenital skin is mostly asymptomatic but can be dry and pruritic. The lesions can be cosmetically disfiguring. Involvement of the genitalia can result in intractable pruritus, leading to the development of dyspareunia in women and phimosis in men. In young females, the initial appearance of lichen sclerosus can have a bruise-like quality (resembling traumatic hemorrhage) and lead to the misdiagnosis of child abuse.

> Bruise-like quality of lichen sclerosus in young females can lead to a misdiagnosis of child abuse.

Physical Examination

Nongenital disease occurs primarily on the trunk and extremities. The initial lesions appear as guttate (i.e., drop-like), white papules that can coalesce into larger plaques (Fig. 18.7). The sclerotic plaques are covered by a finely wrinkled (often referred to as cigarette paper- or parchment-like) epidermis. In women, the vulva and perianal area are often involved, resulting in a figure-of-eight configuration. The initial erythema evolves into a hypopigmented sclerotic plaque that may erode and scar, making sexual intercourse difficult (Fig. 18.8). The corollary in men is foreskin involvement leading to phimosis.

> Guttate white papules are characteristic of early lichen sclerosus.

Differential Diagnosis

The two key differential diagnoses are morphea for nongenital lichen sclerosus and sexual abuse with genital lichen sclerosus in

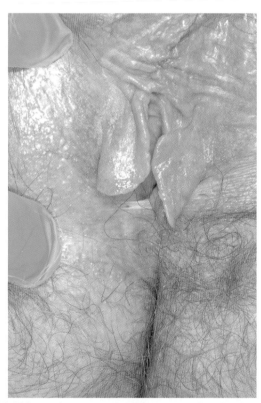

Fig. 18.8 Lichen sclerosus et atrophicus—note the adhesion developing at lower vaginal introitus and faint pinkness. Skin biopsy confirmed the diagnosis.

boys and girls. Early squamous cell carcinoma (erythroplasia of Queyrat) can mimic erosive genital lichen sclerosus (Fig. 18.9), and a biopsy is mandatory.

DIFFERENTIAL DIAGNOSIS FOR LICHEN SCLEROSUS

- Morphea
- Sexual abuse (for genital lichen sclerosus)
- Squamous cell carcinoma (for erosive genital lichen sclerosus)

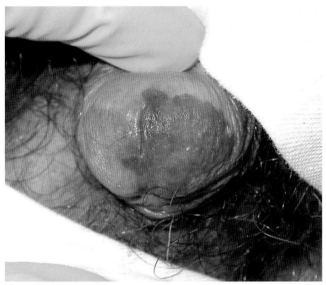

Fig. 18.9 Erosive genital lichen sclerosis—eroded plaque on glans penis; a biopsy is performed to rule out squamous cell carcinoma.

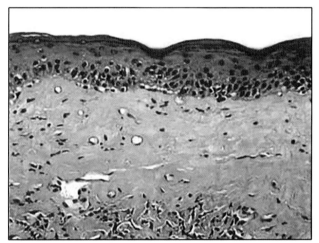

Fig. 18.10 Lichen sclerosus. Epidermis—flattened dermoepidermal junction. Dermis—homogenized (smudgy collagen) in the upper dermis.

> Biopsy erosive lichen sclerosus of the genitals to rule out squamous cell carcinoma.

Laboratory and Biopsy

Lichen sclerosus is not associated with any systemic disease. A biopsy shows a homogenized (smudgy collagen) superficial dermis with a flattened dermoepidermal junction (Fig. 18.10).

Therapy

Emollients and ultrapotent steroids are the treatment of choice in genital lichen sclerosus for both children and adults. Clobetasol propionate 0.05% ointment needs to be applied nightly for 2–3 months followed by a reduced maintenance schedule. Even with long-term use, no major side-effects, including atrophy, have been reported in studies. The authors sometimes recommend topical steroids on alternate days to avoid skin breakdown. Alternatively, topical calcineurin

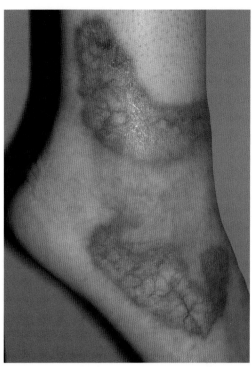

Fig. 18.11 Necrobiosis lipoidica—yellow plaques with atrophic centers and prominent blood vessels.

inhibitors (aka macrolides) used twice daily for 3–6 months have been shown to be effective. For nongenital lichen sclerosus, judicious use of ultrapotent topical corticosteroids is recommended. For severe, generalized disease, acitretin at a dose of 25–50 mg/day for 3–4 months has anecdotally been reported to be effective. Recurrence of disease with treatment discontinuation is always a concern.

THERAPY FOR LICHEN SCLEROSUS

Initial
- Emollients
- Topical ultrapotent steroids (clobetasol propionate 0.05% ointment or cream)

Alternative
- Topical macrolides (tacrolimus or pimecrolimus b.i.d.)
- Acitretin 25–50 mg/day for generalized disease

NECROBIOSIS LIPOIDICA

KEY POINTS

1. Plaques with reddish brown active border and yellowish depressed center with telangiectasias.
2. Involves anterior shins.
3. Two-thirds of patients have abnormal glucose tolerance.

Definition

Necrobiosis lipoidica (NL) is characterized by distinctive, well-circumscribed, yellowish plaques with a yellow center commonly affecting the anterior lower legs (Fig. 18.11). It is often, but not always, associated with diabetes mellitus, hence the use of the alternative term, "necrobiosis lipoidica diabeticorum."

> Necrobiosis lipoidica is strongly associated with diabetes.

Incidence

Necrobiosis lipoidica occurs more commonly in females than in males, with a 3:1 ratio. Approximately 0.3% of patients with diabetes suffer from NL. Young adults are most commonly affected.

History

The plaques of NL evolve slowly over a number of years and are often brought to the attention of the physician because of cosmetic disfigurement. Rarely, the condition ulcerates and becomes painful.

Physical Examination

NL is a brownish red (early) papule that evolves into a plaque. With time, the center of the plaque becomes atrophic, takes on a yellowish hue, and develops prominent telangiectasias. An elevated and sharply defined border is present. The lesion is firm to the touch. Uncommonly, ulcers and erosions develop within the plaques, often following trauma. NL is commonly distributed symmetrically on the anterior shins. Rarely, it appears in a generalized distribution.

> Rarely, ulceration develops within necrobiosis lipoidica following trauma.

Differential Diagnosis

Usually, the clinical appearance is sufficient to make the diagnosis. A skin biopsy is sometimes needed to distinguish between GA and sarcoidosis. Some cases of NL can be confused with stasis dermatitis (Fig. 18.12). Stasis dermatitis has epidermal changes (e.g., scale and crust) that distinguish it from necrobiosis.

> ### DIFFERENTIAL DIAGNOSIS FOR NECROBIOSIS LIPOIDICA
> 1. GA
> 2. Sarcoidosis
> 3. Stasis dermatitis

Laboratory and Biopsy

Abnormal glucose tolerance is detected in two-thirds of patients with NL, hence the historic name of necrobiosis lipoidica diabeticorum. A general rule of thumb to follow for patients with necrobiosis lipoidica is that one-third have diabetes, one-third have abnormal glucose tolerance, and one-third have normal glucose tolerance. A skin biopsy confirms the diagnosis by showing layered granulomatous inflammation in the dermis that is parallel to the epidermis, areas of connective tissue degeneration, and destruction of blood vessels (Fig. 18.13).

> Two-thirds of patients with necrobiosis lipoidica have abnormal glucose tolerance.

Therapy

There is no known effective treatment for NL. The goals of treatment are avoidance of trauma to prevent ulceration and control inflammation to improve appearance. Also, smoking cessation as well as optimizing diabetic control may halt disease progression and decrease the likelihood of ulceration. Potent topical steroids, such as fluocinonide 0.05% cream, and topical calcineurin inhibitors can be applied to the active borders.

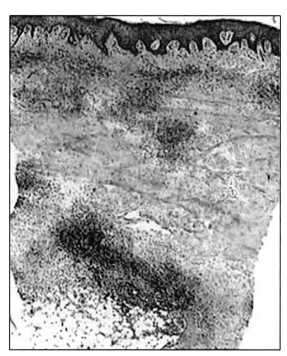

Fig. 18.13 Necrobiosis lipoidica. Epidermis—normal (can be ulcerated). Dermis—layered granulomatous inflammation in the dermis that is parallel to the epidermis, areas of connective tissue degeneration, and destruction of blood vessels

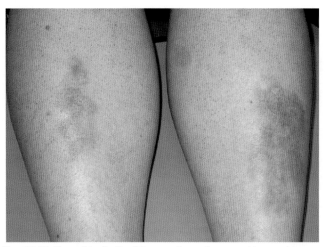

Fig. 18.12 Necrobiosis lipoidica—yellow plaques with atrophic centers on bilateral shins.

Alternatively, intralesional triamcinolone 10 mg/mL can be injected into the active borders to help halt disease expansion. Limited success has been reported with pentoxifylline (Trental; 400 mg b.i.d.) and a host of other agents.

THERAPY FOR NECROBIOSIS LIPOIDICA

Initial
- Optimize diabetic control
- Topical steroid: fluocinonide 0.05% cream b.i.d.
- Topical macrolides (tacrolimus or pimecrolimus b.i.d.)

Alternative
- Intralesional steroids: triamcinolone 10 mg/mL
- Pentoxifylline 400 mg b.i.d.

MORPHEA AND SYSTEMIC SCLEROSIS

KEY POINTS

1. Morphea is sclerosis confined to the skin.
2. Systemic sclerosis (SSc) can be limited (previously called CREST [**c**alcinosis, **Raynaud** phenomenon, **e**sophageal dysfunction, **s**clerodactyly, and **t**elangiectasia]) or diffuse, which involves skin and internal organs, especially the esophagus.
3. Raynaud phenomenon is often present in SSc.
4. Treatment for SSc is supportive but not curative.

Definition

In morphea and SSc, an increase in collagen deposition is found, which results in thickening of the dermis (Fig. 18.14). *Morphea*, previously named localized scleroderma, is confined to the skin. It is distinct from SSc, which is divided into *limited or diffuse* SSc. In both forms, sclerosis starts at the fingers, following a period of nonpitting edema of the hands and Raynaud phenomenon. The sclerosis progresses proximally, and both forms feature facial involvement. In limited SSc, which was formerly called CREST syndrome, sclerosis does not progress past the elbows or knees but also involves the face, esophagus (as reflux with or without dysmotility), and lungs. In diffuse SSc, sclerosis affects the skin more diffusely, extending beyond the elbows and knees, and involves some internal organs, mainly the lungs, heart, esophagus, and kidneys. Lung involvement is usually pulmonary fibrosis in diffuse SSc, and pulmonary hypertension in limited SSc, although either process can be found in both variants. These conditions are all classified as "autoimmune" collagen vascular diseases. The term "scleroderma" was used in various ways to describe all these conditions but led to confusion among patients and clinicians. Standardization of terminology is underway.

> Morphea is localized, confined to the skin; SSc affects the skin and viscera.

Incidence

Both forms of SSc are uncommon. The annual incidence of SSc has been estimated at fewer than three new patients per one million. About 20% of cases occur in children and teenagers. A linear variant of morphea affects children. Otherwise, morphea and SSc are diseases of older adults in the fourth or fifth decades, with women affected three times more often than men.

History

> Morphea is usually asymptomatic; patients present for the treatment because of concern over the appearance of the lesions.

Patients with diffuse or limited SSc frequently have symptoms. Early in the disease, the most common symptom is Raynaud phenomenon, which is characterized by pain and color change of the digits on exposure to cold (Fig. 18.15).

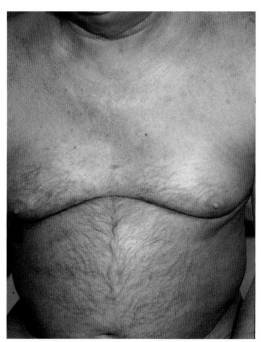

Fig. 18.14 Systemic sclerosis—the epidermis is normal or hyperpigmented, and the dermis is thickened and feels indurated.

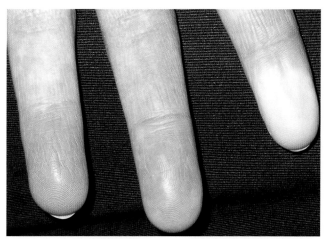

Fig. 18.15 Raynaud phenomenon in a patient with limited systemic sclerosis (CREST syndrome). Note the characteristic red, white, and blue color changes that occurred with exposure to low temperatures.

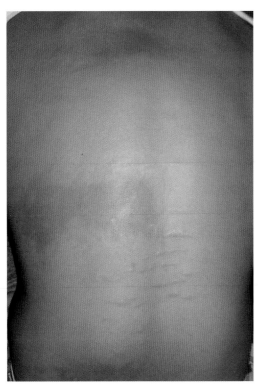

Fig. 18.16 Morphea—indurated, hyperpigmented plaques in mature lesions.

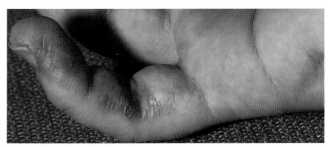

Fig. 18.17 Linear morphea—more common in children.

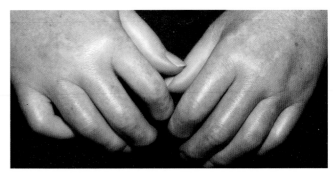

Fig. 18.18 Sclerodactyly in a patient with systemic scleroderma.

The classic color changes are, in sequence, white, purple, and red, but the most important is white, which is caused by cold-induced vasoconstriction. Patients with more advanced disease also notice tightening of the skin, manifested by an inability to open the mouth widely (their dentist may comment on this) and contractures of fingers, causing decreased manual dexterity. Ulcerations of the fingertips also occur frequently. Systemic symptoms include difficulty with reflux, swallowing, joint pain, shortness of breath, or hypertensive crisis.

> White is the most diagnostic color in the Raynaud phenomenon.

Physical Examination

Morphea appears as a sclerotic, asymmetrically distributed, sharply demarcated plaque, which may be flat, slightly elevated, or slightly depressed. Most importantly, it *feels* indurated. Early lesions have a lilac border, indicating inflammatory activity, and a whitish center. Mature lesions are hyperpigmented (Fig. 18.16). Lesions of morphea most often affect the trunk, except for the linear variant, which usually involves the head or an extremity (Fig. 18.17).

The thickened skin in diffuse or limited SSc is not sharply separated from normal skin, although some areas, such as the hands and face (acrosclerosis), may be more thickened than others. Thickened facial skin appears unusually smooth, except around the mouth, where it is furrowed and has a purse-string

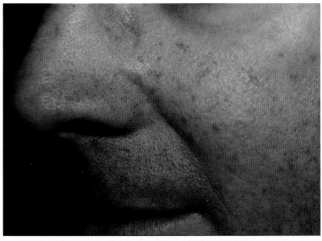

Fig. 18.19 Telangiectasias in a patient with scleroderma.

appearance. Involvement of the digits produces thickened, tapered digits (sclerodactyly; Fig. 18.18). Ulcerations followed by pitted scars occur on the fingertips. In generalized involvement, the skin is often depigmented and may have areas that are speckled light and dark (salt and pepper). Patients with marked generalized thickening of the skin (Fig. 18.14) appear to have the worst prognosis.

Telangiectasia is prominent in some patients, especially in those with limited SSc. It appears as multiple, small, punctate macules that are particularly prominent on the face and hands (Fig. 18.19). Cutaneous calcinosis and impaired esophageal motility also occur in patients with limited SSc, formerly called CREST syndrome.

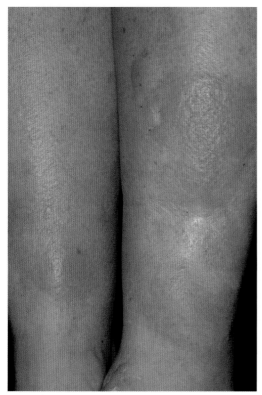

Fig. 18.20 **Myxedema**—indurated red plaques on shins.

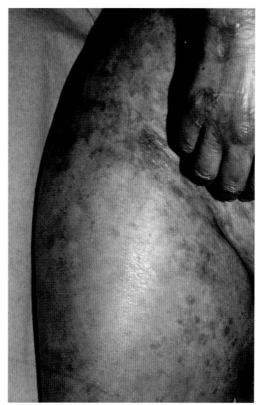

Fig. 18.21 **Chronic graft-versus-host disease**. Note sclerodermoid skin changes.

Differential Diagnosis

The differential diagnosis of morphea includes two uncommon disorders. *Lichen sclerosus* is an idiopathic disorder that appears as a porcelain-white, dermal, indurated plaque with an atrophic, slightly wrinkled epidermis. It most often affects the vulvar area but sometimes occurs in scattered patches on the trunk. Occasionally, lichen sclerosus and morphea coexist. *Necrobiosis lipoidica* occurs most often (but not always) on the lower legs, often in patients with diabetes, as an orange-red, indurated plaque with an atrophic epidermis through which large telangiectatic blood vessels are seen.

The generalized thickened skin in SSc may be confused with several uncommon disorders. In *myxedema* from hypothyroidism, the skin may be markedly thickened, but it feels more doughy than hard (Fig. 18.20). *Scleromyxedema* is a rare disease characterized by mucin deposition in the skin. It can mimic SSc clinically, but the biopsy is diagnostic, and the skin involvement is accompanied by a serum monoclonal immunoglobulin G protein. *Mixed connective tissue disease* is an "overlap" syndrome with features of several rheumatic (i.e., collagen vascular) diseases: SSc, dermatomyositis, and lupus erythematosus. This syndrome is characterized serologically by high levels of antibodies against ribonuclear protein in an extractable nuclear antigen (ENA) testing. In chronic *graft-versus-host disease*, skin manifestations are prominent and may be strikingly similar to those of generalized scleroderma (Fig. 18.21). *Porphyria cutanea tarda* is occasionally accompanied by diffusely thickened, hyperpigmented, "sclerodermoid" skin. The more usual manifestations, however, are blisters and fragility of the skin on the dorsa of the

hands, and hyperpigmentation and hypertrichosis of the upper lateral cheeks.

DIFFERENTIAL DIAGNOSIS OF SCLERODERMA AND MORPHEA

- Lichen sclerosus
- Necrobiosis lipoidica
- Myxedema
- Scleromyxedema
- Mixed connective tissue disease
- Chronic graft-versus-host disease
- Porphyria cutanea tarda

Laboratory and Biopsy

Laboratory tests are not needed in patients with morphea, except for a skin biopsy if the diagnosis is in question. Patients with generalized SSc require laboratory and radiographic evaluation for systemic involvement, which includes a complete blood count, urinalysis, renal function tests, a creatine kinase test (for the evaluation of myopathy), chest radiography, pulmonary function testing, echocardiogram, regular blood pressure testing, and barium swallow. An antinuclear antibody (ANA) test is positive in 95% of patients with SSc. Human epithelial (HEp-2) cells are used as the substrate for the ANA test. The ENA anti-kinetochore (formerly anti-centromere) is strongly associated with limited SSc. Topoisomerase II (formerly anti-Scl-70) antibody is associated with diffuse SSc. These two

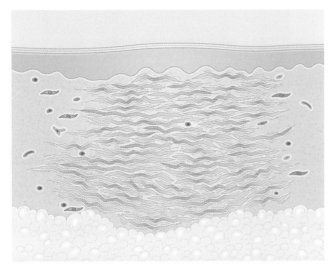

Fig. 18.22 Morphea (early). Epidermis—normal. Dermis—thickened; early morphea appears hypercellular due to inflammatory cell infiltrate, and fibroblasts are actually decreasing in number; collagen bundles are increased in thickness and number.

antibodies are mutually exclusive, but many patients with SSc have neither. Anti-RNA polymerase III antibody is found in patients with rapidly progressive skin involvement and is associated with paraneoplastic disease. There are other serologic tests performed by specialists to assess diagnosis and prognosis.

Laboratory and radiologic tests for SSc:
1. Complete blood count
2. Urinalysis
3. Renal function tests
4. Creatine kinase
5. Chest radiography
6. Antinuclear antibody test
7. Serologic tests (e.g., anti-topoisomerase II, anti-kinetochore antibody, and anti-RNA polymerase III antibody)
8. Pulmonary function tests
9. Echocardiogram
10. Barium swallow

Morphea and SSc show the same histological changes in the skin (Fig. 18.22). Collagen bundles are increased in number and thickness and appear more eosinophilic on hematoxylin and eosin staining. These changes are most marked in the lower two-thirds of the dermis and extend into the subcutaneous fat. Inflammation is present in the early stages, when the diagnosis is easily missed histologically because the collagen changes may not be appreciated. In later stages, the sclerotic process entraps, and finally obliterates, the dermal appendages, with an end result that may resemble a scar. In addition, in the later stages, blood vessels appear thickened, hyalinized, and decreased in number.

Therapy

Treatment of these various conditions is frustrating. Topical, intralesional, and even systemic steroids have been used for morphea, usually with disappointing results. Topical macrolides and calcipotriene have also been used with limited success. For severe cases, especially cosmetically and physically debilitating linear variants, mycophenolate mofetil and methotrexate are often used. Rituximab has also been shown to be effective for severe skin and lung disease. For patients with sclerodactyly and linear variants of morphea, physical therapy should not be overlooked. Daily range-of-motion exercises are important to help limit the flexion contractures that often develop over time. Prompt referral to a specialist who evaluates and treats for organ involvement beyond the skin, mainly the lungs, is important.

THERAPY FOR MORPHEA AND SYSTEMIC SCLEROSIS

Morphea
Initial
- Topical and intralesional steroids (clobetasol 0.05% b.i.d.)
- Topical macrolide (tacrolimus 0.1% b.i.d.)
- Topical calcipotriene with or without steroids

Alternative (for Widespread Disease)
- Systemic steroids
- Mycophenolate mofetil and methotrexate
- Physical therapy for linear variants

Systemic Sclerosis
Initial
- Prednisone
- Mycophenolate mofetil

Alternative
- Rituximab
- Physical therapy (for contractures)

Course and Complications

Morphea is usually limited to a few plaques, although it may be more widespread. Linear morphea in children may be accompanied by the involvement of underlying muscle and even bone, with a resulting atrophy of these tissues. Morphea often "burns out" over time (usually years), with subsequent softening of the affected skin. Residual hypopigmentation or hyperpigmentation is common. Although rare cases of progression to SSc have been reported, in most patients morphea is a benign disease.

SSc is frequently progressive, and death from systemic involvement is not uncommon. Reported 5-year survival rates range from 50% to 90%, depending on the type and extent of visceral involvement. Renal failure, often accompanied by severe hypertension, is a frequent cause of death. Cardiac complications include conduction defects, pericarditis, and heart failure. Pulmonary fibrosis is another serious complication, most commonly in diffuse SSc. Involvement of the smooth muscle of the lower part of the esophagus produces impaired esophageal motility with reflux, causing strictures. Weight loss and malnutrition can result.

The skin thickening often begins with an early, edematous phase followed by hardening and increasing thickening. Cutaneous complications include ulcerations of

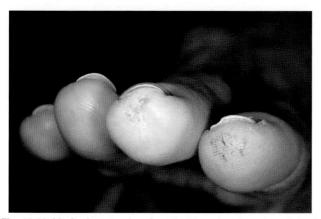

Fig. 18.23 Limited systemic sclerosis. Note the ulceration of the fingertip and the loss of normal contour of the fingertip.

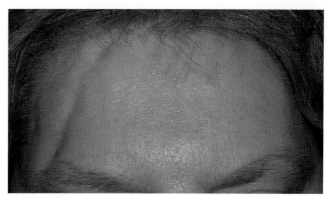

Fig. 18.24 En coup de sabre—indurated linear depression commonly affecting the forehead.

fingertips, sometimes complicated by infection with osteomyelitis (Fig. 18.23). Flexion contractures of the hands and fingers can result from sclerosis.

Pathogenesis

Patients with SSc have an increased rate of collagen biosynthesis in the skin. Although the primary causes are unknown, increasing evidence suggests that the process is immunologically mediated. Several European studies have implicated the spirochete *Borrelia burgdorferi* in the pathogenesis of morphea and have reported success with penicillin treatment in some patients. These results have not been duplicated in the United States. The role, if any, of antinuclear antibodies in the pathogenesis of SSc is unknown. They may be a result, rather than a cause, of the disease.

UNCOMMON CAUSES OF DERMAL INDURATION

En Coup De Sabre

Paramedian sclerotic depressions of the forehead represent a linear variant of morphea (Fig. 18.24). Similar to morphea, purplish borders signal disease activity. It can extend to the eyebrows, nose, or cheek. A severe variant, which can lead to hemifacial atrophy, is called *Parry–Romberg syndrome*. High titers of antinuclear antibodies are frequently present. Treatment is challenging, and methotrexate is often used when cosmetic disfigurement is a concern.

Sarcoidosis

Sarcoidosis is a systemic, granulomatous condition that commonly affects the skin and many organ systems, most often the lungs. The cause remains unknown. Skin lesions can be the first

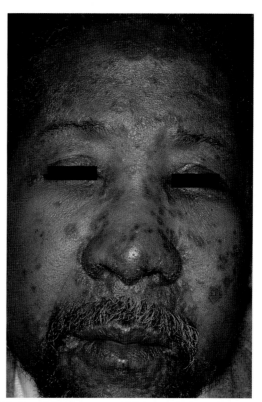

Fig. 18.25 Sarcoidosis—note reddish brown, indurated plaques on the face, a common location.

manifestation of the disease and are characterized by reddish brown papules and plaques, most commonly on the face but can be found at any site (Fig. 18.25). A systemic workup (e.g., assessing for lung involvement) is necessary. A skin biopsy confirms the diagnosis with the demonstration of granulomas mainly in the dermis. Treatment is tailored to the severity of the disease. Topical and systemic steroids, hydroxychloroquine, and antitumor necrosis factor therapy are used based on the severity of the disease.

19

Ulcers

CHAPTER CONTENTS

ABSTRACT

Ulcers have multiple causes, including vascular diseases, neoplasms, hematologic disorders, drug-induced, rheumatic diseases, neurologic disorders, infections, physical etiologies, and idiopathic. The history and physical examination may point to the cause. However, laboratory testing and a skin biopsy are frequently necessary to confirm the diagnosis. Treatment is focused on removing the underlying cause of the ulcer along with good wound care that promotes healing.

KEY POINTS

1. Ulcers have many causes.
2. Good wound care promotes healing.
3. Cure requires resolution of the underlying etiology.

Definition

An ulcer is an open sore that results from the loss of the epidermis and part or all of the dermis (Fig. 19.1). Ulcers have numerous causes (Table 19.1). A detailed history and physical examination are often sufficient to establish a diagnosis; however, laboratory tests and a skin biopsy may be necessary to confirm the initial clinical impression.

Incidence

An ulcer is the chief complaint in 0.5% of the authors' new patients. The frequency of different types of ulcers depends in part on the circumstances of the patient population. For example, decubitus ulcers are a common problem in bedbound patients, whereas leprosy might be considered in a patient from a tropical environment.

History

The history begins with the mode of onset. Is the ulcer acute or chronic? The sudden appearance of severe pain in an extremity suggests *arterial occlusion* due to an embolus or thrombus. The gradual onset of pain with exertion relieved by rest is characteristic of intermittent claudication due to *arteriosclerosis*. A history of lower leg heaviness, aching, and swelling, particularly after periods of inactive standing or sitting, is typical of *venous stasis*.

History:
1. Onset
2. Symptoms
3. Neoplasm
4. Family history
5. Social history
6. Travel
7. Medications

Patients with *neoplastic* ulcers often have a history of a growth that preceded the ulceration. A family history is important in the diagnosis of ulcers caused by *hemoglobinopathies* such as thalassemia and sickle cell anemia.

Factitial ulcers are suspected in patients with a history of certain personality disorders, such as borderline, and typically react to their often dramatic ulcers with indifference. If an ulcer is painless, a *neurotrophic* ulcer should be suspected.

Various *infectious agents* cause ulceration. Acute onset after wildlife exposure in a patient with fever, chills, and malaise suggests a diagnosis of tularemia, *Yersinia pestis* (i.e., plague), or anthrax. Travel history is particularly an important factor in considering tropical diseases, such as amebiasis or leishmaniasis. Sexual history is important if a venereal cause is suspected.

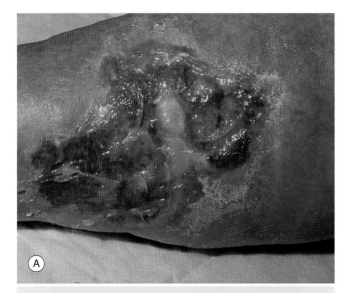

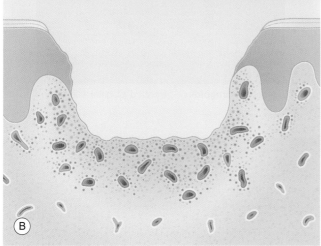

Fig. 19.1 **Stasis ulcer**. (A) Irregularly shaped ulcer surrounded by a red, sclerotic plaque. (B) Epidermis—absent. Dermis—partial loss, chronic inflammation, dilated capillaries.

The *drug* history should not be overlooked. Medications alone, however, are a rare cause of ulcers. More often, ulcers are secondary to drug-induced epidermal necrolysis or vasculitis. Allopurinol, barbiturates, anticonvulsants, and antibiotics may cause these eruptions. The cause of a *physical* ulcer is usually not a diagnostic problem because it is readily apparent to the patient.

Physical Examination

The physical examination should include characteristics of the ulcer (e.g., size, shape, color), its location (e.g., leg, genitals, buttock), and associated physical findings (e.g., surrounding skin, pulses, neurologic findings). Changes in skin color, skin temperature, and pulse pattern suggest *arteriosclerotic* peripheral vascular disease. The skin is purplish red with dependency but changes to pallor when the extremity is elevated. In chronic severe ischemia, the skin and muscles become atrophic in association with hair loss and brittle, opaque nails. The skin is cool, and peripheral pulses are lost. Patients with ischemic leg or ankle ulcers may also have ulceration of the toes.

TABLE 19.1 Etiology of Ulcers

Vascular
- Venous stasis
- Arteriosclerosis
- Thromboangiitis obliterans
- Vasculitis
- Embolic—tumor, infections (subacute bacterial endocarditis)
- Hypertension
- Calciphylaxis
  Alpha-1-antitrypsin deficiency
  Erythema induratum
  Livedoid vasculopathy

Neoplastic
- Carcinoma—cutaneous or metastatic
- Lymphoma—mycosis fungoides
- Sarcoma—Kaposi sarcoma

Hematologic
- Hemoglobinopathy—sickle cell anemia, spherocytosis, thalassemia
- Dysglobulinemia—cryoglobulinemia, macroglobulinemia
  Hypercoagulopathic disorders

Drug Related
- Methotrexate
- Bleomycin
- Ergot
- Coumarin
- Heparin
- Iodine
- Bromine
  Illicit drugs

Rheumatic Disease
- Rheumatoid arthritis
- Lupus erythematosus
- Scleroderma
- Dermatomyositis

Neurologic
- Neuropathic—diabetes, syringomyelia, tabes dorsalis, leprosy, trigeminal trophic syndrome
- Factitial

Infectious
- Bacteria—atypical mycobacteria, tuberculosis, diphtheria, anthrax, tularemia, chancroid, granuloma inguinale, syphilis
- Fungi—blastomycosis, histoplasmosis, chromomycosis, sporotrichosis, cryptococcosis, coccidioidomycosis, aspergillosis
- Protozoa—leishmaniasis, amebiasis
- Virus—herpes

Physical
- Chrome
- Coral
- Beryllium
- Radiation
- Trauma
- Cold
- Heat
- Pressure (decubitus)
- Bites (brown recluse spider)

Unknown
- Pyoderma gangrenosum
- Necrobiosis lipoidica
- Aphtous ulcers
- Behcet disease
- Crohn disease

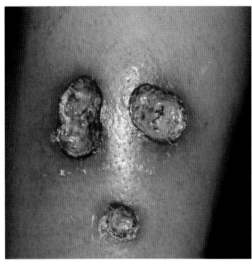

Fig. 19.2 Vasculitis—multiple, punched out ulcers on the leg of a patient with rheumatoid arthritis.

> Physical examination:
> 1. Size, shape, and color of ulcer
> 2. Location
> 3. Associated physical findings

Lower leg edema, induration, brownish discoloration, petechiae, and dermatitis are typical of *venous insufficiency*. Stasis ulcers (Fig. 19.1) rarely occur below the level of the malleolus. Varicose veins may or may not be prominent.

Multiple small ulcers (0.5–2 cm) occurring predominantly on the lower legs suggest *vasculitis* (Fig. 19.2). The ulcer borders are usually purpuric, hemorrhagic, and necrotic. Crusted purpuric papules and nodules also occur.

The development of individual or multiple cutaneous nodules that become ulcerated is characteristic of an underlying *neoplasm* (Fig. 19.3). However, a preceding nodule is not always present in a malignant ulcer. Ulceration of the lower third of the leg above the ankle in a Black adult patient is a major manifestation of homozygous *sickle cell disease* (Fig. 19.4).

Areas of pressure and trauma, particularly in a numb foot, are susceptible to the development of a *neuropathic ulcer* (mal perforans), which occurs mainly in patients with diabetes or leprosy. The ulcer frequently has a significant softened, macerated callus.

Geometric, bizarrely shaped, angular ulcers are characteristic of a self-inflicted *factitial* cause. Genital ulceration is highly suggestive of a venereal cause, which may be *herpes simplex*, *syphilis*, *chancroid*, or *granuloma inguinale*.

The most common physical ulcer (3% of hospitalized patients) is the *pressure sore* or *decubitus ulcer*. Shearing forces, friction, moisture, and pressure contribute to the development of these ulcers. Patients who are mostly confined to their beds or wheelchairs and thus unable to ambulate are most at risk. These patients are usually elderly and frequently incontinent. The most common sites are the sacral and coccygeal areas, ischial tuberosities, and greater trochanter. These ulcers begin as irregular, ill-defined, reddish, indurated areas that resemble

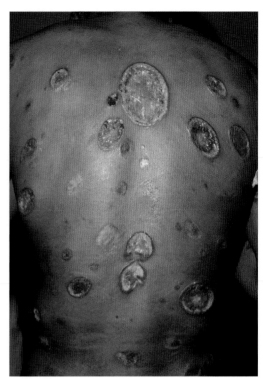

Fig. 19.3 Mycosis fungoides—ulcerated plaques and tumors on the back.

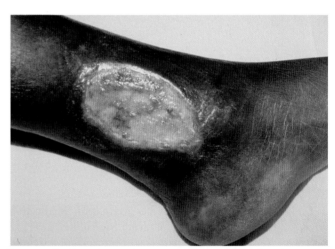

Fig. 19.4 Sickle cell anemia—lower leg ulcer in a Black patient.

abrasions. A full-thickness skin defect develops with extension into the subcutaneous tissue and ultimately, penetration into the deep fascia and muscle.

A rapidly developing, painful ulcer with an undermined edge and gangrenous border is characteristic of *pyoderma gangrenosum* (Fig. 19.5). These ulcers usually occur on the lower legs. Pyoderma gangrenosum is frequently associated with ulcerative and granulomatous colitis, rheumatoid arthritis, and myeloproliferative diseases.

Laboratory and Biopsy

Laboratory tests are necessary to confirm the origin of some ulcers after the history and physical examination. Several *vascular studies* can be used to assess for peripheral vascular disease.

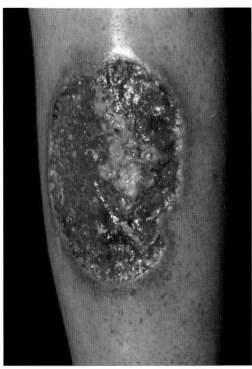

Fig. 19.5 **Pyoderma gangrenosum**—leg ulcer in a patient with inflammatory bowel disease.

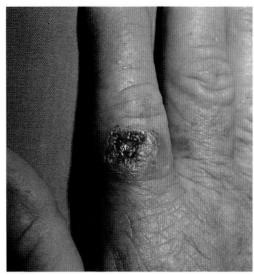

Fig. 19.6 **Sporotrichosis**—finger ulcer developed after traumatic injury while gardening.

Indirect and direct noninvasive testing are used initially to determine arterial competence. The ankle: brachial index is the best screening test to rule out peripheral arterial disease. When limb salvage is indicated, selective arteriography and/or arterial duplex ultrasonography can locate and define the extent of arterial obstruction. Photoplethysmography is performed in patients to delineate venous and arterial pathologic and physiologic abnormalities. In addition, photoplethysmography can be used to determine cutaneous blood perfusion at ulcer margins and thus help to predict the potential for healing. Venous duplex scanning is used to rule out venous insufficiency, deep vein thrombosis, and superficial thrombophlebitis.

Laboratory tests:
1. Vascular studies
2. Blood tests
3. Cultures
4. Biopsy

Several *blood tests* can be helpful in the workup of ulcers. Serologic testing for rheumatic disease is best performed only when other clinical features support suspicion and include tests for antinuclear antibody, rheumatoid factor, anti-DNA antibody, antiphospholipid antibodies, and lupus anticoagulant. Patients with suspected hematologic disorders can be diagnosed with the appropriate tests for sickle cell anemia, spherocytosis, thalassemia, and dysglobulinemias.

Cultures are necessary for diagnosing tropical or unusual infections. Routine cultures of chronic ulcers generally grow out of a mixture of organisms. However, antibiotic therapy for secondarily infected ulcers without treatment of the underlying cause does not result in healing. Diagnostic radiography is indicated when underlying osteomyelitis is a potential complication.

A *biopsy* is indicated for all chronic ulcers of unknown origin and is particularly helpful in ruling out neoplasms. Vascular causes of ulcers, including venous stasis and vasculitis, have characteristic histologic changes. Infectious ulcers are diagnosed by skin biopsy, with special stains used to demonstrate the causative organism. In addition, a portion of the biopsy specimen is sent to the microbiology laboratory for culture (Fig. 19.6).

Biopsy chronic ulcers of unknown origin, to rule out cancer.

Therapy

Appropriate treatment depends on correctly identifying and removing the cause. Venous or arterial insufficiency is the most common cause of ulceration in the ambulatory patient, and correcting the underlying vascular abnormality, if possible, is paramount. For example, *stasis ulcers* are unlikely to heal in a patient with persistent edema caused by incompetent veins. External compression of venous-diseased legs is the most effective therapy. Initially, stasis ulcers and edema are treated with a compressive boot that is changed weekly. After healing, knee-high, medium-pressure elastic compression stockings are used to prevent recurrent stasis ulcers.

Surgery, chemotherapy, and radiotherapy are used to treat *neoplastic ulcers*. The most important treatment for *neuropathic* ulcers and *pressure sores* is prevention of pressure, friction, and trauma. Pressure is relieved with mechanical devices, such as orthotic shoes for a diabetic patient with a foot ulcer. *Infection* requires appropriate antibiotic therapy. Removal of the offending *drug* is the obvious remedy for ulcers caused by drugs.

The general management of ulcers includes measures that promote wound healing, such as medical or surgical debridement, occlusive dressings, treatment of infection, and good nutrition. Numerous agents are used to remove devitalized and purulent tissue from wounds, including moist to dry dressings with normal saline.

Occlusive dressings made from various polymers (e.g., polyethylene, polyurethane) have made a significant contribution to ulcer therapy. These dressings keep the ulcer moist, a feature that promotes epidermal repair through the migration of epithelial cells over the ulcer. Initially, large amounts of exudate form under the occlusive dressing, which remove crust and necrotic debris through a process of autolytic digestion. The dressing must be changed every 2–3 days because of exudate buildup, but with healing, the dressing may be changed less frequently (i.e., every 5–7 days). Another characteristic of occlusive dressings is significant pain relief.

The use of oral and topical antibiotics is often ineffective because of the development of resistant bacteria. Antibiotics should be reserved for ulcers that are complicated by cellulitis, lymphangitis, or septicemia.

Surgical intervention (bypass graft or thromboendarterectomy) is required in patients with peripheral vascular disease. In venous ulcers that have failed to respond to more conservative therapy, skin grafting is often necessary.

THERAPY FOR ULCERS

Initial

Correct or Treat the Underlying Cause
- Venous insufficiency—compression boot or stocking
- Arterial insufficiency—surgery
- Neoplasm—surgery, chemotherapy, radiotherapy
- Infection—antibiotics, antifungals, antivirals
- Neuropathic or decubitus ulcer—remove pressure
- Vasculitis or pyoderma gangrenosum—prednisone, dapsone, immunosuppressants, biologics, treatment of associated disease

Promote Wound Healing
- Cleanse and/or debridement—surgical, enzymes
- Dressings—nonadherent, occlusive, or moist to dry

Alternative
- Secondary infection control—antibiotics
- Skin grafting

Course and Complications

The healing rate of ulcers is related directly to successful treatment of the cause and aggravating factors, as well as prevention of complications. For example, a venous stasis ulcer may persist for years if treated inadequately. Removal of aggravating factors such as secondary infection and necrotic debris promotes ulcer healing. Complications such as cellulitis, lymphangitis, septicemia, and osteomyelitis may complicate healing and prolong the duration of the ulcer.

Complications:
1. Cellulitis
2. Lymphangitis
3. Septicemia
4. Osteomyelitis

Pathogenesis

Infectious agents, toxic chemicals, physical injury, and loss of nutrition from interruption of the cutaneous vasculature cause cell death, tissue loss, and ulceration. As long as cell death continues, the ulcer will persist.

Ulcer healing is a complex biological process that requires an intact vascular supply, inflammation, and proliferation of fibroblasts, endothelial cells, and keratinocytes. Dermal integrity depends on the synthesis of collagen, elastin, and proteoglycans (ground substances) by fibroblasts. Epidermal repair requires the proliferation and migration of keratinocytes over a fibrin–fibronectin support matrix. Inflammation always accompanies the wound healing process, in which the macrophage is the essential and most important cell. Various growth factors (e.g., epidermal, platelet-derived, fibroblast, and transforming growth factor-β) appear to have a role in wound healing by enhancing reepithelialization and granulation tissue.

SELF-ASSESSMENT

Case 1—Ulcer Behind the Ear (Fig. 19.7)
What Is Your Differential Diagnosis of This Ulcer?

The differential diagnosis of an ulcer is extensive. Neither the history nor the physical examination gives us a clue to its origin. However, a negative medical history and normal general physical examination make a vascular, hematologic, neurologic, drug, connective tissue disease, or physical cause of this ulcer less likely. This leaves a neoplastic, infectious, or unknown origin.

What Would You Do Now?

The next step is a biopsy of the ulcer.

What Is the Best Treatment?

The biopsy revealed a basal cell carcinoma. Treatment was the excision of the tumor with the Mohs technique, which conserves as much normal skin as possible and ensures the greatest potential for cure.

IMPORTANT POINTS
1. Ulcers of unknown origin must be examined by biopsy to rule out neoplasm.
2. Appropriate therapy is dictated by the correct identification of the cause.

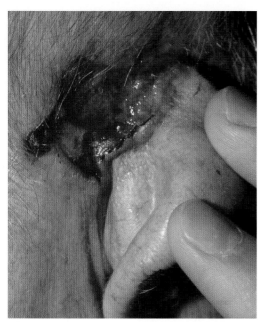

Fig. 19.7 This 60-year-old man had a 1-year history of a nonhealing ulcer. He had otherwise been in excellent health and had no previous history of ulcers. The general physical examination was normal. The skin examination revealed a fair-skinned Caucasian man with a 6-cm shallow ulcer behind his ear. The base of the ulcer was clean, and the surrounding skin appeared normal. The patient had used a number of topical preparations and had been treated with systemic antibiotics without success.

Case 2—Lip Ulcer (Fig. 19.8)
How Would You Complete the Physical Examination?

Palpate the lesion and feel for local lymph nodes. This lesion felt firm and indurated. The patient's head and neck were examined for lymphadenopathy, but none was found.

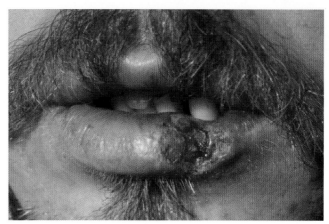

Fig. 19.8 This 33-year-old man presented with a lesion on the lower lip that started with a "cigarette burn" 1 year earlier. He remained a heavy smoker. On examination, you see a crusted and scaling ulcer.

What Is Your Most Likely Diagnosis?

For a chronic mucous membrane ulcer, squamous cell carcinoma is the favored diagnosis. The suspicion is heightened by the finding of induration.

How Would You Confirm It?

A biopsy is required. In this case, it confirmed the diagnosis of squamous cell carcinoma. The lesion was totally excised subsequently.

IMPORTANT POINTS

1. Smoking is a risk factor for the development of mucous membrane squamous cell carcinoma.
2. Biopsy is required for all chronic ulcers, especially when these lesions are indurated.

20

Hair Disorders

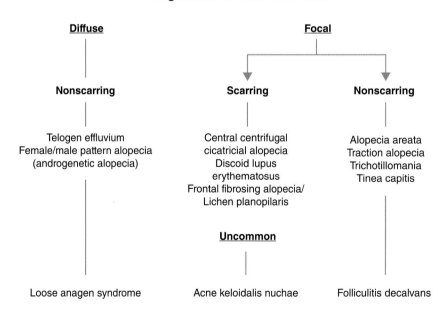

Algorithm for Hair Disorders

ABSTRACT

The evaluation of a patient with hair loss requires a detailed history, physical examination, and, in some cases, laboratory tests and biopsy (Table 20.1). Important elements of the history include the time of onset, medications taken, recent emotional or physical stress, diet, grooming techniques, and family history of baldness or hair disorders.

The physical examination is helpful in making an accurate diagnosis by observing the pattern (patchy or diffuse) of

TABLE 20.1   Alopecia

	Incidence (%)[a]	History	Physical Examination	Scarring	Pattern	Differential Diagnosis	Laboratory Test (Biopsy)
Alopecia areata	0.9	Acute onset	Exclamation point hairs	Absent	Circular patches	Trichotillomania Secondary syphilis Fungal infection	None
Discoid lupus erythematosus	<0.1	Photosensitivity Other symptoms of lupus	Erythema Follicular plugs	Present	Patchy	Fungal infection Lichen planopilaris Neoplasm	Biopsy
Traction alopecia	30 in Black women and girls	Tight, repetitive hair styling	Fringe sign	Absent early in condition	Patchy	Frontal fibrosing alopecia, alopecia areata, trichotillomania	None
Androgenetic (male and female pattern hair loss)	0.6	Family history of thinning	Normal scalp	Absent	Patterned	Androgen excess in women	None
Central centrifugal cicatricial alopecia	6–15 in Black women	Frequent manipulation of hair through styling, family history	Bald patch usually on crown, radiating outward across scalp	Present	Patchy	Female pattern, discoid lupus, lichen planopilaris	Biopsy
Telogen effluvium	1.0	Physical or emotional stress 2–3 months previously	Positive hair pull >25% telogen hair	Absent	Diffuse	Female pattern hair loss Identify trigger or cause	None
Trichotillomania	0.1	Emotional problems	Broken hair	Absent	Patchy	Alopecia areata Tinea capitis	None
Tinea capitis	0.1	Schoolmates with hair loss	Scaling, erythema, pustules	Absent	Patchy	Seborrheic dermatitis Alopecia areata Bacterial infection Trichotillomania	KOH preparation, culture

KOH, Potassium hydroxide.
[a]Percentage of new dermatology patients with this diagnosis seen at the Hershey Medical Center Dermatology Clinic, Hershey, Pennsylvania.

hair loss and whether scarring is present as evidenced by the loss of follicular openings. Patchy hair loss is readily apparent. However, diffuse hair loss may not be noticeable until the patient has more than 50% hair loss. The presence or absence of scarring is important diagnostically and prognostically. In nonscarring alopecia, the diagnosis is usually made without a biopsy. In scarring alopecia, a biopsy is useful in establishing a prognosis and diagnosis and should be performed. Nonscarring alopecia may be a temporary phenomenon, whereas scarring indicates permanent hair loss.

KEY POINTS

1. Diagnosis requires a detailed history.
2. Diagnose the pattern as patchy or diffuse.
3. Determine whether hair loss is scarring or nonscarring.

Observe the pattern of hair loss and whether scarring is present.

ALOPECIA AREATA

KEY POINTS

1. An autoimmune disorder
2. Acute onset of well-circumscribed, oval patches of nonscarring alopecia
3. No cure but treatments are available

Definition

Alopecia areata is an idiopathic disorder characterized by well-circumscribed, round or oval patches of nonscarring hair loss (Fig. 20.1).

Incidence

The incidence in the United States is about 2% across a lifetime. Alopecia areata affects both sexes equally, with onset occurring most often in early adulthood. Almost 1% of the authors' new patients had this diagnosis.

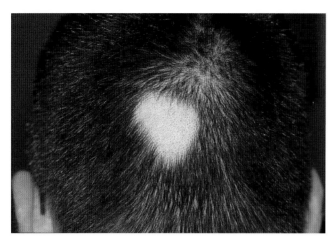

Fig. 20.1 Alopecia areata—characteristic round patch of nonscarring alopecia.

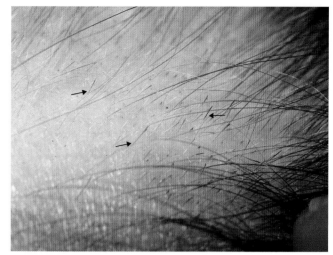

Fig. 20.2 Alopecia areata—note exclamation point hairs at the periphery of alopecia. (black arrows)

History

Alopecia areata has an acute onset. It is sometimes associated with emotional stress, but in most patients, the emotional stress seems to be caused by the hair loss. Approximately 25% of patients have other autoimmune disorders, such as type 1 diabetes mellitus, thyroid disease, and vitiligo. Atopic dermatitis is especially common in alopecia areata. Patients are generally healthy otherwise. Some 20%–25% of patients have a family history of alopecia areata. In a study on monozygotic twins, both twins had alopecia areata in 42% of the pairs who were researched.

Physical Examination

The disorder is characterized by well-circumscribed, round or oval patches of hair loss, leaving a smooth, normal-appearing scalp. Erythema and slight tenderness may be present early in the course. Characteristically, the periphery of the patches of hair loss is studded with *exclamation point hairs*, which are so named because of their resemblance to the printed punctuation mark (Fig. 20.2). These fractured hairs are 2–3 mm long and tapered at the base.

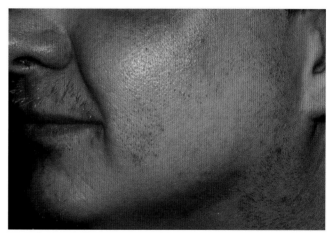

Fig. 20.3 Alopecia areata in beard area—patch of nonscarring alopecia extending from chin to cheek.

> Alopecia areata is characterized by nonscarring circular patches of alopecia with exclamation point hairs.

Alopecia areata most often affects the scalp, frequently with several 2- to 3-cm patches of hair loss. The eyebrows, eyelashes, and beard may also be affected, as may hair elsewhere on the body (Fig. 20.3). Approximately 1%–2% of patients develop loss of all scalp hair (*alopecia totalis*) or loss of all body hair (*alopecia universalis*) (Fig. 20.4). Fine stippling and pitting of the nails are associated findings and occur in about 10%–20% of patients. Nail findings are associated with more severe disease.

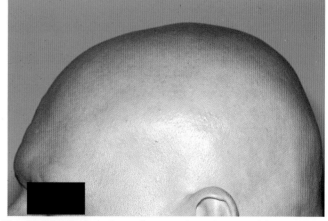

Fig. 20.4 Alopecia universalis—complete absence of hair on scalp, eyebrows, and eyelashes.

Differential Diagnosis

Other nonscarring forms of alopecia need to be considered in the differential diagnosis. *Secondary syphilis* can be ruled out by an appropriate serologic examination. *Trichotillomania* and *tinea capitis* should also be considered. Ill-marginated, irregular patches of alopecia containing the stubble of broken hairs are typical of trichotillomania (Fig. 20.5). If doubt exists, a biopsy helps to differentiate trichotillomania from alopecia areata.

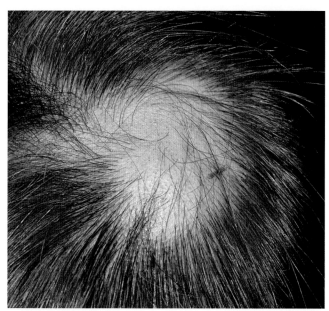

Fig. 20.5 **Trichotillomania**—note hairs of uneven length and "black dots," which represent snapped off anagen hairs. This child was mistakenly diagnosed as having alopecia areata.

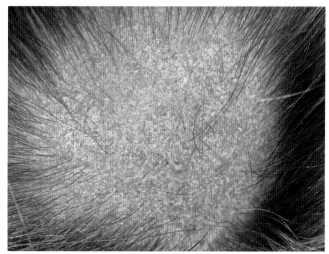

Fig. 20.6 **Tinea capitis**—circular patch of alopecia with typical scale and "black dot" hairs due to the breakage of weakened hair shafts from fungal invasion.

A potassium hydroxide (KOH) preparation and culture, and clinical evidence of redness and scale enable the diagnosis of a fungal infection (Fig. 20.6).

DIFFERENTIAL DIAGNOSIS FOR ALOPECIA AREATA

- Secondary syphilis
- Trichotillomania
- Tinea capitis

Laboratory and Biopsy

Histopathological examination of alopecia areata reveals the presence of small, dystrophic hair structures. A lymphocytic infiltrate surrounds the early anagen hair bulbs like a "swarm of bees" (Fig. 20.7).

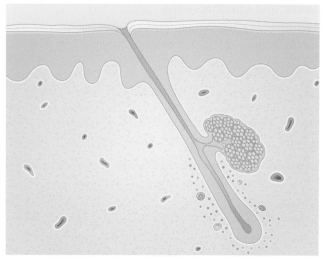

Fig. 20.7 **Alopecia areata**. Dystrophic follicle without a hair shaft. Dermis—lymphocytes surrounding the hair bulb.

Therapy

The treatment of alopecia areata depends on the extent of involvement and the patient's emotional need for regrowth of hair. There is no cure for alopecia areata. In localized disease, topical potent steroids such as clobetasol (Temovate) gel or intralesional injections of triamcinolone (Kenalog-10) are sometimes effective. In widespread disease, the Janus kinase (JAK) inhibitor, baricitinib (Olumiant), can be used. It is the first systemic treatment approved by the US Food and Drug Administration (FDA) for adults with severe alopecia areata and is given orally. Another oral JAK inhibitor FDA approved for ages 12 and older is ritlecitinib (Litfulo) for severe disease. Other oral JAK inhibitors, tofacitinib (Xeljanz) and ruxolitinib, have also been shown to be effective for severe alopecia areata in adolescents and adults but are not FDA approved. Patients must be screened and monitored for potentially severe side-effects while on JAK inhibitors. Topical formulations of JAK inhibitors have also been used with mixed results. Systemic steroids are sometimes used, but their hazards must be considered before starting treatment. Prompt hair loss after discontinuation of oral steroids is discouraging. Other modes of therapy include immunotherapy by induction of allergic contact dermatitis (aka contact sensitization), phototherapy, topical minoxidil, and oral cyclosporine. Patients with alopecia areata need psychological support, and all patients should visit the National Alopecia Areata Foundation's website (http://www.naaf.org) or Children's Alopecia Project (www.childrensalopeciaproject.org). A wig is recommended when the hair loss is extensive and medical therapies have failed.

THERAPY FOR ALOPECIA AREATA

Initial
- Steroids
- Topical—clobetasol twice daily
- Intralesional—triamcinolone 5 mg/mL every 4–6 weeks
- Topical-minoxidil 5% foam or solution daily
- Oral - for severe disease, baricitinib 2–4 mg once daily, ritlecitinib 50 mg once daily

Alternative
- Contact sensitization
- Systemic—prednisone (short course only)

Course and Complications

Alopecia areata has a variable, unpredictable course. Most patients with localized disease have spontaneous recovery. However, relapses are not uncommon. Duration of more than 1 year and extensive hair loss are poor prognostic signs. Spontaneous regrowth of hair in alopecia totalis (scalp) and alopecia universalis (total body) may occur but is uncommon; fewer than 5% of patients show any tendency toward hair regrowth. Statistics will hopefully improve with newer therapies.

> Poor prognosis:
> 1. Long duration
> 2. Large areas of alopecia

Pathogenesis

The pathogenesis of alopecia areata remains poorly understood, although an immunological process is favored. Research has shown the common initiation of the autoimmune response in alopecia areata, celiac disease, rheumatoid arthritis, and diabetes. A lymphocytic inflammatory infiltrate surrounds the affected bulbs and presumably has a role in the disease. In response to this autoimmune process, the hair matrices become arrested but retain the capacity for normal hair regrowth after months or years.

LUPUS ERYTHEMATOSUS

KEY POINTS

1. Alopecia can be scarring or nonscarring.
2. Biopsy confirms the diagnosis.
3. Treat aggressively to prevent permanent hair loss.

Definition

Lupus erythematosus is an autoimmune disorder that often affects the scalp and causes alopecia. Hair loss may be diffuse and nonscarring (systemic lupus erythematosus [SLE]) or patchy and scarring (discoid lupus erythematosus [DLE]). A general discussion of lupus erythematosus is found in Chapters 9 and 14.

Physical Examination

Diffuse nonscarring alopecia of the scalp in the form of a telogen effluvium accompanies the acute phases of SLE in more than 20% of patients. In addition, short, broken hairs (lupus hairs) may be present, particularly on the frontal margin.

> SLE—nonscarring
> DLE—scarring

DLE is characterized by oval, scarring areas of alopecia. A typical plaque has an active erythematous margin and a white, atrophic, inactive center (Fig. 20.8). Within the plaques, telangiectasia and dilated keratin-filled follicles are present.

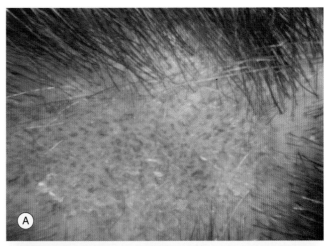
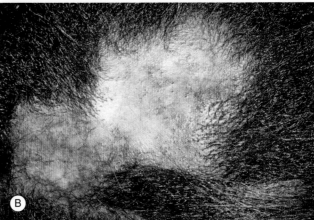

Fig. 20.8 Discoid lupus erythematosus. (A) Early lesion showing erythema and scarring. (B) Late lesion showing hyperpigmentation and hypopigmentation within scarring alopecia in dark skin.

Similar discoid lesions may be found on the ears, face, trunk, and extremities.

Differential Diagnosis

For the nonscarring alopecia caused by SLE, other causes of telogen effluvium, such as hypothyroidism, may be considered. However, in most patients with SLE, other manifestations of the disease are almost always evident.

Scarring alopecia caused by DLE must be differentiated from alopecia caused by *lichen planopilaris* (LPP), a form of lichen planus, *fungal infection*, or *neoplasm* (Fig. 20.9). A biopsy helps to differentiate DLE from LPP and neoplasm. A KOH preparation and culture enable the diagnosis of a fungal infection.

DIFFERENTIAL DIAGNOSIS FOR SLE AND DLE INVOLVING SCALP

- Telogen effluvium
- Lichen planopilaris
- Fungal infection
- Neoplasm

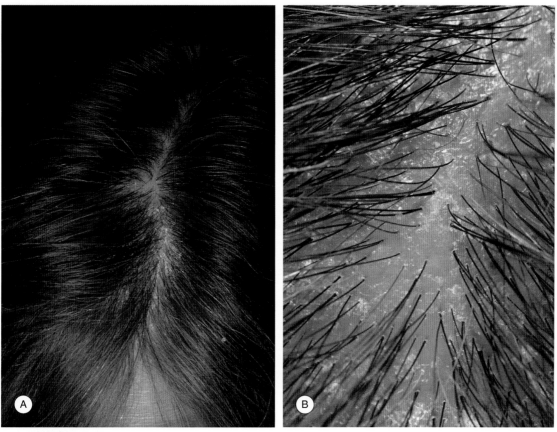

Fig. 20.9 Lichen planopilaris. (A) Note the thinning on the crown; initially, the diagnosis was female pattern hair loss. (B) Close inspection reveals permanent alopecia (e.g., follicular dropout) and perifollicular redness and scale.

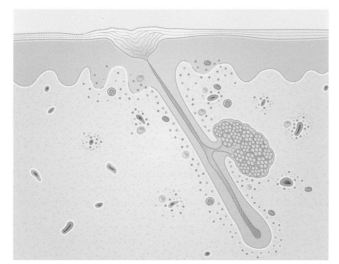

Fig. 20.10 Discoid lupus. Epidermis—dystrophic follicle without a hair shaft; hyperkeratosis. Dermis—lymphocytic infiltrate at the dermal–epidermal junction and around hair follicles and blood vessels.

Laboratory and Biopsy

A biopsy of the scalp for routine histological examination is usually diagnostic of DLE. Atrophic epidermis, keratotic plugging of the follicles, hydropic degeneration of the basal cells, and patchy perivascular and perifollicular lymphocytic infiltrate are characteristic (Fig. 20.10). The lupus band test (direct immunofluorescence) is positive but is usually not necessary to make the diagnosis. Appropriate laboratory tests, starting with a complete blood count, platelet count, antinuclear antibody test, renal profile, and urinalysis, should be ordered to rule out SLE.

Therapy

The goal of treatment in DLE is to prevent the follicular destruction that results in permanent alopecia. In many cases, the process can be arrested by the use of potent topical (clobetasol, Temovate gel) or intralesional corticosteroids (triamcinolone, Kenalog-10). Topical macrolides can also be tried. When this therapy fails, the addition of an antimalarial agent (hydroxychloroquine, Plaquenil) or immunosuppressant (e.g., mycophenolate mofetil) is indicated. While not FDA approved for DLE, an agent approved for SLE, anifrolumab (Saphnelo), appears promising for treatment in severe or refractory disease.

THERAPY FOR DISCOID LUPUS ERYTHEMATOSUS

Initial
- Sun protection
- Steroids
  - Topical—clobetasol twice daily
  - Intralesional—triamcinolone 10 mg/mL every 4–6 weeks
- Topical macrolides—tacrolimus 0.1% twice daily

Alternative
- Hydroxychloroquine 200 mg twice daily
- Immunosuppressants

Course and Complications

Chronic scarring of DLE causes permanent alopecia, whereas the diffuse alopecia associated with SLE is temporary and improves when the condition improves.

Pathogenesis

The pathogenesis of lupus erythematosus is discussed in Chapters 9 and 14.

TRACTION ALOPECIA

KEY POINTS

1. The result of chronic tension on the hair
2. Usually involves the frontotemporal region of the scalp
3. Begins as a nonscarring hair loss but can progress to permanent loss

Definition

Traction alopecia is a type of nonscarring hair loss that occurs after chronic, repeated tension on the hair shaft, usually from hair styling practices. It occurs most commonly in women and girls of African descent but can occur in anyone who wears tight hairstyles over time (e.g., ballerina buns, braids, high and tight ponytails). Early detection is critical because over time, untreated traction alopecia leads to permanent hair loss.

Incidence

The exact incidence is unknown for traction alopecia; however, it is known to be found more commonly in women and girls of African descent, likely because of the cultural practices of wearing high-tension hairstyles in this population (e.g., corn-row braids, hair weaves, locs). In addition, African-textured hair tends to be drier with more twists and turns in the coiled strands of hair, which can lead to stress points that make the phenomenon of hair loss and breakage easier to occur.

History

The process can begin at any age, and the hair loss is usually gradual but can be noticed acutely during the removal of braids and weaves. Patients should be asked about hair styling practices at initial visits, including preferred hairstyles and general hair care practices. Ask the patient how long high-tension hairstyles are left in place (with a longer time increasing the risk), and if pain medication is needed before or after initial hair styling. If a patient answers in the affirmative about the use of pain medication around hair styling, that is an important clue for traumatic hair care practice that could result in traction alopecia. Hair styling should never be a painful process and yet pain with styling has often been normalized. This pain equates to damage to the hair follicle. The risk of traction alopecia is higher when patients combine styling techniques. For example, if a patient states that they regularly chemically relax their hair *and* wear tight hairstyles, that combination would increase the likelihood of traction alopecia.

Physical Examination

Look at the overall appearance, texture and style of the hair, which can clue the clinician into the patient's susceptibility to

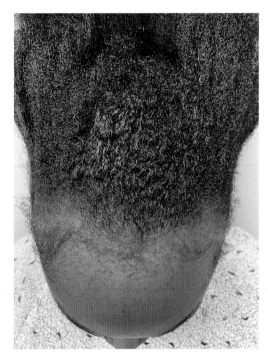

Fig. 20.11 Traction alopecia—loss of hair along the frontal scalp from tight, repetitive hairstyles. The "fringe sign" is diagnostic, where one can appreciate a rim of vellus hairs, followed by a bald patch, followed by normal-thickness hair.

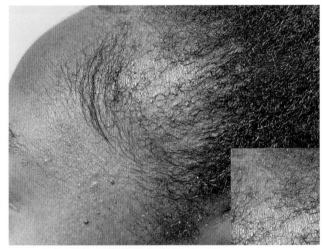

Fig. 20.12 Traction alopecia—On close inspection of the patient (inset), clinicians can appreciate follicular papules and pustules from tight traction on the hair follicle.

traction alopecia. The hair loss characteristically occurs along the frontal and temporal margins of the scalp. Importantly, look for an area of intact, small-caliber or fine hairs, behind which will be an area of loss, followed by normal-thickness hair behind the area of hair loss. This pattern is called the "fringe sign" and is diagnostic of traction alopecia (Fig. 20.11). Evaluate the affected area for follicular pustules, follicular erythema or violaceous color, red papules, and scale, all of which indicate inflammation and early signs of hair loss (Fig. 20.12).

The "fringe sign" is diagnostic for traction alopecia.

Differential Diagnosis

The differential diagnosis includes frontal fibrosing alopecia, alopecia areata, and trichotillomania. In frontal fibrosing alopecia, look for facial papules around the temples, lateral eyebrow hair loss, and the "lonely hair sign" instead of the "fringe sign." For alopecia areata, look for smooth, round bald patches over the scalp, and a lack of history of high-tension hairstyles, as well as other autoimmune history. Trichotillomania is a traumatic, self-induced alopecia. To differentiate from traction, look for irregular shapes of hair loss, hairs at various stages of growth, and the patient history of other similar disorders (e.g., nail biting, anxiety, eating disorders). If there is any doubt left, a biopsy would help distinguish between these diagnoses.

> ### DIFFERENTIAL DIAGNOSIS FOR TRACTION ALOPECIA
>
> - Frontal fibrosing alopecia
> - Alopecia areata
> - Trichotillomania

Laboratory and Biopsy

Generally, no laboratory examination or biopsy is needed, and the diagnosis can be made based on the history and physical examination. A biopsy of early traction alopecia would show mild dermal inflammation and trichomalacia (i.e., twisted and deformed anagen bulbs). Late-stage traction alopecia would show follicular miniaturization, follicular "dropout," fibrous tracts replacing terminal follicles, and minimal inflammation of the dermis.

Therapy

The most important treatment is centered on patient behavior modification and discontinuing traumatic hairstyles, which is the first-line therapy for children and young people. Care should be taken to discuss the importance of reducing high-tension styles and that if stopped early, regrowth is expected. It should be noted that many styles that may cause hair loss are personally or culturally relevant to patients and complete discontinuation of the styles may not be feasible. In this case, clinicians must encourage looser styles and altered styling methods that minimize tension. Loose buns, low ponytails, and frequent changes of tighter styles are important to review with patients.

All other options are based on expert opinion, and there are no large clinical trials for treatment. For adult patients with traction alopecia, in addition to minimizing traumatic hair styling, most experts recommend minoxidil 5% foam or solution be applied once daily to reduce the rate of hair loss and prolong the anagen (growth phase) of hair follicles. Alternatively, 2% minoxidil solution can be used twice daily. Both options are available commercially, and patients should be advised that it can take up to 1 year to see results. If there are signs of active inflammation, topical steroids (clobetasol solution) and oral tetracyclines are warranted. Intralesional corticosteroids at a dose of 2.5–10 mg/mL

can be used; however, patients should be informed of possible hypopigmentation as a side-effect.

For late-stage traction alopecia in which hair cannot be recovered in a cosmetically acceptable way, the area can be covered with the help of a stylist adept at using the remaining hair to camouflage the loss or with camouflaging products such as hair protein fibers (Toppik), sprays, powders, scalp tattoos, or wigs. Patients can also be referred to surgeons specializing in hair transplantation for treatment.

> ### THERAPY FOR TRACTION ALOPECIA
>
> **Initial**
> - Discontinuing or minimizing traumatic hair styling practices
> - Minoxidil 2% solution twice daily or 5% solution/foam daily
> - Oral Tetracyclines (Doxycycline, Minocycline 100 mg twice daily)
> - Super-potent topical or intralesional steroids
>   - Topical—clobetasol once to twice daily
>   - Intralesional—triamcinolone 5–10 mg/mL every 4–8 weeks
>
> **Alternative**
> - Camouflaging options (hair-building proteins, powders, sprays, tattoos, wigs)
> - Surgery (hair transplant)

Course and Complications

Treatment for traction alopecia is about time. If caught early in the process, it can be fully reversible with styling changes and proper education about the condition. Educating hair stylists in the community is an excellent way to prevent and treat early signs of traction alopecia. However, over time and without modifying hair styling practices and treating the associated inflammation, traction alopecia can result in permanent hair loss. Early intervention is critical.

Pathogenesis

The pathogenesis is not fully known. It is thought that tension on the hair follicles induces inflammation and folliculitis. As a result, follicules start to shrink and arrest, leading to thinner hairs and reduced density. The "fringe sign" is typically due to smaller hairs around the frontal scalp not being long enough to be incorporated into the tight style. These "baby hairs," as they are colloquially known, are usually laid down with gel or another product along the edges of the forehead; thus, tension is not placed, and the hairs remain intact.

> Treating early traction alopecia leads to the reversal of hair loss and subsequent regrowth.

MALE AND FEMALE PATTERN HAIR LOSS (ANDROGENETIC ALOPECIA)

> ### KEY POINTS
>
> 1. Nonscarring hair loss occurs in a patterned distribution
> 2. Occurs most often in genetically predisposed men and women
> 3. In males, dihydrotestosterone causes hair miniaturization

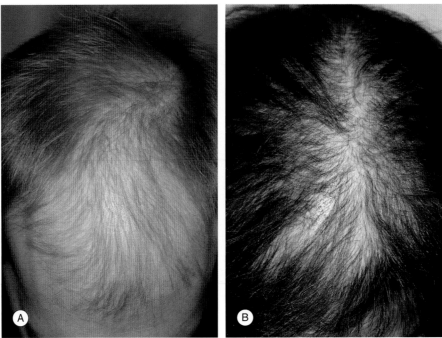

Fig. 20.13 Male and female pattern hair loss. (A) Frontal and vertex alopecia in a male. (B) Diffuse thinning on the crown with an intact frontal hairline in a woman.

Definition

Male and female pattern hair loss (MPHL and FPHL, respectively) represents postpubertal replacement of terminal hairs by miniaturized hairs and eventually completely atrophic follicles (Fig. 20.13). It occurs in individuals, both males and females, who are genetically predisposed. Clinically, the disorder is nonscarring and involves the vertex and frontotemporal regions of the scalp.

Incidence

Male and female pattern hair thinning is the most common cause of hair loss. It is estimated that 50% of men and women are affected by the condition by the age of 50 years.

History

The process begins at any age after puberty, but temporal recession is often noticed between the ages of 20 and 30 years. Women can note the onset of hair thinning in their 20s and 30s or around menopause. The onset and progression are gradual. Women often report see-through hair where scalp skin is noticeable. The patient usually has a family history of baldness.

Physical Examination

In areas of baldness, the coarse, dark terminal hairs are replaced by finer, miniaturized (i.e., vellus-like) hairs, which then become atrophic, leaving a smooth, shiny scalp with barely visible follicular orifices (Fig. 20.14). The number of hair follicles remains unchanged. Baldness characteristically occurs in a distinctive pattern that spares the posterior and lateral margins of the scalp. In men, the process begins with bitemporal recession, followed by balding of the vertex and/or reshaping of the frontal hairline. In women, FPHL is most often manifest by diffuse thinning

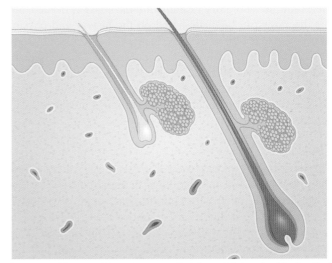

Fig. 20.14 Male and female pattern hair loss. Miniaturized (vellus-like) hair (*left*) is found in the areas of thinning. Terminal hair (*right*) is shown for comparison.

over the top of the scalp (e.g., the crown) and by an intact frontal hairline. The earliest sign in women is a gradual widening of the part width on the crown of the scalp when compared with the back of the scalp. Women experience thinning of hair, not baldness. In areas of baldness, the scalp appears completely normal, with no evidence of scarring or inflammation.

> Miniaturized hairs replace thicker terminal hairs in androgenetic alopecia.

Differential Diagnosis

In men, the diagnosis is usually straightforward. In women, the diagnosis of FPHL may be more difficult. Telogen effluvium affects the entire scalp equally and does not result in patterned hair loss. Permanent alopecia, like LPP, can occur in a patterned distribution on biopsy, and close clinical inspection of follicular dropout are distinguishing factors. *Hormonal abnormality* should be considered in women who have menstrual irregularities, hirsutism, rapidly progressive patterned thinning, and infertility.

Laboratory and Biopsy

Ordinarily, no laboratory examination or biopsy is done. Biopsy would show increased numbers of miniaturized hairs. Androgen excess in women can be screened for with measurements of serum-free and total testosterone and dehydroepiandrosterone sulfate.

Therapy

Minoxidil, 5% foam/2% solution (Women's Rogaine) and 5% solution/foam (Men's Rogaine) applied twice daily (except for Women's 5% Rogaine foam, which is applied once daily) is a moderately effective treatment for men and women with androgenetic alopecia. It stops or reduces the rate of hair loss and reverses the process of hair miniaturization by prolonging anagen or the growth phase of hair follicles. After 1 year of treatment, 20%–40% of men achieve moderate-to-dense regrowth of terminal hairs with the 2% solution and some increased effectiveness with the 5% solution. Up to 60% of women experience hair regrowth with the 2% solution or 5% foam after 6 months of treatment. This new hair growth is not permanent. Cessation of treatment results in the loss of hair within a few months. Even with continued therapy, hair regrowth plateaus after 1 year and slowly declines over subsequent years. Despite FDA approval for treating vertex thinning, minoxidil solution and foam also work on the frontal scalp in both men and women but not on the bitemporal recession seen in men. Oral minoxidil, while an old drug used for hypertension, has recently been used in treating androgenetic hair loss. Patients appreciate the ease of use, minimal side-effect profile, and similar efficacy to topical minoxidil. It should be noted that oral minoxidil is not FDA approved for hair loss. Patients typically take 1.25–5 mg daily. Side-effects are usually mild but include transient pretibial edema, hypertrichosis of body hair, elevated heart rate at rest, small changes in blood pressure, orthostatic hypotension, and rare cases of pericardial effusion. Patients should be screened for hypotension and cardiac history prior to use. Increased hair growth appears to be dose dependent; however, lowering the dose might mitigate undesirable side-effects.

Finasteride, 1 mg (Propecia), a type II 5a-reductase inhibitor, is given once daily. Five-year data show that 90% of men maintain their present hair and two-thirds of men experience some degree of hair regrowth. Side effects are uncommon and include sexual dysfunction and depressed mood. Finasteride is contraindicated in women of childbearing potential because of its teratogenic effects on male offspring.

For women who can tolerate it, oral antiandrogens are used (spironolactone) either initially with topical minoxidil or as an adjunct. Spironolactone has been shown to have some benefits for FPHL. Treatment is started at 50 mg twice daily and can be titrated up to 200 mg daily in divided doses. Side-effects include headaches, breast tenderness, menstrual irregularities, diuresis, orthostatic hypotension, hyperkalemia, and theoretical concern for teratogenicity for the male fetus (i.e., feminization of genitalia); therefore, women should not get pregnant while on spironolactone.

Extensive areas of baldness can be covered with a hairpiece or wig. For selected patients, surgical treatment with hair transplantation is successful.

Course and Complications

The balding process is usually gradual and most evident between the ages of 30 and 50 years. Thereafter, it is much slower, although hair thinning continues into later life.

Pathogenesis

The development of common baldness is genetically predetermined and androgen-dependent. Castration of males before puberty prevents the development of baldness. However, when testosterone is administered, a predisposed eunuch becomes bald. It seems contradictory that androgens cause scalp baldness but stimulate hair growth on the chest, face, and genital regions. This phenomenon may be explained by regional differences in androgen metabolism. Hair follicles in bald areas of the scalp have increased the levels and activity of 5a-reductase, which causes increased levels of dihydrotestosterone that shortens the hair cycle and miniaturizes scalp follicles.

Common baldness is androgen-dependent in males.

CENTRAL CENTRIFUGAL CICATRICIAL ALOPECIA

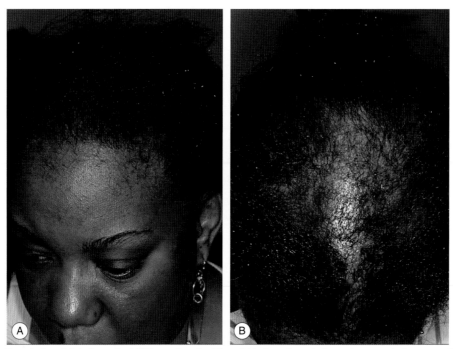

Fig. 20.15 Central centrifugal cicatricial alopecia. (A) The patient is able to hide her alopecia from the casual observer with styling. (B) Parting the hair on physical examination reveals a bald patch at the crown of the scalp, radiating outward.

Definition

Central centrifugal cicatricial alopecia (CCCA) is a scarring (cicatricial) hair loss that often affects the crown of the scalp and expands outward, or centrifugally, eventually causing an irreversible alopecia. It is typically accompanied by signs of inflammation such as redness, pustules, scale, and bogginess of the scalp. CCCA is most commonly seen in women of African descent.

Incidence

The true incidence of CCCA is likely higher than what is documented because there are a few large, epidemiological studies providing precise numbers, but the condition has been found to be 6%–15% in women of African descent across several reports.

History

Hair loss occurs gradually, usually starting on the vertex scalp and radiating in an outward fashion from the center (centrifugally). Most patients are Black who may or may not have a history of chemical hair styling, the use of heat to straighten the hair, tight braids, glued in wigs or weaves, or a family history of similar findings in related women. The patient may experience tingling, burning, or a pulling sensation in the affected area, which may prompt the first visit. Sometimes, patients are asymptomatic.

Physical Examination

This condition often begins as a patch of thinned hair on the vertex scalp (the central back portion of scalp or crown) (Fig. 20.15). The earliest sign of this condition can be also broken hairs in the same distribution (Fig. 20.16). Over time, the hair loss increases in a centrifugal pattern. While the central scalp is often most commonly affected, there are reports of atypical locations of hair loss outside of

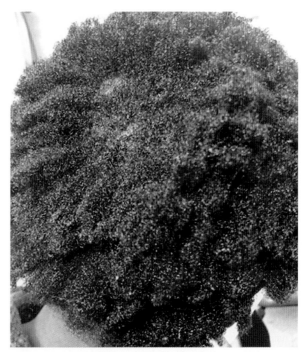

Fig. 20.16 Central centrifugal cicatricial alopecia—The first sign of condition may be only broken hairs at the crown.

the vertex scalp, and the authors have seen these atypical manifestations of CCCA in our clinics. Unfortunately, many patients arrive at dermatology clinics at later stages of the disease, with large areas of scarring hair loss on evaluation, making medical treatment almost impossible.

> Unexplained broken hairs on the central scalp can be a presenting sign. Early detection is critical to halt the scarring process.

Differential Diagnosis

FPHL is perhaps the most common differential diagnosis for CCCA. FPHL is typically asymptomatic, and more importantly, is nonscarring. A scarring alopecia that must be differentiated from CCCA is LPP, a form of lichen planus. It is in a similar distribution on the scalp and can present with perifollicular scale and erythema. Discoid lupus presents with scaly, red plaques and follicular plugging. A biopsy helps differentiate CCCA from these other diagnoses. The histopathological findings of FPHL would show a nonscarring process, LPP would demonstrate a lichenoid pattern, and discoid lupus would show classic signs of lupus (i.e., superficial and deep lymphocytic infiltrate) on pathology.

> ### DIFFERENTIAL DIAGNOSIS FOR CCCA
> - FPHL
> - LPP
> - Discoid lupus

Laboratory and Biopsy

A biopsy of the scalp for routine histological examination is usually diagnostic of CCCA. Premature desquamation of the inner root sheath, particularly in slightly or uninflamed hair follicles, is characteristic of CCCA, as well as eccentric thinning of the follicular epithelium, perifollicular concentric lamellar fibroplasia, and a perifollicular lymphocytic infiltrate (Fig. 20.17). There are no classic laboratory tests for this condition to date.

Therapy

The goal of treatment in CCCA is to alleviate symptoms and prevent the follicular destruction, which results in permanent alopecia. There are no standardized guidelines or large clinical trials for treatment, and therapy is based on expert opinion. In mild cases, treatment includes the use of highly potent topical (clobetasol, Temovate) or intralesional corticosteroids (triamcinolone, Kenalog 5–10 mg/mL). Topical macrolides (tacrolimus, Protopic) can also be used to minimize the side-effects of the steroids while still treating the inflammation. Oral tetracycline antibiotics are often utilized

> ### THERAPY FOR CENTRAL CENTRIFUGAL CICATRICIAL ALOPECIA
>
> **Initial**
> - Super-potent topical or intralesional steroids
>   - Topical—clobetasol once to twice daily
>   - Intralesional—triamcinolone 5–10 mg/mL every 4–8 weeks
> - Topical macrolides (tacrolimus 0.1% ointment twice daily)
> - Oral tetracyclines
>   - Doxycycline 100 mg once to twice daily
> - Behavioral modifications
>   - Looser hairstyles and minimized hair manipulation
>   - Less chemical processing
>
> **Alternative**
> - Hydroxychloroquine 200 mg twice daily
> - Immunosuppressants
> - Wigs

for their antiinflammatory properties. When more conservative therapy fails, the addition of an antimalarial agent (hydroxychloroquine, Plaquenil) or immunosuppressant (e.g., mycophenolate mofetil, CellCept) is indicated. Many clinicians also recommend that patients alter their hair styling practices, such as opting for looser hairstyles that avoid excessive tension and increasing the time between applying relaxers if patients choose to wear their hair chemically straightened. Finally, if treatment is not effective or the loss is too advanced, clinicians should discuss camouflaging techniques (e.g., wigs, hair transplants) with patients.

Course and Complications

CCCA over time causes permanent alopecia.

Pathogenesis

The pathogenesis of CCCA is not clear. In the past, this condition was known by names related to the styling practices common among Black women (e.g., hot comb alopecia, chemically induced cosmetic alopecia). One theory is that CCCA may be a fibroproliferative disorder that is characterized by long-term, low-grade inflammation, irritation, and eventual fibrosis. This theory is supported by studies that have shown an association with uterine fibroids in patients with CCCA. Another theory posits that premature desquamation of the inner root sheath in the hair follicle is the predisposing factor. Normally, the inner root sheath (IRS) guides the hair shaft out of the follicle at the level of the isthmus during the anagen (growth) phase of the hair cycle. In CCCA, the IRS is desquamated prematurely leading to the hair shaft pressing against and eventually perforating through the deeper layers of the follicular unit abnormally, causing an inflammatory cascade that leads to scarring. Perhaps the premature desquamation of the IRS is triggered by chemicals and styling, but this has not been fully elucidated.

TELOGEN EFFLUVIUM (STRESS-INDUCED ALOPECIA)

> ### KEY POINTS
> 1. Identify triggers for increased shedding of telogen hairs.
> 2. Triggering event occurs 3–6 months before the onset of hair shedding.
> 3. Gentle hair pull is positive for telogen hairs.

Definition

Marked emotionally or physiologically stressful events may result in an alteration of the normal hair cycle and diffuse hair loss. The scalp is made up of a mosaic of anagen (growing) and telogen (resting) hairs. Telogen effluvium is characterized by the excessive and early entry of hairs into the telogen phase. Causes of telogen effluvium include high fever, childbirth, chronic illness, major surgery, anemia, severe emotional disorders or stress, crash diets and nutritional deficits, hypothyroidism, and medications such as birth control pills (starting, stopping, or changing).

> Telogen effluvium occurs most often postpartum.

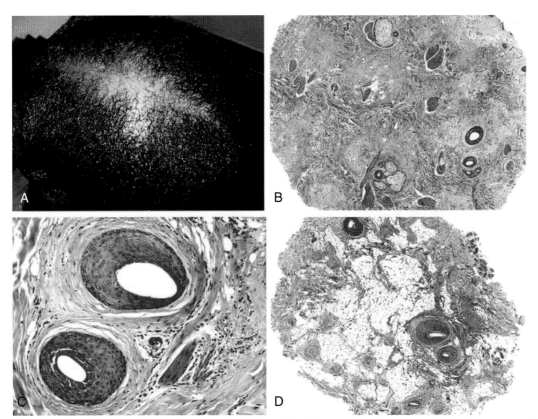

Fig. 20.17 Central Centrifugal Cicatricial Alopecia. Note the eccentric thinning of the follicular epithelium, the perifollicular concentric fibroplasia (scarring), and the perifollicular lymphocytic infiltrate surrounding the follicle.

Incidence

The incidence of telogen effluvium is probably greater than that seen by the dermatologist because most episodes are transient and minor.

History

Hair loss occurs 2–4 months after the physical or mental stress. Most patients are women who have diffuse hair thinning postpartum. They are concerned about going bald and characterize their hair loss as coming out by "handfuls" after combing and shampooing. They may bring photos of their shower drain or hair brush, or bring in bags of hair. If the patient has not recently given birth, a history of other physical or emotional stress, dietary habits, and medications should be sought.

Physical Examination

The patient has diffuse thinning of the hair that at first is not readily apparent to the examiner (Fig. 20.18). The scalp is normal, with no scarring or erythema. The part width on the crown is equal in coverage compared to the back of the scalp. The remainder of the skin examination, including hair elsewhere on the body, is normal. Gentle pulling of the hair (hair-pull test) verifies excessive hair shedding. The hair pull is done by grasping a small lock of hair and applying gentle traction from the base to the tip of the lock of hair. Normally, fewer than three hairs are pulled out with this maneuver. Pulling out more than

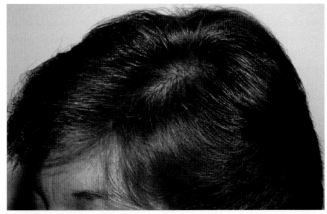

Fig. 20.18 Telogen effluvium—thinning of hair not readily apparent to a casual observer.

three hairs consistently from different scalp areas confirms that excessive shedding is present (Fig. 20.19).

> The excessive loss of telogen hairs is characteristic and manifested by a positive hair-pull test.

In stress-induced alopecia, the number of telogen hairs is increased from a normal percentage of 10%–20% to more than 25%. This results in as many as 400–500 lost hairs daily. Normally, fewer than 100 hairs are lost daily.

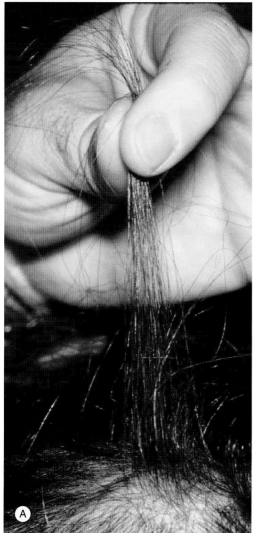

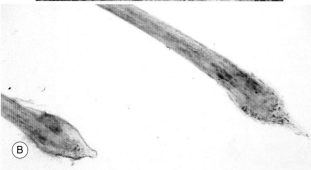

Fig. 20.19 (A) Demonstration of gentle hair-pull test. (B) Microscopic examination shows telogen or club hairs.

Differential Diagnosis

The challenge is to search for a cause of the telogen effluvium. In women, FPHL is most often confused with telogen effluvium. Telogen effluvium is distinguished by having equal part widths on the crown and occipital scalp and by having a positive pull test. The part width is wider on the crown compared to the occiput scalp in FPHL. *Abnormal thyroid function*, particularly hypothyroidism, produces hair that is dry and sparse diffusely, often with the loss of the lateral third of each eyebrow. *Nutritional deficiencies* (e.g., lack of an essential fatty acid, biotin, or zinc), rarely seen in practice, also cause a telogen effluvium.

Toxic drugs, particularly alkylating agents, cause loss of hair in the anagen phase, and this is called anagen effluvium.

DIFFERENTIAL DIAGNOSIS FOR TELOGEN EFFLUVIUM

- FPHL
- Identify the causes of telogen effluvium

Laboratory and Biopsy

The history and clinical examination are usually diagnostic. Minimum laboratory tests include complete blood count, thyroid-stimulating hormone, and iron studies, including ferritin to assess for total body iron storage. Biopsy is rarely performed but would show an increased percentage (>25%) of telogen hairs in a 4-mm punch biopsy submitted for horizontal sectioning.

Therapy

In most patients, the stressful event has passed, and reassurance that the patient will not go bald is the mainstay of treatment. In other patients, pinpointing the underlying condition that triggered the hair loss is required, and ordering the laboratory tests mentioned will be helpful. Camouflaging techniques can be shared with the patient while the hair loss resolves and regrowth begins (e.g., scalp coloring, hair-building protein fibers). Some patients may need an additional psychological support, which can be provided in part with clinical follow-up evaluations.

THERAPY FOR TELOGEN EFFLUVIUM

Initial
- Reassurance

Course and Complications

This condition is usually a self-limiting, reversible problem that resolves within 2–6 months. It may be prolonged for years if the underlying stress continues. A chronic telogen effluvium lasting for up to 5 years has been described to occur, particularly in middle-aged women, without a recognizable initiating factor.

Pathogenesis

The normal hair cycle is disturbed in telogen effluvium. Growing anagen hairs are prematurely converted to resting telogen hairs, which are subsequently shed. The mechanism for this alteration of the normal hair cycle is unknown, but it is thought that some physiological event stimulates a change in follicular cycling after an insult occurs on the anagen bulb.

TINEA CAPITIS

KEY POINTS

1. Superficial fungal infection (*Trichophyton tonsurans*) of the scalp, most common in children
2. Diagnosis confirmed by KOH and fungal culture
3. Treatment with systemic antifungals

Definition

Tinea capitis is a superficial fungal infection of the scalp (Fig. 20.20). The three most common dermatophytes that cause

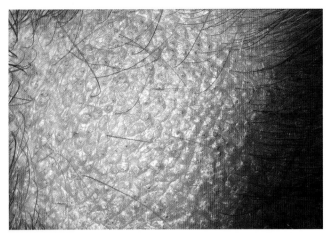

Fig. 20.20 Tinea capitis—nonscarring patch of alopecia with black dots (broken hairs), erythema, and scale.

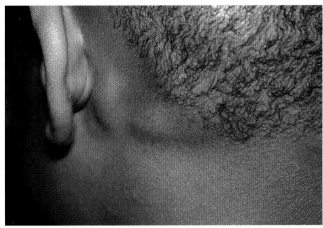

Fig. 20.21 Tinea capitis—lymphadenopathy in conjunction with patches of alopecia is a typical sign.

tinea capitis are *Trichophyton tonsurans*, *Microsporum canis*, and *Microsporum audouinii*. The disease varies from noninflamed scaling patches to inflamed, pustule-studded plaques (kerion) that may leave scars.

Incidence

Epidemic tinea capitis occurs worldwide, mostly in school-aged children. Males and females are equally affected. *T. tonsurans* is the predominant cause of tinea capitis. *M. canis*, typically transmitted by pets, is seen less frequently.

History

Often, the patient has a history of a family member, friend, or pet with hair loss.

Physical Examination

Tinea capitis can appear as seborrheic-like dermatitis with minimal inflammation, patchy alopecia with broken hair shafts, leaving residual black stumps ("black dot" ringworm). Occipital lymph nodes are often present (Fig. 20.21). A more severe infection with indurated, boggy plaques (kerion) covered with pustules and crusting, accompanied by lymphadenopathy, can result in scarring.

Tinea capitis causes:
1. Seborrheic-like dermatitis
2. "Black dot" ringworm
3. Kerion

Differential Diagnosis

Alopecia areata, *seborrheic dermatitis*, *bacterial scalp infection*, and *trichotillomania* should be considered in the differential diagnosis of tinea capitis. A KOH preparation or fungal culture confirms the diagnosis of tinea capitis.

DIFFERENTIAL DIAGNOSIS FOR TINEA CAPITIS

- Alopecia areata
- Seborrheic dermatitis
- Bacterial scalp infection (e.g., folliculitis)
- Trichotillomania

Laboratory and Biopsy

In the past, the Wood's lamp examination was a simple method of screening for tinea capitis. Hairs infected with *M. audouinii* and *M. canis* fluoresce bright green with this long-wave ultraviolet light. The Wood's lamp, however, has become much less useful because most cases of tinea capitis are now caused by nonfluorescing *T. tonsurans*.

The diagnosis is made by KOH microscopic examination and a culture of broken hairs. The KOH preparation reveals spores surrounding the hair shaft (ectothrix), characteristic of *Microsporum* spp., or within the shaft (endothrix), characteristic of *T. tonsurans*. Although biopsy is not usually performed, histopathological sections that are stained with periodic acid–Schiff or silver reveal spores and hyphae in the stratum corneum and hair shaft (Fig. 20.22).

Therapy

Topical agents are ineffective in treating tinea capitis. For children, microsize griseofulvin (Grifulvin V tablets or suspension), 20–25 mg/kg daily for 6–8 weeks, is the treatment of choice. In addition, shampooing with 2.5% selenium sulfide (Selsun) twice a week helps to reduce viable fungal spores and probably should be used by asymptomatic family members to reduce the carrier state. Oral terbinafine (Lamisil), fluconazole (Diflucan) and itraconazole (Sporanox) are alternative drugs if treatment with griseofulvin fails.

THERAPY FOR TINEA CAPITIS

Initial
- Griseofulvin—20–25 mg/kg daily

Alternative
- Terbinafine
  - <20 kg: 62.5 mg daily
  - 20–40 kg: 125 mg daily
  - 40 kg: 250 mg daily
- Fluconazole
  - 6 mg/kg daily for 3–4 weeks
  - 6 mg/kg once weekly for 6–12 weeks
- Itraconazole
  - <20 kg: 5 mg/kg daily
  - 20–40 kg: 100 mg daily
  - 40 kg: 200 mg daily

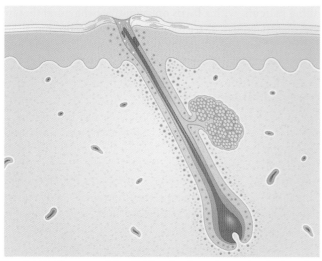

Fig. 20.22 **Tinea capitis**. Epidermis—hyperkeratosis, broken hair; spores and hyphae in the stratum corneum and hair shaft. Dermis—perifollicular inflammation.

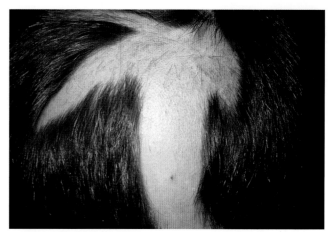

Fig. 20.23 **Trichotillomania**—bizarre patch of broken hairs.

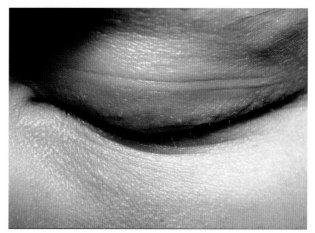

Fig. 20.24 **Trichotillomania**—plucked eyelashes in a child.

Course and Complications

With treatment, tinea capitis is cured in 1–3 months in most cases. Without treatment, the course is variable. In some children, particularly those with inflammatory tinea capitis, the course is self-limiting, with resolution within a few months. In others, the disease lasts for years, with resolution at puberty. Scarring and permanent hair loss may be the sequelae of a kerion, but often the permanent damage is surprisingly little, given the intense inflammation.

Pathogenesis

Epidemic tinea capitis is transmitted by human-to-human spread of the dermatophytes *M. audouinii* and *T. tonsurans*. Fungi have been cultured from fallen hairs, scales, and shared combs, hats, and brushes. *M. canis* spreads from animals (cats and dogs) to humans.

After an incubation period of several days, the fungal hyphae grow into the hair shaft and follicle. This growth causes broken hair, scaling, and a host of inflammatory responses. The infection spreads centrifugally for 8–10 weeks, involving an area of the scalp up to 7 cm in diameter. Spontaneous cure ensues, or a host–parasite equilibrium is maintained that results in a smoldering infection.

TRICHOTILLOMANIA

KEY POINTS

1. Self-induced alopecia from compulsive hair pulling
2. Bizarre patterns of nonscarring alopecia
3. Poor prognosis in adults and better prognosis in children

Definition

Trichotillomania is a traumatic, self-induced alopecia caused by patients obsessively or compulsively pulling, plucking, twisting, and rubbing their own hair, causing broken or epilated hair shafts. It is thought to be used as a coping mechanism to relieve stress or other emotions (Fig. 20.23).

Incidence

Trichotillomania occurs in both children and adults and may affect up to 4% of the general population. The highest incidence is in children and adolescence, equally affecting boys and girls, but with age, women are more frequently diagnosed. Adult males may be affected more than previously realized as they may disguise the condition as MPHL or shaving.

History

A history of emotional problems may be elicited, often with difficulty.

Physical Examination

The scalp is affected most often; less often, the eyebrows and eyelashes are plucked (Fig. 20.24). Ill-marginated, irregular, patchy areas of alopecia characterize trichotillomania. The scalp is normal, without inflammation or scarring. The patient has numerous twisted and broken hairs, which have a characteristic feel of coarse stubble.

Coarse-feeling and broken hairs are the characteristics of trichotillomania.

Differential Diagnosis

Alopecia areata and *tinea capitis* should be considered in the differential diagnosis of trichotillomania. Exclamation point hairs, if present, are diagnostic of alopecia areata. Biopsy findings are also discriminating. KOH examination and fungal culture enable the diagnosis of fungal infection.

DIFFERENTIAL DIAGNOSIS FOR TRICHOTILLOMANIA

- Alopecia areata
- Tinea capitis

Laboratory and Biopsy

The biopsy (usually not required) reveals increased numbers of catagen (e.g., regressing) follicles, empty hair follicles in a non-inflammatory dermis, and traumatized follicles with broken hair matrixes and perifollicular hemorrhage (Fig. 20.25).

Therapy

Treatment is based on the degree of underlying emotional disturbance. In children, the condition is usually self-limiting and is best termed "trichotill," because the habit of hair pulling is often not associated with psychiatric illness. When insight and reassurance are given to the child and parents, the process often resolves. In adults, the habit may be much more difficult to stop. Gentle probing into the stresses and anxieties that have led to the hair pulling can be explored. Referral for psychiatric evaluation should be considered for

---

THERAPY FOR TRICHOTILLOMANIA

Initial
- Emotional support
- Behavioral counseling

Alternative
- Referral to psychiatry
- Selective serotonin reuptake inhibitors (e.g., fluoxetine)

---

willing patients, with a focus on cognitive behavioral therapy over pharmacological treatments. Selective serotonin reuptake inhibitors are occasionally used. Small data sets have utilized N-acetylcysteine.

Course and Complications

Trichotillomania is generally chronic and may be resistant to treatment, especially in adults, in whom it can be a serious problem. Symptoms may be severe enough to interfere with daily life; a patient's appearance may be sufficiently embarrassing to result in social isolation. Other comorbidities exist with trichotillomania, such as nail biting (onychophagia), nail picking (habit tic deformity), acne excoriee, lip biting, and cheek chewing. Trichobezoar, or undigested hair balls in the gastrointestinal (GI) tract, is a rare but potentially serious complication from patients with trichotillomania ingesting the pulled hair (trichophagia). Patients may complain of GI distress, and the condition can cause bowel obstruction or perforation. In most children, hair pulling is a "phase," which improves and clears with time. Follow-up is required to establish rapport and to determine whether trichotillomania is a symptom of a serious underlying psychiatric disorder.

Pathogenesis

The obsessive urge to pull out one's own hair has been attributed to various psychodynamic conflicts. In children, problems at home or school, sibling rivalry, developmental delay, and hospitalization can be psychosocial triggers for trichotillomania.

UNCOMMON HAIR DISORDERS

ACNE KELOIDALIS NUCHAE

This often pruritic condition occurs on the nape of the neck, most commonly in men who have darkly pigmented skin and coiled hair. Early lesions appear as dome-shaped papules with a central hair. Later, the papules may coalesce into large hypertrophic scars (Fig. 20.26). Multiple hairs entrapped by scar tissue

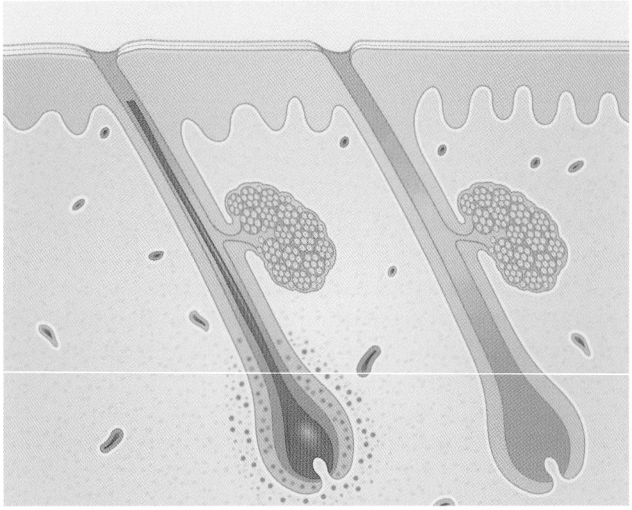

Fig. 20.25 Trichotillomania—broken hair; empty follicle. Dermis—perifollicular hemorrhage.

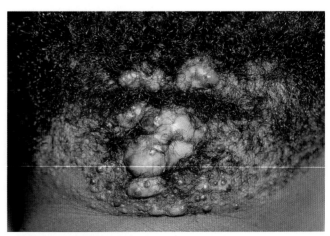

Fig. 20.26 Acne keloidalis nuchae. Note dome-shaped papules on the periphery and larger hypertrophic scars centrally.

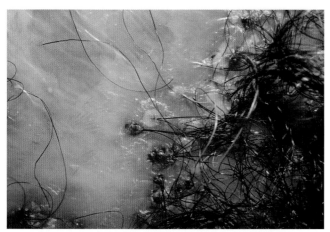

Fig. 20.27 Folliculitis decalvans—scarring alopecia characterized by loss of follicular openings (*slick surface*) expanding centrifugally on the crown of the scalp. Note pustules at the periphery.

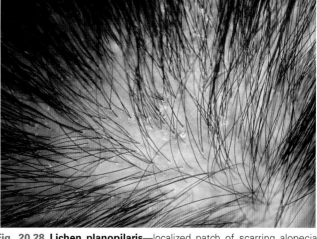

Fig. 20.28 Lichen planopilaris—localized patch of scarring alopecia. Note widened spaces between follicles, and perifollicular erythema and scale.

can be seen exiting a single follicular opening (tufting). Despite common belief, acne keloidalis nuchae is not caused by ingrown hairs and most likely represents an abnormal inflammatory reaction to hairs. Antiinflammatory treatments include intralesional and topical corticosteroids, and topical and oral antibiotics. Refractory treatment includes surgery, oral isotretinoin, and laser therapy.

FOLLICULITIS DECALVANS

Folliculitis decalvans is characterized by an expanding patch of scarring alopecia with pustules at the periphery (Fig. 20.27). It occurs predominantly on the crown of the scalp. *Staphylococcus aureus* is often cultured from the pustules and may play a pathogenic role. Treatment is difficult and includes appropriate systemic antibiotics.

LICHEN PLANOPILARIS

This scarring alopecia occurs more commonly in women than in men. Physical examination shows permanent loss of follicular openings, and perifollicular erythema and scale (Fig. 20.28). The condition can be localized or widespread. Changes in lichen planus can be seen on glabrous skin and mucous membranes 50% of the time. A biopsy confirms the diagnosis. LPP is relatively resistant to treatment (e.g., antimalarial medications, oral and topical corticosteroids). Spontaneous resolution occurs on average in 18 months.

LOOSE ANAGEN SYNDROME

Loose anagen syndrome typically presents in a young girl with short blond hair (Fig. 20.29). The child seldom needs a haircut

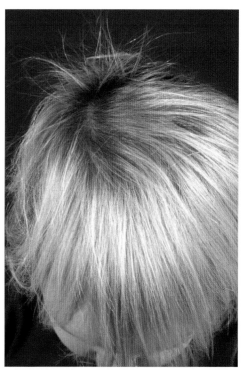

Fig. 20.29 Loose anagen syndrome—a 2-year-old girl with the classic phenotype of short blond hair that will not grow; in this case, hair thinning was diffuse.

because the "hair will not grow." The hair thinning may be diffuse or patchy. Diagnosis is confirmed by the painless extraction of microscopically confirmed anagen hairs through gentle hair pulling. The cause remains unknown. Improvement occurs with age. The differential diagnosis includes telogen effluvium and trichotillomania.

SELF-ASSESSMENT

Case 1—Hair Loss (Fig. 20.30)

What Is Your Differential Diagnosis?

The differential diagnosis of nonscarring alopecia includes stress-induced alopecia, androgenic alopecia, trichotillomania, alopecia areata, lupus erythematosus, and fungal infection. The patchy nature of the hair loss ruled out stress-induced, androgenic alopecia and SLE. This was not DLE because the patient had no scarring or follicular plugging. Alopecia areata and trichotillomania do not scale. The inflammation and scaling of the scalp favored a fungal infection.

What Would You Do Now?

A KOH preparation of several plucked broken hairs was positive for spores and hyphae. If the KOH preparation had been negative or equivocal, a fungal culture would have been done. A biopsy with special stains also enables the diagnosis of a fungal infection but is usually not needed.

How Would You Treat This Patient?

The patient should be treated with oral griseofulvin or terbinafine for at least 4–6 weeks. Treatment is continued until the scalp appears normal, new hair regrowth appears, and the KOH preparation is negative.

IMPORTANT POINTS

1. KOH preparations for tinea capitis require plucked hairs. The scale may be negative. When in doubt, do a fungal culture.
2. Treatment of tinea capitis requires oral preparations; topical antifungals are ineffective.

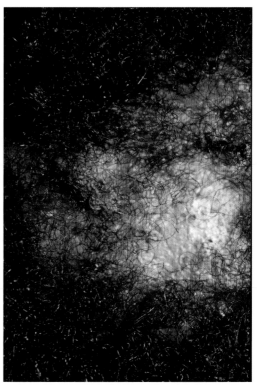

Fig. 20.30 This 7-year-old Black girl developed itching of the scalp and progressive areas of hair loss 6 weeks before she was seen in the dermatology clinic. The use of an antiseborrheic shampoo, oral erythromycin, and a topical antifungal agent had not helped. The physical examination revealed circular areas of nonscarring alopecia. The scalp was erythematous, crusted, and scaling in the patches of hair loss.

Nail Disorders

CHAPTER CONTENTS

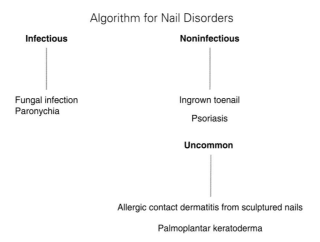

Algorithm for Nail Disorders

Infectious — Fungal infection / Paronychia

Noninfectious — Ingrown toenail / Psoriasis

Uncommon — Allergic contact dermatitis from sculptured nails / Palmoplantar keratoderma

ABSTRACT

The nail is a specialized keratinized appendage found on the dorsum of each finger and toe. It protects the distal phalanx against trauma, is used for fine grasping and scratching, and has an esthetic value. The diagnosis of nail diseases can be difficult because a single disease can cause widely varying changes in the nail and, conversely, because a given nail malformation can be the expression of a variety of diseases. Numerous disorders may affect the nail, including cutaneous and systemic diseases, tumors, infections, hereditary disorders, physical factors, and drugs. In this chapter, the four most common causes of nail disease are discussed: fungal infection, psoriasis, paronychia (Table 21.1), and ingrown toenail.

KEY POINTS

1. Appearance alone is usually not sufficient to make the diagnosis.
2. Therapy is often difficult or unsuccessful.

The physical appearance of the nail cannot be used reliably to make a diagnosis.

FUNGAL INFECTION

KEY POINTS

1. Confirm the diagnosis with periodic acid–Schiff (PAS) stain, culture, or potassium hydroxide (KOH) preparation
2. Cure requires oral therapy

Definition

Onychomycosis and tinea unguium are synonyms for infection of the nail with dermatophytic fungi. The most common etiologic dermatophytes are *Trichophyton rubrum* and *Trichophyton mentagrophytes*.

Incidence

The prevalence of onychomycosis is 22 per 1000 population. Some 20% of people in the United States between 40 and 60 years of age have onychomycosis. The most common sites of infection are the toenails, especially in the elderly.

History

The onset of onychomycosis is slow and insidious. The condition is often asymptomatic, but it can also cause pain in the affected

TABLE 21.1 Nail Disorders

	Physical Examination				Laboratory Test	
	Frequency (%)[a]	Pits	Brown Stains	Differential Diagnosis	PAS/KOH	Culture
Fungal infection	0.4	Absent	Present	Psoriasis Trauma Aging Secondary to eczema	Positive	Positive
Psoriasis	<0.1	Present	Present	Fungus Trauma Aging Secondary to eczema Alopecia areata (pits)	Negative	Negative
Paronychia	0.3	Absent	Absent	Herpes simplex	Negative Positive	Bacterial Candida albicans

KOH, potassium hydroxide; PAS, periodic acid–Schiff stain.
[a]Percentage of new dermatology patients with this diagnosis seen at the Hershey Medical Center Dermatology Clinic, Hershey, Pennsylvania.

toe, nail-trimming problems, discomfort when wearing shoes, and embarrassment because of the nail's distorted appearance.

Physical Examination

Toenail infection is more frequent than fingernail infection, and it is uncommon for all 10 nails to be involved. Dermatophytes most often infect the distal nail bed and undersurface of the distal nail, resulting in the discoloration (white, yellow, or brown) of the nail plate and the accumulation of subungual debris with separation of the plate from the nail bed (Fig. 21.1A). Less often, dermatophytes infect the top surface of the nail plate and cause a white, crumbly surface (superficial white onychomycosis) to develop. Neither type of infection produces much inflammatory reaction. Proximal white subungual onychomycosis, an infection of the proximal nail plate, is a marker of HIV infection.

> Onychomycosis is associated with tinea pedis and tinea manuum.

Differential Diagnosis

Often, the nail changes of onychomycosis cannot be distinguished clinically from those of nail dystrophy caused by psoriasis, eczema of the digits, trauma, and aging. Associated skin findings and fungal studies differentiate these entities.

Laboratory and Biopsy

The most sensitive method of confirming the diagnosis of onychomycosis is a PAS stain of nail clippings.

DIFFERENTIAL DIAGNOSIS OF ONYCHOMYCOSIS

- Psoriasis
- Eczema
- Trauma
- Aging

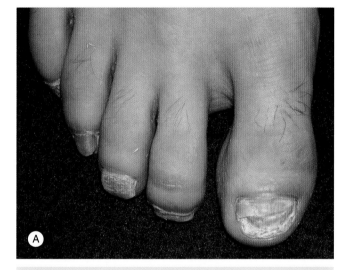

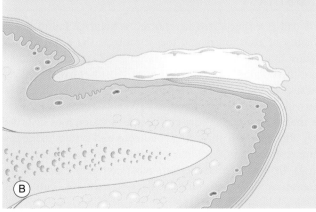

Fig. 21.1 Onychomycosis. (A) White, thick, and crumbly nail plate. (B) Nail plate—irregular, thick, and containing fungal hyphae.

A KOH preparation or fungal culture can alternatively be done. Compared with skin scrapings, more time must be allowed for the KOH to dissolve thin nail specimens before microscopic examination. If the infection is in the nail bed or the deeper portion of the nail plate, scrapings should be obtained from as far back under the nail as possible (Fig. 21.1B).

Therapy

Topical antifungal agents (ciclopirox, tavaborole, azoles) are usually ineffective (<20% clearing) in treating onychomycosis. Oral therapy with terbinafine (Lamisil) or itraconazole (Sporanox) should be given. Studies suggest that terbinafine is the most effective agent. The nail will not look completely normal at the end of treatment. Because terbinafine and itraconazole remain in the nail for months after therapy, retreatment should not be considered for approximately 6 months for fingernails and 12 months for toenails. In many individuals with asymptomatic onychomycosis of the toenails, systemic therapy is neither requested nor suggested. The risks and costs may outweigh any possible benefit.

> Asymptomatic onychomycosis of toenails needs no treatment.

THERAPY FOR ONYCHOMYCOSIS

Initial
- Terbinafine: 6 weeks for fingernails, 12 weeks for toenails
  - <20 kg: 62.5 mg daily
  - 20–40 kg: 125 mg daily
  - >40 kg: 250 mg daily

Alternative
- Itraconazole: 2 pulses for fingernails, 3 pulses for toenails
  - <20 kg: 5 mg/kg daily for 1 week/month
  - 20–40 kg: 100 mg daily for 1 week/month
  - >40–50 kg: 200 mg daily for 1 week/month
  - >50 kg: 200 mg b.i.d. for 1 week/month

Course and Complications

Onychomycosis is a chronic infection that is difficult to eradicate permanently. Even with oral therapy, failure rates for treating toenail infections are 20%–30%. Residual fungal spores present in the patient's shoes and environment are probably responsible for the recurrence of the infection. For this reason, a topical antifungal (e.g., tolnaftate, miconazole, clotrimazole, or terbinafine) applied to the feet every week may be helpful for long-term prophylaxis.

Pathogenesis

Superficial fungal infection of the nail is probably a direct extension of involvement of the surrounding digital skin. Invasion and deformity of the nail are facilitated by fungal keratinases, which disrupt the keratin structure of the plate.

INGROWN TOENAIL

KEY POINTS

1. Ingrown toenail causes a foreign body reaction.
2. Nail avulsion and matrix destruction are curative.

Definition

Ingrown toenail occurs when the lateral portion of the nail plate grows into the lateral nail fold, resulting in an inflammatory response.

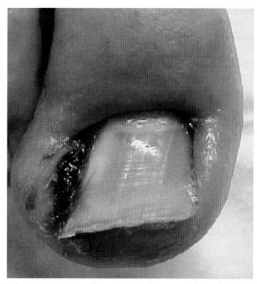

Fig. 21.2 **Ingrown toenail**—red, swollen, and lateral nail fold with granulation tissue.

Incidence

Ingrown toenail is a fairly common occurrence, with the great toenails most commonly affected.

History

Pain and swelling are the symptoms that cause patients to seek medical attention. Usually, the problem has been present for weeks or months with an acute flare, which may signal a secondary infection.

Physical Examination

The lateral nail fold is red, swollen, and usually has weeping granulation tissue (Fig. 21.2). The nail plate is penetrating into the lateral nail fold.

Differential Diagnosis

The diagnosis of ingrown toenail seldom causes difficulty because of its typical presentation.

Laboratory and Biopsy

Because the diagnosis is straightforward, laboratory testing or biopsy is not necessary.

Therapy

For mild-to-moderate ingrown toenail, wearing sufficiently wide shoes, trimming the nail plate straight across, antiseptic application, and inserting a cotton pledget under the nail edge may be successful. Operative intervention is necessary when conservative treatment fails or for severely ingrown toenails. Partial or total nail plate avulsion followed by surgical or chemical (85% aqueous phenol) nail matrix destruction is usually curative. Granulation tissue can be excised or cauterized.

THERAPY FOR INGROWN TOENAIL

Initial
- Well-fitting shoes
- Trim nail plate straight across
- Topical antiseptics
- Cotton pledget insertion

Alternative
- Nail avulsion with matrix destruction

Course and Complications

Ingrown toenail is a chronic process that causes pain and swelling, which interfere with ambulation. Occasionally, cellulitis of the toe can be a complication.

Pathogenesis

The ingrown nail plate acts as a foreign body, causing an inflammatory reaction in the lateral nail fold.

PARONYCHIA

KEY POINTS
1. Acute paronychia is a primary bacterial infection.
2. Chronic paronychia is a secondary candidal infection.

Definition

Paronychia is an inflammatory process of the nail fold (Fig. 21.3A). Acute paronychia is most often the result of a bacterial infection, commonly from *Staphylococcus aureus*. Chronic paronychia is usually caused by *Candida albicans*. The predisposing factor in the production of chronic paronychia is trauma or maceration, producing a break in the seal (cuticle) between the nail fold and the nail plate. This break produces a pocket that holds moisture and promotes the growth of microorganisms.

Acute paronychia is usually caused by *Staphylococcus aureus*; chronic paronychia is caused by *Candida albicans*.

Incidence

Chronic paronychia occurs in children who habitually suck their thumbs and in adults who do "wet" work. Particularly vulnerable are adults (nondiabetic, 3.4%; diabetic, 9.6%) who are exposed to a wet environment while they perform the chores of childrearing and housework. Bartenders, janitors, and other workers in wet occupations are also at risk.

History

Acute paronychia develops rapidly, leading to marked tenderness of the nail fold. Chronic paronychia develops insidiously and initially often goes unnoticed by the patient. A history of manicuring or wet work in adults or of finger sucking in children is common.

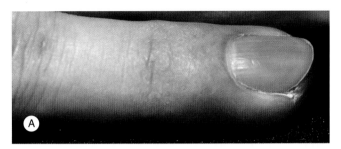

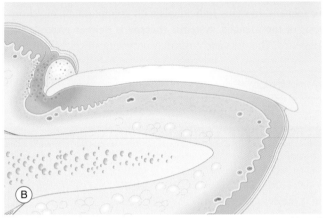

Fig. 21.3 (A) **Acute paronychia**—red and swollen nail fold. (B) **Chronic paronychia**—edema and inflammation, deformed cuticle with pocket of pus, and candidal hyphae.

Physical Examination

Although any finger may be involved with paronychia, the second and third digits are the most commonly affected. Acute paronychia is painful, red, and swollen, and may be accompanied by an abscess or cellulitis.

Chronic paronychia is characterized by loss of the cuticle, slight tenderness, swelling, erythema, and, sometimes, separation of the nail fold from the plate. A purulent or "cheesy" discharge and deformity of the nail plate are frequently seen.

Differential Diagnosis

Acute bacterial paronychia can be confused with herpetic whitlow. Polymerase chain reaction, Tzanck preparation, and cultures help to distinguish the two. Chronic paronychia is a distinctive clinical entity and should not be confused with other inflammatory processes.

Differential diagnosis of acute bacterial paronychia is herpetic whitlow.

Laboratory and Biopsy

Acute paronychia that does not respond to appropriate antibiotic therapy should be cultured and possibly radiographed, to rule out osteomyelitis. For chronic paronychia, a candidal origin can be confirmed with a KOH examination of debris taken from under the cuticle (Fig. 21.3B). Culture, if taken, often reveals mixed flora, including bacteria and *Candida* species.

Therapy

Acute paronychia should be incised and drained when it is fluctuant. Appropriate antibiotic therapy for the causative agent should be instituted. In most cases, this therapy consists of cefalexin, erythromycin, or dicloxacillin.

Chronic paronychia requires the avoidance of prolonged exposure to wetness. Wearing gloves is mandatory, preferably cotton under rubber or vinyl gloves. Frequent washings and manicures should be avoided. An anticandial and antiinflammatory topical preparations such as clotrimazole plus betamethasone dipropionate (Lotrisone) applied twice daily is helpful.

> Trauma and exposure to water must be stopped to cure chronic paronychia.

THERAPY FOR PARONYCHIA

Acute
- Cefalexin: 25–50 mg/kg daily in oral suspension, 500 mg b.i.d.
- Erythromycin: 30–50 mg/kg daily in oral suspension, 500 mg b.i.d.
- Dicloxacillin: 500 mg b.i.d.

Chronic
- Avoid trauma, water, and irritants
- Clotrimazole plus betamethasone dipropionate cream b.i.d.

Course and Complications

Acute paronychia is usually not a precursor of chronic paronychia. It resolves after appropriate antibiotic therapy and, if needed, incision and drainage.

By definition, chronic paronychia continues for a long time because repeated mechanical trauma and exposure to water predispose to the chronic infectious and inflammatory process.

Pathogenesis

Chronic paronychia is caused by microorganisms that produce swelling and inflammation of the nail fold. Interruption of the cuticle and wetness create an environment that fosters the growth of yeast and bacteria. These microorganisms also cause inflammation of the nail matrix, resulting in abnormal nail formation and subsequent nail dystrophy.

PSORIASIS

KEY POINTS
1. Psoriatic nails can mimic onychomycosis.
2. Treatment is unsatisfactory.

Definition

Nail dystrophy caused by psoriasis is the result of abnormal keratinization of the nail matrix and bed secondary to the involvement of these structures with psoriasis.

Incidence

Nail involvement in patients with psoriasis is common. Reported incidences range from 10% to 50%.

History

Psoriasis of the nail is usually asymptomatic. However, involvement of the fingernails may be a significant cosmetic liability, and deformity of the toenails may cause pain secondary to pressure from shoes.

Physical Examination

In psoriasis, fingernails are affected more often than toenails. All, or a few, nails may be involved. It is unusual for psoriasis to involve only the nails; fewer than 5% of patients have involvement of the nails alone without cutaneous disease. The examiner should look elsewhere to confirm the diagnosis, especially in other areas frequently affected by psoriasis: the scalp, elbows, knees, and intergluteal fold. In the nails, the most characteristic lesions are small, multiple pits produced by punctate psoriatic lesions in the nail matrix. Involvement of the nail bed produces brownish discoloration (oil stain), thickening of the nail plate, separation of the nail plate from the nail bed (onycholysis), distal crumbling, and splinter hemorrhages (Fig. 21.4A).

> Psoriatic nails have:
> 1. Pits
> 2. Oil stain
> 3. Onycholysis
> 4. Thickening

Differential Diagnosis

The differential diagnosis of psoriasis of the nails includes onychomycosis, trauma, aging, and dystrophy secondary to eczema

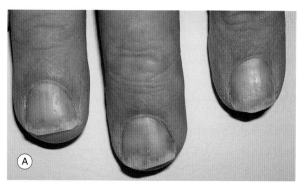

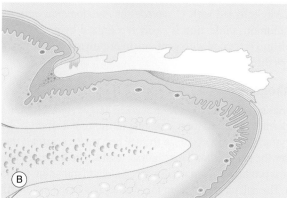

Fig. 21.4 Psoriasis. (A) Brown, discolored nail with distal separation. (B) Nail plate—thick and pitted. Epidermis—thick, hyperkeratosis.

or some other inflammatory process in the nail fold area. Fungal infections of the nail can be ruled out by a PAS stain of nail clippings, KOH preparation, and culture. Otherwise, psoriatic nails can be diagnosed with confidence only when other typical lesions of psoriasis are found elsewhere. Although nail pitting is the finding most characteristic of psoriasis, it is also occasionally associated with alopecia areata.

DIFFERENTIAL DIAGNOSIS OF NAIL PSORIASIS

- Onychomycosis
- Trauma
- Aging
- Eczema

Laboratory and Biopsy

Nails are rarely examined by biopsy to confirm the diagnosis of psoriasis (Fig. 21.4B).

Therapy

Treatment of psoriasis of the nails is difficult and usually unsatisfactory. Consequently, therapy is often not recommended. Injection of steroids into the proximal nail fold is painful, and the results are often disappointing. Topical preparations are ineffective.

Systemic medications used for psoriasis often help with nail involvement, but nail disease alone does not justify the use of these potent therapies. Trimming and paring of deformed nails reduce discomfort caused by pressure. Fingernails may be cosmetically improved by the use of sculptured plastic nails and the application of fingernail polish.

THERAPY FOR NAIL PSORIASIS

- Trimming
- Cosmetics

Course and Complications

Psoriasis of the nail is a chronic condition and has a waxing and waning course. Frequently, distal interphalangeal joint arthritis is associated with nail involvement. The nail is sometimes secondarily infected with *C. albicans* or *Pseudomonas aeruginosa*. Pseudomonas infection is easily recognized by green discoloration and is treated with gentamicin or polymyxin B, one or two drops three times daily.

Pathogenesis

Psoriasis is characterized by a marked acceleration of the rate of epidermal cell replication, resulting in the proliferation of keratinocytes. When this occurs in the nail bed, excess keratin is trapped under the nail plate and onycholysis results. The "oil stain" appearance is produced by keratinous debris and inflammation in the nail bed. The nail pits result from the involvement of the nail matrix, in which the psoriasis presumably produces small defective foci in the nail plate. As the nail plate advances, these defective portions fall out, leaving behind the characteristic pits.

UNCOMMON NAIL DISORDERS

ALLERGIC CONTACT DERMATITIS TO ACRYLIC NAILS

The artificial nail is made by mixing a liquid monomer with a powder polymer and then molding this acrylate compound onto the natural nail. Polymerization of these acrylate plastics can be initiated by ultraviolet light, which is frequently used in nail salons; however more recently, kits have been sold for at-home use. The acrylate monomer is the sensitizer that causes red, pruritic, and painful paronychial inflammation a day or two after application. The resulting nail bed inflammation causes nail dystrophy as well as removal of the artificial nail (Fig. 21.5).

PALMOPLANTAR KERATODERMA

Palmoplantar keratoderma is a rare hereditary disorder caused by keratin gene mutations. It appears as diffuse, thick, yellow hyperkeratosis of the palms and soles which has a red base and border. The nails may be affected by marked dystrophy—thickened, discolored, and crumbling (Fig. 21.6). Treatment can be difficult. However, keratolytic preparations with salicylic acid, propylene glycol, or urea may be helpful, as well as retinoids.

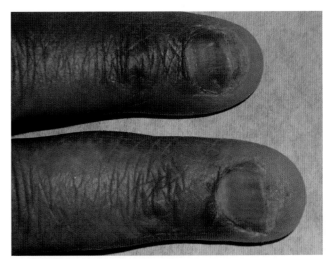

Fig. 21.5 Allergic contact dermatitis—to artificial nails, causing nail dystrophy.

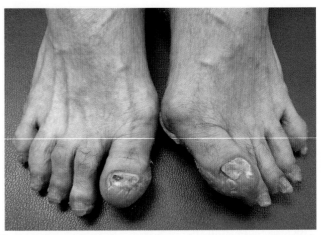

Fig. 21.6 Palmoplantar keratoderma nail dystrophy. Note the margins of the soles and toes with marked hyperkeratosis and inflammation.

Mucous Membrane Disorders

CHAPTER CONTENTS

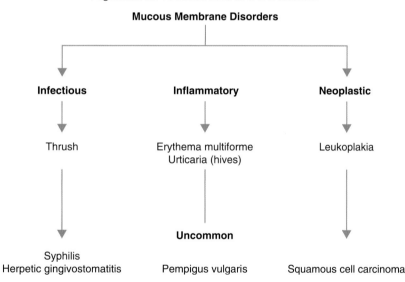

Algorithm for Mucous Membrane Disorders

ABSTRACT

Examination of the oral cavity can provide important diagnostic information for dermatologic diagnosis and therefore should be included in every skin examination. A variety of skin disorders can be accompanied by mucous membrane involvement. For example, erythema multiforme and systemic lupus erythematosus can cause erosions in the mouth, nose, or eyes. However, this chapter focuses on disorders either exclusively or predominantly confined to mucous membranes, usually of the oral cavity.

Mucous membrane disorders that can be infectious, inflammatory, and neoplastic are divided into two broad morphologic categories: (1) erosions and ulcerations and (2) white lesions (Table 22.1). Erosions are lesions in which the mucosal epithelium is partly denuded. Ulcerations extend through the epidermis into the underlying tissue, which in mucous membranes is called *lamina propria* rather than dermis. Erosive and ulcerative diseases range in frequency from common (aphthous stomatitis) to rare (pemphigus), and their causes are idiopathic, immunologic, infectious, and malignant.

Categorization of mucous membrane disorders:
1. Erosions and ulcerations
2. White lesions

TABLE 22.1 Mucous Membrane Disorders

	Etiology	History	Physical Examination	Differential Diagnosis	Laboratory Test
Ulcers					
Aphthous stomatitis (common cause)	Unknown	Recurrent disease	Sharply demarcated, round, yellowish surrounded by erythema	Herpes simplex Behçet disease Inflammatory bowel disease	–
Pemphigus and pemphigoid (uncommon causes)	Autoimmune	May have associated skin lesions	Ragged erosions and ulcerations; intact blisters are rarely present	Aphthous stomatitis Erythema multiforme	Biopsy with immunofluorescence
Viral infections	Primary herpes simplex Coxsackievirus	Fever, malaise	Gingivitis, blisters also on the lips	Aphthous stomatitis Erythema multiforme	PCR assay
		Fever	Vesicles in the posterior oral cavity	Aphthous stomatitis	–
Syphilis	Treponema pallidum	Sexual contact	Indurated, painless ulcer	Malignancy	Serological test for syphilis
Deep fungal infection	Histoplasmosis	Immunosuppressed	Systemically ill, indurated ulcer	Malignancy	Biopsy with culture
Malignancy		Nonhealing ulcer	Indurated ulcer	Major aphthous ulcer	Biopsy
White Lesions					
Thrush	Candida albicans	Found in newborns and immunosuppressed patients	"Curd-like" papules, easily scraped off	Lichen planus Geographic tongue	KOH preparation
Lichen planus	Unknown	Chronic disease; it may have associated skin lesions	Reticulated white lines; sometimes erosions are present	Candidiasis Leukoplakia Secondary syphilis	Biopsy
Leukoplakia	Chronic irritation	Smoking Denture trauma	White patches and plaques	Lichen planus Secondary syphilis White sponge nevus Leukokeratosis	Biopsy
Squamous cell carcinoma		Smoking Alcohol Prior leukoplakia	*Indurated* or *ulcerated* plaque	Leukoplakia Major aphthous ulcer Erosive lichen planus Chancre Deep fungal infection	Biopsy

KOH, Potassium hydroxide; *PCR*, polymerase chain reaction.

White spots are hyperkeratotic lesions of the oral mucosa. The thickened stratum corneum of mucous membranes appears white because of maceration from continuous wetness. Malignancy must be ruled out as a cause.

> White lesions represent hyperkeratosis.

APHTHOUS STOMATITIS

KEY POINTS

1. Most common cause of recurrent oral ulcers.
2. Ulcers have a yellow base and peripheral erythema.
3. Multiple therapies indicate a lack of effective treatment.

Definition

Aphthous stomatitis is a common, recurrent, idiopathic disorder of the mouth, most often manifest by multiple small, "punched out" ulcers (Fig. 22.1).

Incidence

Recurrent aphthous stomatitis is a common disease, occurring in 20%–60% of the general population. It is most common in young adults; a 60% prevalence was found in a survey of students attending professional schools.

History

A history of previous episodes is invariable. Recurrences are sometimes precipitated by trauma from biting or misguided toothbrushes. Some patients correlate outbreaks with emotional

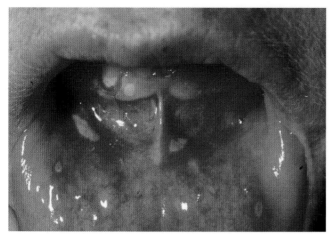

Fig. 22.1 **Aphthous stomatitis**—round, punched out ulcer with a white-yellow necrotic surface.

stress. Lesions are usually preceded by a 1-day prodrome of discomfort in the area of involvement. The ulcers are painful and sometimes interfere with eating.

Physical Examination

Lesions in aphthous stomatitis appear as 2- to 5-mm, round, punched out ulcers with a yellowish necrotic surface and surrounding erythema. Lesions may be single but are more often multiple. The buccal and labial mucosae are the most common locations.

> Aphthous stomatitis is the most common cause of oral ulceration.

Differential Diagnosis

Recurrent aphthous stomatitis is most often confused with *herpes simplex infection*. Recurrent herpes simplex occurs rarely inside the mouth. When it does, it appears as grouped small vesicles or erosions on an erythematous base. Polymerase chain reaction assay is the preferred method for diagnosing herpes infections, being it is rapid, specific, and sensitive.

> Herpes simplex recurs rarely inside the mouth.

The oral ulcerations in *Behçet disease* are indistinguishable from those of aphthous stomatitis. However, Behçet disease is distinguished by its extraoral manifestations. The classic triad consists of oral ulcerations, genital ulcerations, and ocular inflammation (iridocyclitis) (Fig. 22.2). Erythema nodosum, thrombophlebitis, arthritis, and neurologic and intestinal involvement may also occur. Patients with inflammatory bowel disease, particularly *ulcerative colitis*, occasionally have oral ulcerations that resemble aphthous stomatitis.

> Oral ulcerations in Behçet disease look like aphthous stomatitis.

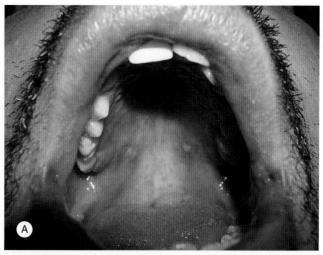
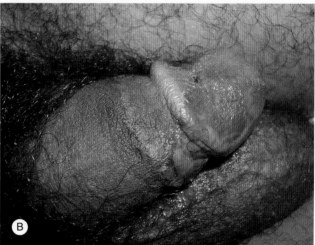

Fig. 22.2 **Behçet disease**. (A) Oral ulcers on hard palate. (B) Erosions on the penis.

DIFFERENTIAL DIAGNOSIS FOR APHTHOUS STOMATITIS

- Herpes simplex infection
- Behçet disease
- Oral ulcers from inflammatory bowel disease

Laboratory and Biopsy

Usually, a biopsy is not required. If a biopsy is performed, the findings will not be diagnostic and will show only ulceration and nonspecific inflammation, composed primarily of lymphocytes. The only other laboratory test to consider is a complete blood count to screen for the questionable association of iron or folate deficiency anemia in some patients with aphthous stomatitis.

Therapy

The variety of therapies that have been recommended for this disease indicates that a highly successful treatment is lacking. If an underlying iron or folate deficiency is detected, it should be corrected. The ulcerations are usually treated topically. Tetracycline suspension (250 mg/5 mL) "swished and swallowed" four times daily helps in some patients. Patients in whom tetracycline therapy fails are treated with topical steroids in a gel (e.g., fluocinonide, Lidex gel) or a special adherent base (e.g., triamcinolone, Kenalog in Orabase) applied three times daily or with a spray preparation (e.g., beclomethasone, Vanceril) applied three to four times daily. Intralesional steroids (triamcinolone, Kenalog-10) are useful in patients with large aphthous ulcerations. Oral prednisone is effective in aphthous stomatitis but should be used for only a short course in patients with severe, incapacitating disease. Colchicine, pentoxifylline (Trental), anti–tumor necrosis factor (TNF)-alpha biologics, apremilast, and dapsone have also been reported to be helpful in preventing recurrent disease, but the clinical trials were not controlled.

Pain relief can be obtained with topical anesthetics such as dyclonine hydrochloride (Dyclone liquid) or topical lidocaine (viscous Xylocaine) used 20 minutes before meals. These preparations numb the entire mouth, including the taste buds, for 1–2 hours and allow for pain-free, albeit taste-free, dining.

THERAPY FOR APHTHOUS STOMATITIS

Initial
- Topical steroids
  - Fluocinonide gel 0.05%
  - Triamcinolone in Orabase
  - Beclomethasone spray
- Tetracycline "swish and swallow"
- Dyclonine hydrochloride 1% solution
- Lidocaine jelly 2%

Alternative
- Intralesional triamcinolone
- Systemic treatment (colchicine/pentoxifylline/apremilast/dapsone/anti-TNF-alpha biologics/prednisone)

Course and Complications

For minor aphthous stomatitis, spontaneous healing occurs within 4–14 days. Large aphthous ulcers (major aphthous ulcers) take as long as 6 weeks to heal. Individual ulcers lasting much longer than that should be examined by biopsy to rule out malignancy. Recurrences are common and range in frequency from occasional to almost continuous. In most patients, the disease eventually remits, but the time course is highly variable—from 5 to 15 years or longer.

Pathogenesis

Factors implicated in the pathogenesis include emotional and physical stress, hormones, infection, and autoimmunity. An immune mechanism is the most favored cause. Circulating T lymphocytes that are cytotoxic against oral mucosa have been identified and appear to play a role.

LEUKOPLAKIA

KEY POINTS

1. White plaques can signify cancer.
2. Indurated white plaques require biopsy.
3. Smoking is the most frequent cause.

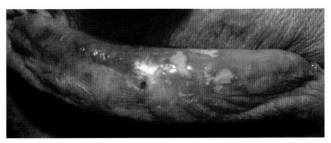

Fig. 22.3 **Leukoplakia**—white patch or plaque that requires biopsy to rule out malignancy.

Definition

Leukoplakia literally means "white plaque" (Fig. 22.3). Some clinicians simply use that as the definition of the disease, defining leukoplakia as "a white patch or plaque that cannot be characterized clinically or pathologically as any other disease." Others use the term *leukokeratosis* to describe a white patch that is histologically benign and reserve the term *leukoplakia* for a white patch or plaque in which epithelial dysplasia is present pathologically. The authors prefer the second definition. Either way, the important point to remember is that, for white plaques on mucous membranes, a dysplastic change should be considered a possible cause.

The white color is due to macerated hyperkeratosis, which, in most cases, is caused by chronic irritation. Smoking tobacco is the most frequent origin, but physical irritation from dentures or ragged teeth may also be causative.

Smoking is a frequent cause.

Incidence

Leukoplakia is an uncommon disorder affecting primarily middle-aged and elderly adults. The incidence depends, of course, on the definition. The disease is about one-tenth as common when dysplastic histological changes are the required criteria.

History

The onset is gradual and usually asymptomatic. Accordingly, leukoplakia is sometimes an incidental finding during a routine physical examination. Some patients seek medical attention because of irritation, which may be the original cause of the problem. Many patients are smokers or have used smokeless tobacco.

Physical Findings

Leukoplakia appears as a white patch or plaque on the mucous membrane. The surface may be flat or verrucous, and the color varies from pure white to gray. It can be located anywhere in the mouth, including the lips. The tongue is a common location, but leukoplakia can occur on the tonsils, pharynx, or larynx. Leukoplakia may also be found on the genital mucosa.

All white lesions should be palpated for induration. Induration and ulceration are important physical findings that strongly suggest carcinoma (Fig. 22.4). Sometimes, only part of

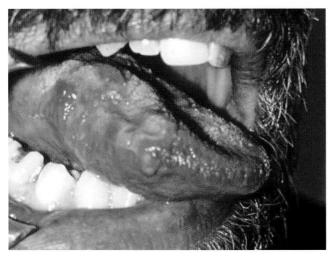

Fig. 22.4 Squamous cell carcinoma of the tongue—the surface of this large nodule is white (hyperkeratotic) and ulcerated, and the base feels hard and indurated.

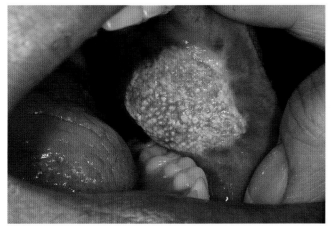

Fig. 22.5 White sponge nevus—"spongy" white plaque on buccal mucosa.

a white plaque is indurated, and this area should be examined by biopsy to rule out cancer.

> All white plaques should be palpated; indurated areas must be examined by biopsy to rule out cancer.

Differential Diagnosis

The differential diagnosis of white lesions in the mouth is given in Table 22.1. The reticulated form of oral *lichen planus* is usually clinically distinctive. Mucous patches in *secondary syphilis* are accompanied by other manifestations of the disease, including skin rash and constitutional symptoms. *White sponge nevus* is a hereditary condition that begins in childhood and results in a white lesion that appears "spongy" (Fig. 22.5). *Leukokeratosis* is a diagnosis of exclusion that clinically does not fit another known entity and histopathologically shows no dysplastic changes. The diagnosis then often rests with the biopsy.

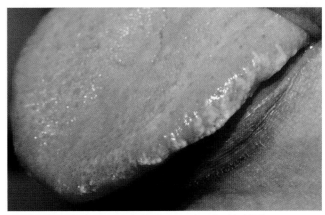

Fig. 22.6 Oral hairy leukoplakia is associated with AIDS.

> Diagnosis depends on the biopsy.

Oral hairy leukoplakia affects the sides of the tongue with white papules and plaques that sometimes have a filiform (hairy) surface (Fig. 22.6). This disorder occurs almost exclusively in patients with AIDS and may be the first sign of HIV infection. It is asymptomatic, not premalignant, and is now known to be caused by infection with Epstein–Barr virus. Treatment with acyclovir and other antiviral agents can cause the condition to regress. With advances in treatment for HIV infection, this disease is rarely seen in the United States.

DIFFERENTIAL DIAGNOSIS FOR LEUKOPLAKIA

- Oral lichen planus
- Secondary syphilis
- White sponge nevus
- Oral hairy leukoplakia

Laboratory and Biopsy

The histopathologic findings include hyperkeratosis, acanthosis, and underlying inflammation in the lamina propria composed of lymphocytes and plasma cells (plasma cells are common in inflammatory reactions of mucous membranes). In leukoplakia, the epithelial dysplastic changes are similar to those found in actinic keratosis and include cellular pleomorphism, increased numbers of mitotic figures, and derangement of the usual orderly architectural pattern of stratified epithelium. The dysplastic changes may be mild, moderate, or severe. When they are severe (carcinoma in situ), the entire thickness of the epithelium is involved in marked dysplastic changes. Invasion of these cells into the underlying lamina propria signifies squamous cell carcinoma.

Therapy

The goals of therapy are to eliminate the cause and surgically remove persistent lesions. Smoking or the use of smokeless tobacco should be eliminated, and sources of physical trauma should be corrected. Lesions may then resolve spontaneously, particularly when only mildly dysplastic. For lesions that are persistent or more severely dysplastic, active intervention is recommended. Superficial mucosal lesions can be removed with cryosurgery, carbon dioxide laser ablation, or shave excision. Medical therapies include topical bleomycin and systemic retinoids. Lesions suggestive of squamous cell carcinoma should be excised.

THERAPY FOR LEUKOPLAKIA

Initial
- Biopsy
- Cessation of tobacco use
- Elimination of sources of physical trauma
- Excision (if cancer is suspected)

Alternative
- Ablation of superficial lesions
  - Cryosurgery
  - Carbon dioxide laser
  - Shave excision
- Topical bleomycin
- Systemic retinoids

Course and Complications

Spontaneous involution may occur, especially when the aggravating factors are withdrawn. Some lesions may become stationary, whereas others progress to squamous cell carcinoma.

The frequency of the development of squamous cell carcinoma in lesions of leukoplakia depends in part on the definition. If dysplasia is among the diagnostic criteria, approximately 30% of leukoplakia lesions will progress to squamous cell carcinoma. If the broader definition (not requiring dysplasia) is used, invasive carcinoma will occur in only 3%–6%.

> Squamous cell carcinoma develops in 30% of patients with "dysplastic leukoplakia."

Pathogenesis

Usually, leukoplakia appears to be induced by chronic, mild irritation from physical, chemical, or inflammatory processes. Smoking is the most frequent and important cause. Chemical agents in smoking include polycyclic hydrocarbons and phenolic oils. Heat may also contribute. Physical trauma from ill-fitting dentures, long-term use of toothpicks, and irritation from jagged teeth can also cause leukoplakia. Also, human papillomavirus infection has been implicated in the pathogenesis of some cases of leukoplakia.

LICHEN PLANUS

KEY POINTS
1. Characteristic lace-like pattern on the buccal mucosa
2. Diagnosis confirmed by biopsy
3. Resistant to treatment

Definition

Oral lesions in lichen planus occur alone or in association with skin lesions. The oral lesions are characterized by inflammation and hyperkeratosis, which appear clinically as white lesions, most commonly in the form of reticulated papules and lines that assume a lace-like pattern (Fig. 22.7). *Erosive lichen planus* is a less common variant. The origin of lichen planus is unknown.

Incidence

Lichen planus is probably the most common cause of white lesions in the mouth. It has been found in 0.5%–1% of patients in dental clinics. The highest incidence occurs in adults aged 40–60 years.

> Lichen planus is the most common cause of white lesions in the mouth.

History

Drugs can also cause a lichen planus type of eruption in the mouth. Most often implicated drugs are quinidine, quinacrine, sulfonylureas, and tetracycline.

> Drugs can be causative.

Usually, no symptoms are associated with the hyperkeratotic type of oral lichen planus. Erosive lichen planus is painful and may make eating difficult. If the patient has accompanying skin lesions, they are usually pruritic.

Physical Examination

Patches of oral lichen planus usually appear as white lines and puncta in a reticulated (lace-like) pattern. Occasionally, these patches become confluent, producing a solid plaque. Blisters and erosions occur less often and are the result of an intense dermal inflammatory reaction occurring at the epidermal–lamina propria junction.

> The reticulated (lace-like) pattern is characteristic.

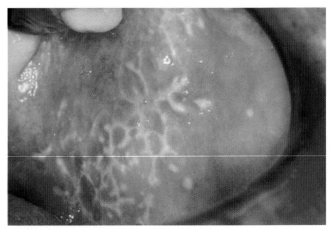

Fig. 22.7 Lichen planus—reticulate, lace-like pattern of lines and papules on the buccal mucosa.

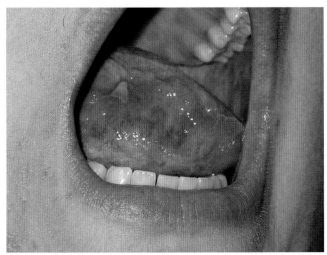

Fig. 22.8 Lichen planus—ulcer on the tongue must be biopsied to rule out squamous cell carcinoma.

The most common site of involvement is the buccal mucosa, which is affected bilaterally in virtually 100% of patients. The tongue, gingiva, and lips may also be affected (Fig. 22.8). Skin lesions (described in Chapter 11) accompany oral lichen planus in 10%–40% of cases.

Differential Diagnosis

Candidiasis is distinguished from lichen planus by the ease with which white material can be scraped off and by finding hyphae on potassium hydroxide (KOH) examination. The two conditions can coexist, so a scraping is often worthwhile because the candidal component is easily treatable. *Leukoplakia* and *malignancy* should be considered in patients with the plaque form of lichen planus—a biopsy enables distinction between the two. Mucous patches in *secondary syphilis* are usually accompanied by other manifestations of this disease (e.g., rash, fever, lymphadenopathy), and the disease is diagnosed with a serologic test for syphilis.

> ### DIFFERENTIAL DIAGNOSIS FOR ORAL LICHEN PLANUS
> - Candidiasis
> - Leukoplakia/malignancy
> - Secondary syphilis

Laboratory and Biopsy

The diagnosis is generally made clinically for lesions in the usual reticulate pattern. If doubt exists or if the patient has plaques, blisters, or erosions, a biopsy is diagnostic. The histologic findings are similar to those in lichen planus in the skin. Even a thin keratinized layer represents *hyper*keratosis in areas that are not normally keratinized, such as the buccal mucosa. In addition, a dense, band-like, inflammatory infiltrate in the lamina propria obscures the basement membrane zone and is accompanied by degenerative changes in the basal cell layer. If the reaction is intense, separation may occur at this area and may result in blisters and erosions.

> Biopsy is diagnostic.

Therapy

Oral lesions in lichen planus tend to be even more resistant to therapy than skin lesions. Asymptomatic involvement requires no therapy. In patients with symptoms (e.g., those with erosive disease), various agents have been tried with limited success. Some patients benefit from twice-daily applications of a potent (e.g., Lidex) topical steroid gel or ointment. Long-term use, however, predisposes to candidiasis and causes tissue atrophy. Intralesional triamcinolone (Kenalog) in a concentration of 5 mg/mL can be injected into local lesions, sometimes with a long-lasting effect. Systemic corticosteroids are effective but should be generally avoided for this chronic disease. Topical tretinoin (Retin-A) gel 0.025%, applied twice daily, helps occasionally. A higher success rate is achieved with the orally administered retinoid, acitretin, at a dose of 25 mg daily. This drug is associated with many side-effects, so its use should be reserved for patients with severe, refractory disease. Such patients have also been successfully treated with oral cyclosporine. Improvement has also been reported with the use of a cyclosporine "swish and spit" regimen at a dose of 5 mL (500 mg) three times daily. The extraordinary expense of this therapy can be reduced by applying smaller amounts of the medication directly to the lesions. Several studies have demonstrated clinical improvement with the off-label use of the oral phosphodiesterase IV inhibitor, apremilast

> ### THERAPY FOR ORAL LICHEN PLANUS
> **Initial**
> - Topical therapy
>   - Steroids (e.g., fluocinonide gel 0.05%)
>   - Pimecrolimus/tacrolimus
>
> **Alternative**
> - Topical
>   - Tretinoin gel 0.025%
>   - Cyclosporine solution
> - Intralesional steroids
> - Systemic therapy (reserved for extremely severe disease)
>   - Prednisone
>   - Acitretin
>   - Cyclosporine

Course and Complications

The course is measured in terms of months to decades. In patients with white lesions, approximately 50% experience remittance within 2 years and, of these, approximately 20% experience recurrence. The course is more prolonged in patients with blistering and erosive diseases.

> The course is usually chronic.

Secondary candidal infection occurs in some patients with oral lichen planus. Cases of squamous cell carcinoma have been reported in association with the oral lichen planus. Although this complication is uncommon, it appears to be more than coincidental. Therefore patients with chronic erosive oral lichen planus should be followed; if an indurated lesion develops, a biopsy should be performed to rule out squamous cell carcinoma.

> Patients with erosive oral lichen planus are at risk for squamous cell carcinoma.

Pathogenesis

The pathogenesis of lichen planus is discussed in Chapter 11.

THRUSH (ORAL CANDIDIASIS)

KEY POINTS

1. Common in newborns and immunosuppressed adults
2. Appears as white patches that easily scrape off
3. Treat with topical or oral antifungals

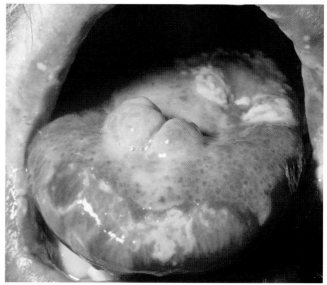

Fig. 22.9 Thrush—white, curd-like plaques that are easily scraped off.

Definition

Thrush is caused by infection of the oral epithelium with *Candida albicans*. The infected epithelium appears white and can be scraped off, leaving an inflamed base (Fig. 22.9).

Incidence

Thrush is most common in newborns, with one-third of neonates affected by the first week after birth. In adults, this disorder is uncommon and usually occurs in denture-wearing patients or in the setting of local or systemic immunosuppression. For example, oral candidiasis used to be a frequent finding in patients with AIDS; in these patients, it may extend to involve the esophagus. Thrush also occurs in patients with chronic mucocutaneous candidiasis, a rare disorder in which chronic mucous membrane infection is accompanied by skin and nail involvement, most likely secondary to a T-cell defect (Fig. 22.10).

> Thrush is most common in newborns and immunosuppressed patients.

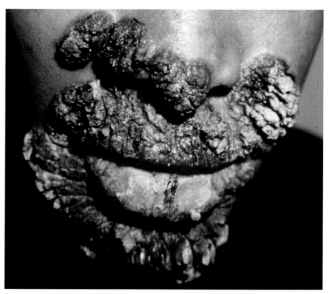

Fig. 22.10 Chronic mucocutaneous candidiasis—warty, hyperkeratotic plaques; culture grew *Candida*.

History

Mothers of infected newborns usually have a history of vaginal candidiasis during the latter part of their pregnancy. For older patients acquiring thrush, predisposing factors include the following: dentures; intraoral steroids, such as the aerosolized preparations used to treat asthma; broad-spectrum systemic antibiotics; systemic immunosuppression from disease or drugs, including systemic corticosteroids; and diabetes.

> Predisposing factors:
> 1. Dentures
> 2. Steroids
> 3. Antibiotics
> 4. Immunosuppression
> 5. Diabetes

Physical Examination

The lesions appear as white, curd-like papules and patches that sometimes resemble "cottage cheese." Much of this material can be scraped off, leaving an erythematous base. The tongue and buccal mucosa are affected most often. In denture-wearing patients, the mucosal surfaces under the dentures are involved, so the dentures must be removed for the mucosa to be evaluated. The angles of the mouth also may be involved (*angular cheilitis*), particularly when this area remains moist, such as in patients with ill-fitting dentures that cause excessive overlap of the upper lip (Fig. 22.11).

> The curd-like material can be scraped off easily.

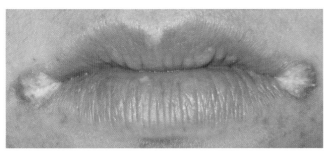

Fig. 22.11 Angular cheilitis—moist white papules at corners of mouth; potassium hydroxide confirms clinical suspicion.

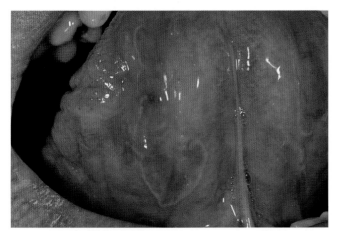

Fig. 22.12 Geographic tongue—red patches with white, scalloped borders on the underside of the tongue in a patient with psoriasis.

Differential Diagnosis

Lichen planus may be confused with thrush. However, thrush is differentiated from this and the other white lesion diseases in that the white material in thrush is scraped off easily. *Geographic tongue* is characterized by red patches with white, scalloped borders, usually on the dorsal and lateral tongue. This disorder is most commonly seen in patients who have psoriasis; its cause is unknown, and it is not infectious. The white borders do not scrape off, a distinguishing factor from thrush (Fig. 22.12).

DIFFERENTIAL DIAGNOSIS FOR ORAL CANDIDIASIS
• Lichen planus
• Geographic tongue

Laboratory and Biopsy

The diagnostic test is a KOH examination of material from a scraping. With thrush, there is usually no difficulty in finding hyphae and pseudohyphae. These same elements would be found in the surface epithelium were a biopsy to be done, but because the KOH preparation is diagnostic, biopsy is not required. A culture is not helpful because *C. albicans* may be found in normal flora in the mouth. Candidiasis affecting

adults who do not have predisposing factors, such as dentures, antibiotics, corticosteroid use, or diabetes, should prompt consideration of immunosuppressive conditions, such as AIDS.

The KOH examination is diagnostic.

Therapy

Infants are treated with nystatin suspension by applying 1 mL (100,000 units) to each side of the mouth four times daily for 5–7 days. Adults can be treated with a "swish and swallow" nystatin suspension in a dose of 5 mL (500,000 units) four times daily. An alternative topical therapy is clotrimazole (Mycelex) troches dissolved in the mouth five times daily for 1–2 weeks. Itraconazole (Sporanox) solution can also be used in a "swish and swallow" regimen. Other systemic therapies include fluconazole (Diflucan) and itraconazole (Sporanox), taken for 1–2 weeks.

THERAPY FOR THRUSH
Infants and Children
Initial
• None
• Nystatin suspension 2 mL (200,000 units) q.i.d.
Alternative
• Fluconazole oral suspension 2–3 mg/kg daily
Adults
Initial
• "Swish and swallow"
• Nystatin suspension 5 mL (500,000 µL) q.i.d.
• Itraconazole solution 10 mL (100 mg) b.i.d.
• Clotrimazole troches 10 mg five times per day
Alternative
• Oral
• Fluconazole 100 mg daily
• Itraconazole 200 mg twice daily

In denture-wearing patients, candidal colonization of the dentures also must be treated. Acrylic dentures can be soaked overnight in a dilute (1:10) sodium hypochlorite (Clorox) solution, and a 0.12% chlorhexidine solution (Peridex) can be used for soaking metal plates.

Course and Complications

In newborns, thrush often clears spontaneously, but healing is hastened with therapy. In immunosuppressed patients, the disease can become recurrent and chronic. The most chronic infections are encountered in patients with the syndrome of chronic mucocutaneous candidiasis who are deficient in cellular immunity for *C. albicans*. Even in those patients, however, systemic therapy results in clearing, although recurrences usually follow cessation of therapy.

Complications are uncommon. In severely immunosuppressed patients, esophageal involvement can occur; rarely, the infection spreads systemically, causing disseminated candidiasis, which is frequently a fatal infection.

Pathogenesis

The pathogenesis of candidal infections is discussed in Chapter 12.

UNCOMMON CAUSES OF ORAL ULCERS

Numerous uncommon causes of oral ulcerations exist; several are listed in Table 22.1. Causes include autoimmunity, infection, and malignancy.

AUTOIMMUNE DISEASES

Pemphigus vulgaris and mucous membrane pemphigoid are autoimmune chronic blistering diseases with prominent or predominant mucosal involvement. Some 90% of patients with *pemphigus vulgaris* have oral involvement, and in 50% of patients, the disease begins in the mouth (Fig. 22.13). Fragile blisters are easily broken, so erosion is the usual finding. The erosions are larger than those of aphthous stomatitis and are present continuously. Further details of this disease are discussed in Chapter 10. *Cicatricial pemphigoid* is a subepidermal blistering process confined to mucous membranes (Fig. 22.14A). Mucosae of the mouth, eyes, and conjunctivae are most frequently affected. Eye involvement may lead to scarring and blindness (Fig. 22.14B).

In both diseases, autoantibodies are directed against mucosal epithelia and are detected by direct immunofluorescence of biopsied mucosa (Fig. 22.14C) or by indirect immunofluorescence of serum. In pemphigus vulgaris, the antibodies are deposited between the cells in the epithelium; in mucous membrane pemphigoid, as in bullous pemphigoid, the deposition occurs in the basement membrane zone.

CANCER

Malignant tumors inside the mouth can erode and result in ulceration. Characteristically, these lesions are indurated. The most common cause is *squamous cell carcinoma*, but lymphomas and leukemias can also cause oral ulcers (Fig. 22.15). A biopsy is diagnostic. Intraoral squamous cell carcinoma is of high risk and more likely to metastasize than cutaneous squamous cell carcinoma.

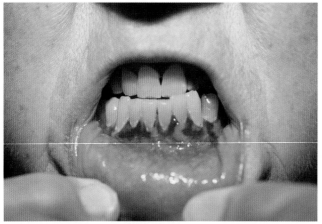

Fig. 22.13 **Pemphigus vulgaris**. Erosive and inflamed gingiva present.

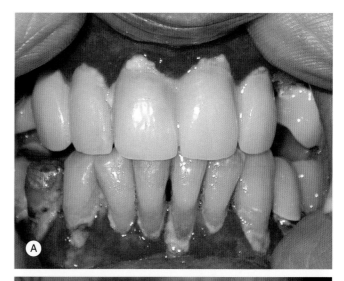

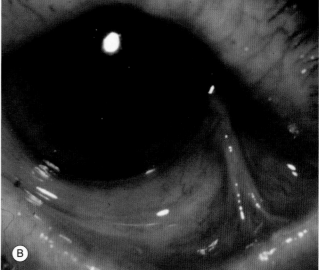

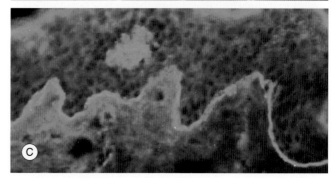

Fig. 22.14 **Cicatricial pemphigoid (mucous membrane pemphigoid)**. (A) Shallow, inflamed ulcerations of gingiva. (B) Eye involvement can lead to scarring and symblepharon formation. (C) Immunoglobulin G deposition at the basement membrane zone.

INFECTIONS

Infectious diseases causing oral ulcerations include, in decreasing order of frequency, viruses (herpesvirus and coxsackievirus), *Treponema* (syphilis), and systemic fungi (histoplasmosis). As already mentioned, herpes simplex rarely recurs inside the mouth, but the initial episode often involves the oral mucosa

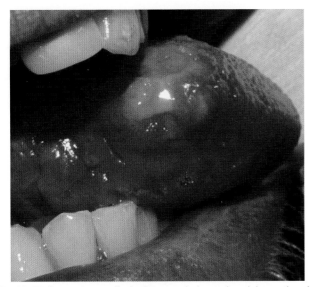

Fig. 22.15 Squamous cell carcinoma—indurated nodule on the side of the tongue; a biopsy is mandatory.

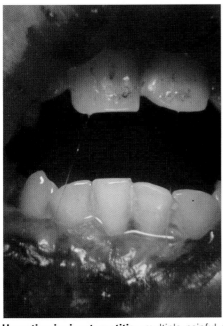

Fig. 22.16 Herpetic gingivostomatitis—multiple painful erosions on labial mucosa and inflamed gingiva.

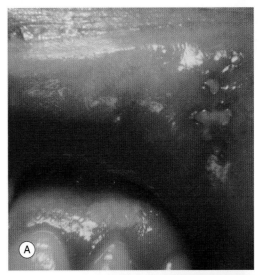

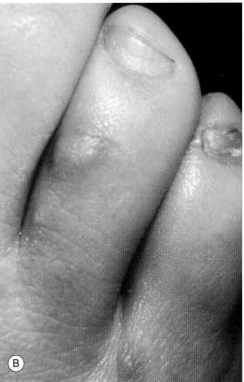

Fig. 22.17 Hand, foot, and mouth disease. (A) Erosions on the upper labial mucosa. (B) Pustule with a red flare on the toe.

with *herpetic gingivostomatitis*. Erosive gingivitis is characteristic of primary oral herpetic infection and is usually accompanied by lesions on the lips and perioral skin (Fig. 22.16). It is accompanied by fever and regional lymphadenopathy and lasts for 2–3 weeks. Infection with coxsackievirus A-4 causes *herpangina*, which appears as a vesicular eruption in the posterior oral cavity lasting 7–10 days. Coxsackievirus A-16 causes *hand, foot, and mouth disease* and is a distinctive disorder characterized by small vesicles in the posterior portion of the mouth and accompanied by similar lesions on the palms and soles (Fig. 22.17).

The lesion in primary *syphilis* is a *chancre*, which appears as a single, painless, punched out ulcer and characteristically feels indurated. A darkfield examination of an oral chancre must be interpreted with caution because nontreponemal spirochetes

normally colonize the mouth. If doubt exists, a serologic test for syphilis should be performed. If the result is negative, the test should be repeated in 1 month.

Indurated oral ulcerations occur rarely in patients with disseminated systemic fungal infections such as *histoplasmosis*. A biopsy with special stains and cultures confirms the diagnosis.

KEY POINTS

1. Often present as white lesions or ulcers/erosions
2. Biopsy white lesions and nonhealing ulcers/erosions to rule out malignancy

23

Skin Signs of Systemic Disease

ABSTRACT

The skin can be the window to systemic diseases. The presenting cutaneous symptoms and signs will lead the clinician to a more focused differential diagnosis and thus aid in the ordering of laboratory tests. In some cases, for example, lymphoma, a skin biopsy is diagnostic.

FEVER AND RASH

KEY POINTS

1. Characterize the rash to limit the differential diagnosis
2. Do laboratory tests based on the history and physical examination

A wide spectrum of diseases can present with fever and rash, including infections, drug reactions (e.g., DRESS; Fig. 23.1), rheumatic diseases and so on. These causes are listed in Table 23.1, according to the primary cutaneous lesions: macules and papules, purpura, nodules and plaques, vesicles and bullae, and pustules. Some of these diseases (e.g., meningococcemia; Fig. 23.2) are life-threatening and require prompt diagnosis and treatment.

The methods used to diagnose the cause of fever and rash are similar to those used for fever of unknown origin. Clues are sought in the history and physical examination (e.g., Sweet syndrome) (Fig. 23.3). The type of eruption is particularly important, as noted in Table 23.1.

Diagnostic laboratory tests are directed by the history and physical examination. Simple procedures such as a potassium hydroxide preparation, a Gram stain, and a Tzanck smear should not be overlooked. These "bedside" tests can quickly establish an infectious cause. A skin biopsy with appropriate stains and cultures may be diagnostic. Further workup is dictated by the clinical setting.

ITCHING PATIENT

KEY POINTS

1. Primary lesions suggest a dermatologic disorder.
2. No primary lesions suggest a systemic cause.

Because itching is a common symptom, it is often not diagnostically discriminatory. Chronic pruritus has a significant negative impact on quality of life similar to pain. Table 23.2 lists two general categories in which itching is important: skin rashes in which itching is a *prominent* complaint, and systemic conditions causing generalized pruritus without primary skin lesions. For the itching patient, therefore, one must first decide whether the itching is caused by a skin disorder or a systemic disorder.

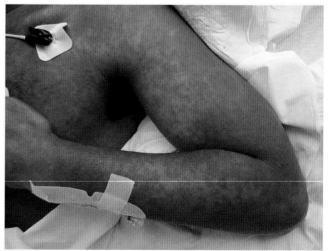

Fig. 23.1 DRESS—drug reaction with eosinophilia and systemic symptoms.

TABLE 23.1 Fever and Rash

Macules and Papules (Erythematous Rashes)
- Infections
  - Viral
    Measles (rubella, rubeola)
    Adenovirus
    Echovirus
    Infectious mononucleosis
    HIV
    West Nile
    Ebola
    Chikungunya
    Zika
  - Bacterial
    Staphylococcus—toxic shock syndrome
    Streptococcus—erysipelas, rheumatic and scarlet fever
    Typhoid fever
    Typhus—endemic
    Rat-bite fever
  - Treponemal
    Erythema migrans (Lyme disease)
    Secondary syphilis
  - Fungal
    Cryptococcosis
- Drug reaction with eosinophilia and systemic symptoms (DRESS)
- Rheumatic disease
    Systemic lupus erythematosus
    Dermatomyositis
    Juvenile rheumatoid arthritis
    Adult Still disease
- Erythema multiforme
- Kawasaki syndrome
- Tumor necrosis factor receptor–associated periodic syndrome (TRAPS)
- Familial Mediterranean fever
- Hyperimmunoglobulinemia D syndrome (HIDS)
- Interferonopathies

Purpura
- Infections
  - Viral
    Ebola
    Enterovirus
    Dengue
    Hepatitis
  - Bacterial
    Gonococcemia
    Meningococcemia
    Pseudomonas septicemia
    Bacterial endocarditis (Osler nodes, Janeway lesions)
    Ehrlichiosis
  - Rickettsial
    Typhus—epidemic
    Rocky Mountain spotted fever

- Fungal
    Candidal septicemia
- Drug reaction
- Vasculitis
- Rheumatic disease
    Systemic lupus erythematosus
    Rheumatoid arthritis
- Thrombotic thrombocytopenic purpura

Nodules and Plaques
- Infections
  - Bacterial
    Tuberculosis
  - Fungal
    Histoplasmosis
    Blastomycosis
    Coccidioidomycosis
- Lymphoma
- Erythema nodosum
- Sweet syndrome

Vesicles and Bullae
- Infections
  - Viral
    Herpes simplex (primary, disseminated)
    Herpes zoster (disseminated)
    Coxsackie (hand, foot, and mouth syndrome)
    Varicella
    Mpox
    Orf
    Smallpox
  - Rickettsial
    Rickettsialpox
  - Bacterial
    Staphylococcal scalded skin syndrome
    Drug reaction (toxic epidermal necrolysis [TEN])
- Erythema multiforme

Pustules
- Infections
  - Viral
    Herpes simplex and zoster
    Varicella
  - Treponemal
    Congenital syphilis
  - Bacterial
    Gonococcemia
  - Fungal
    Candidal septicemia
    Blastomycosis
- Drug eruption (acute generalized exanthematous pustulosis [AGEP])
- Pustular psoriasis

For skin disorders, primary lesions are present, and the type of primary lesion is used to identify the cause. Of the skin disorders listed, scabies (Fig. 23.4) is missed most often because of its nonspecific eczematous appearance and the difficulty in finding a mite. Dermatitis herpetiformis, a rare disorder, is also overlooked because the intensely pruritic vesicles are excoriated, leaving only nonspecific crusts. Xerotic (dry) skin is one of the most common causes of itching, along with eczema and psoriasis.

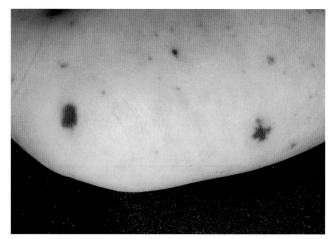
Fig. 23.2 Meningococcemia—purpura in an acutely ill patient.

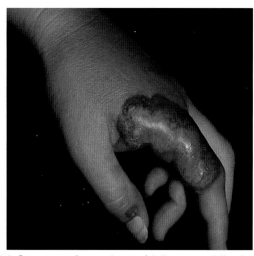
Fig. 23.3 Sweet syndrome (acute febrile neutrophilic dermatosis) manifest by a bullous-appearing hemorrhagic plaque. This patient had fever, neutrophilia, and acute myelogenous leukemia.

TABLE 23.2   Pruritus

Primary Lesion (Skin Disease)	No Primary Lesion (Systemic Disease)
Macules	Endocrine
Urticaria pigmentosa (hives when stroked)	Hyperthyroidism
Erythroderma (Sézary syndrome)	Diabetes mellitus[a]
Drug eruptions	Hypothyroidism[a]
Papules and plaques	Hepatic
Scabies	Biliary obstruction
Lichen planus	Renal
Atopic dermatitis	Uremia
Psoriasis	Hematologic
Essential dermatitis	Lymphoma (especially Hodgkin disease)
Insect bites	Polycythemia vera
Miliaria (heat rash)	Leukemia[a]
Drug eruption	Anemia[a]
Dry skin	Carcinomas[a]
Vesicles	Lung
Chickenpox	Gastrointestinal
Dermatitis herpetiformis	Breast
Urticaria	Neuropsychogenic/neuropathic
	Delusions of parasitosis
	Neurodermatitis
	Infections
	Intestinal parasites

[a]Not well-documented.

In pruritus resulting from systemic disease, primary skin lesions are absent (e.g., Hodgkin disease; Fig. 23.5), although excoriations may be found. For patients with generalized pruritus, take their medical history and perform a physical examination. Screening tests include a complete blood count with differential, liver and renal function tests, thyroid profile, and chest radiography. Sometimes, however, a primary cutaneous or systemic cause is not found.

SKIN SIGNS OF AIDS

KEY POINTS
1. Chronic or unusual infection
2. Kaposi sarcoma

Skin disorders are frequent in patients with AIDS. A generalized erythematous exanthem may accompany a febrile illness that occurs 3–6 weeks after the primary inoculation with HIV. This symptomatic primary infection occurs in only

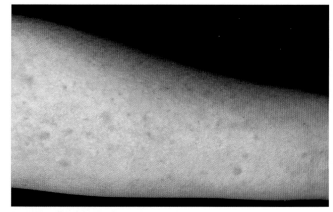
Fig. 23.4 Scabies—markedly pruritic, nonspecific-appearing, pink, papules.

approximately 10%–20% of patients and is not diagnostic of early HIV infection. Skin signs are more frequent and more diagnostic later in the course of the disease. Immunosuppression predisposes to infections and probably also to some of the neoplastic manifestations. For example, infection with type 8 herpes simplex virus is strongly associated with Kaposi sarcoma

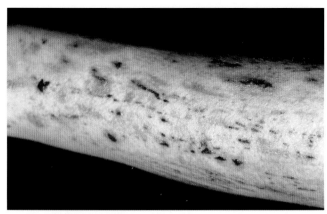

Fig. 23.5 Hodgkin disease—excoriations with no primary lesions in this patient with severe generalized pruritus.

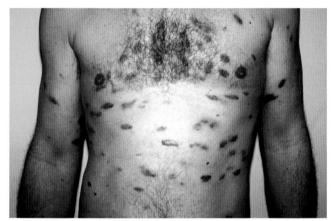

Fig. 23.6 Kaposi sarcoma—diffuse purple plaques in a patient with AIDS.

TABLE 23.3   Skin Signs of AIDS

Skin Sign	Condition
Viral infection	Herpes simplex, chronic ulcerative[a]
	Herpes zoster, severe
	Oral hairy leukoplakia
	Genital warts
	Molluscum contagiosum, extensive
Fungal infection	Candidiasis (esophageal, tracheal, pulmonary)[a]
	Papules and nodules from systemic fungal infection[a]
	Seborrheic dermatitis (Malassezia), severe
Bacterial infection	Staphylococcal abscesses, recurrent and severe
	Papules, nodules, abscesses from mycobacterial infection[a]
	Bacillary angiomatosis
Neoplasm	Kaposi sarcoma[a]
	Oral and rectal squamous cell carcinoma
	Lymphoma
Miscellaneous	Psoriasis, explosive and severe
	Acquired ichthyosis
	Pruritic papules/folliculitis

[a]AIDS-indicator conditions (mucocutaneous findings that are diagnostic for AIDS).

(Fig. 23.6), and human papillomavirus 16 has been implicated in oral squamous cell carcinoma. The cause of the miscellaneous disorders in patients with AIDS is unknown.

As noted in Table 23.3, some of the mucocutaneous findings are diagnostic for AIDS, as defined by the Centers for Disease Control and Prevention. HIV-infected individuals are diagnosed as having AIDS if they have any of the following mucocutaneous AIDS indicator conditions: Kaposi sarcoma; herpes simplex ulcers lasting for more than 1 month; candidiasis of the esophagus or pulmonary tree; or extrapulmonary (e.g., skin) coccidioidomycosis, cryptococcosis, histoplasmosis, cytomegalovirus infection, or infection with a mycobacterial organism.

Of the disorders listed in Table 23.3 that are not diagnostic for AIDS, oral hairy leukoplakia is the most suggestive because 83% of these patients develop AIDS within 3 years. For the other nondiagnostic disorders, such as severe and explosive-onset psoriasis (Fig. 23.7), the possibility of AIDS should be raised. For the confirmation of HIV infection, blood testing is performed.

SKIN SIGNS OF CANCER

KEY POINTS
1. Hard dermal nodules
2. Chronic chest "cellulitis"

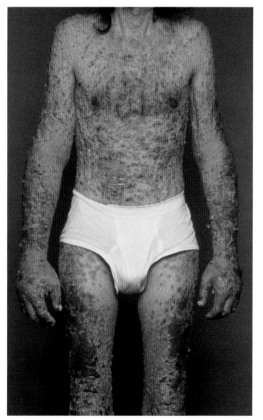

Fig. 23.7 Psoriasis—severe and explosive onset in a patient with AIDS.

TABLE 23.4 Skin Signs of Cancer

Skin Sign	Condition
Dermal nodules	Metastases—carcinoma, lymphoma, leukemia, myeloma
Erythema, macular, and generalized	Flushing—carcinoid
	Exfoliative erythroderma—cutaneous lymphoma
Erythema, localized plaques or nodules	"Cellulitis"—inflammatory breast carcinoma
	Subcutaneous fat necrosis—pancreatic carcinoma
Erythema with scaling patches	Erythema gyratum repens—carcinoma
	Neurolytic migratory erythema—glucagonoma
	Dermatomyositis—carcinoma
Pigmentation, macular and generalized	Addisonian pigmentation—ACTH/MSH-producing tumor
	Slate-gray pigmentation—melanoma
Pigmented patches and plaques	Acanthosis nigricans—carcinoma
	Eruptive seborrheic keratoses (Leser–Trélat)—carcinoma
Bullae/"juicy" plaques	Sweet syndrome—leukemia
	Paraneoplastic pemphigus—lymphoma, thymoma
Scaling (acquired ichthyosis) Excoriations (from generalized pruritus)	Lymphoma (especially Hodgkin disease)
	Lymphoma (especially Hodgkin disease)

ACTH, Adrenocorticotropic hormone; *MSH*, melanocyte-stimulating hormone.

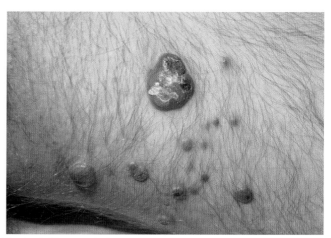

Fig. 23.8 Metastatic lymphoma—hard dermal nodules and papules with some crusts.

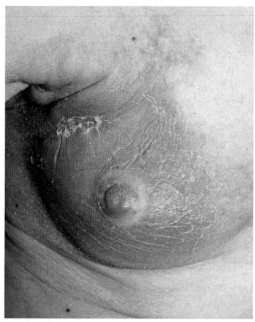

Fig. 23.9 Inflammatory breast carcinoma—cellulitic-appearing plaque.

Numerous internal cancers have cutaneous manifestations that may be a clue to an underlying malignancy (Table 23.4). These lesions are produced by three mechanisms: infiltration of the skin with cancer, changes in the skin produced by secretory products from the tumor, and unknown. The two most common infiltrative presentations of metastatic cancer are *hard* dermal nodules (e.g., lymphoma) (Fig. 23.8) and chest "cellulitis" from inflammatory breast carcinoma (Fig. 23.9). Examples of tumors with secretory products that cause skin changes include carcinoid tumors that produce vasoactive substances causing the classic flush, and tumors (most commonly small cell carcinomas of the lung) that produce polypeptides with melanocyte-stimulating activity. The necrolytic skin lesions that develop in patients with glucagon-secreting pancreatic tumors may be caused by the accompanying low levels of circulating amino acids that are normally needed for skin maintenance and repair. Acanthosis nigricans and acquired ichthyosis are examples of skin signs of cancer in which the pathogenesis is unknown.

SUN SENSITIVITY

KEY POINTS

1. Sun-exposed distribution.
2. The primary lesion helps to narrow the diagnosis.

Table 23.5 outlines the small but important differential diagnosis for patients with photosensitivity. The eruption characteristically occurs on sun-exposed skin: the face, the "V" of the neck and chest, and the dorsal aspects of the arms and hands. A clear history of exacerbation by sunlight is present in all of these diseases except porphyria cutanea tarda.

Lupus erythematosus (Fig. 23.10), phototoxic drug eruption (Fig. 23.11), and polymorphous light eruption are the most frequent causes of photosensitivity. Lupus erythematosus, whether cutaneous or systemic, has a diagnostic biopsy and patients with

TABLE 23.5 Sun Sensitivity

Skin Sign	Condition
Macules, papules, plaques	Lupus erythematosus[a]
	Phototoxic—thiazide, quinidine, griseofulvin, doxycycline
	Photoallergic—sunscreens, fragrances
	Polymorphous light eruption—idiopathic[a]
Hives	Solar urticaria
Bullae	Porphyria cutanea tarda

[a]Most common causes.

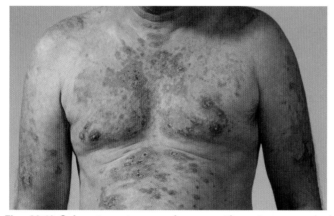

Fig. 23.10 Subacute cutaneous lupus erythematosus—marked photosensitive, red, patches and plaques.

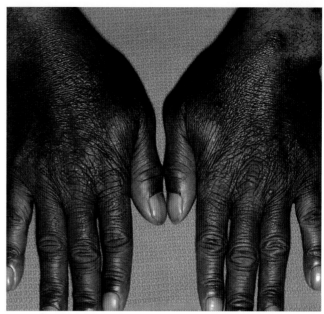

Fig. 23.11 Phototoxic drug eruption–hyperpigmented patches in sun-exposed skin caused by doxycycline.

systemic lupus have positive serologic test results. The diagnosis of a phototoxic drug eruption is suggested by the history and confirmed by resolution of the eruption when the offending medication is discontinued. Polymorphous light eruption is a diagnosis of exclusion. It is an idiopathic disorder in which eczematous papules and plaques develop within 24 hours after sun exposure and persist for a couple of days, despite sunlight avoidance. The skin biopsy has characteristic findings suggesting polymorphous light eruption. With repeated sunlight exposure, the eruption becomes less prominent, a phenomenon called "hardening."

Photoallergic contact dermatitis is an uncommon adverse effect of sunscreens. Photopatch testing can confirm this diagnosis. Solar urticaria is a rare idiopathic disorder that has a characteristic history of urticaria occurring within minutes of sun exposure and disappearing in approximately an hour with sunlight avoidance. Porphyria cutanea tarda typically presents as blisters and fragile skin affecting the dorsum of the hands (see Chapter 10).

INDEX

Note: Page numbers followed by *f* indicate figures, *t* indicate tables and *b* indicate boxes.